SEXOLOGY RESEARCH AND ISSUES

SEXUAL DYSFUNCTIONS

RISK FACTORS, PSYCHOLOGICAL IMPACT AND TREATMENT OPTIONS

SEXOLOGY RESEARCH AND ISSUES

Additional books in this series can be found on Nova's website
under the Series tab.

Additional e-books in this series can be found on Nova's website
under the e-book tab.

SEXUAL DYSFUNCTIONS

RISK FACTORS, PSYCHOLOGICAL IMPACT AND TREATMENT OPTIONS

FRÉDÉRIQUE COURTOIS
EDITOR

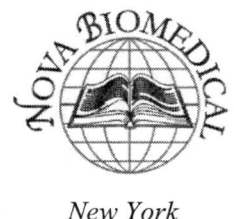

New York

Library of Congress Cataloging-in-Publication Data

ISBN: 978-1-62808-765-9

Library of Congress Control Number: 2013945779

Published by Nova Science Publishers, Inc. † New York

CONTENTS

PREFACE

Sexual dysfunctions in men and women cover a wide range of disorders that can affect any phases of the human sexual response and that can originate from a variety of etiologies. Identifying the sexual dysfunction and its symptomatology is the first step to understanding the patient's complaint, but the etiology of the dysfunction can also participate to the treatment options and influence their relative effectiveness (eg. sexual dysfunctions secondary to neurological conditions or treatment options that can be offered in palliative care units). This book is designed to help understanding the basics of human sexual function and the impact of various pathologies on the development and treatment of sexual dysfunctions.

In men, sexual dysfunctions can range from erectile to ejaculation disorders, to anorgasmia and painful ejaculation. They can originate from a variety of conditions including (but not restricted to) neurological, vascular and psychological or psychiatric conditions, diabetes, and lower urinary tract diseases, and prostatic conditions, all of which are covered in this book. In women, sexual dysfunctions range from hypoactive sexual desire to sexual aversion, arousal disorder, anorgasmia, vaginismus and dyspareunia. While aging and its associated menopause can influence the emergence of sexual dysfunctions in women, other etiologies including neurological, psychiatric conditions and urogynecological disorders can, as in men, participate to the emergence of sexual disorders.

This preface provides a definition of the various sexual dysfunctions diagnosed in men and women, and which can be affected by the various etiologies covered throughout the chapters of the book.

Erectile dysfunction (ED) in men is usually defined as a persistent or recurring inability to achieve or maintain an erection of sufficient quality to achieve intercourse. It can include a deficient or absent tumescence, or the ability to achieve an erection but of insufficient quality (tumescence and rigidity) to allow penetration. ED can also include the inability to sustain an erection for a sufficient duration to complete sexual activity (ruling out the loss of erection due to premature ejaculation). As for any of the next disorders, ED can be life-long and described by individuals who never reported proper function, or acquired and appearing at some point in time, as a consequence of known factors (eg. medical conditions, stress, depression), or as a sign of an emerging condition (eg. diabetes, metabolic syndrome). ED and other sexual disorders can be generalized and occur upon any stimulation condition, or situational and only occur under specific conditions (eg. during intercourse, but not masturbation). Statistically most men experience some degree of erectile dysfunction at some point in their lives (Porst, 2012). While life-long ED usually (but not necessarily) suggests organic etiology, acquired ED can result from psychological and/or pathological conditions (and their treatments), all of which needs to be investigated.

Erectile problems can also include priapism, which contrary to ED, results from a sustained erection, lasting for more than 4 hours despite ejaculation, or cessation of sexual stimulation (Porst &Cruz, 2012). Two types of priapism are known: low flow or ischemic priapism, which is a medical emergency, and high flow or non-ischemic priapism, which is a vascular condition usually of no gravity. Low flow priapism results from a venous occlusion, often following intracavernous injections, where blood is trapped in the penile cavities and where the latter can be damaged by the lack of circulation. High flow is an arterial condition where blood remains (but is not trapped) in the penile cavities despite the end of sexual stimulation. Treatment is not necessary, and when it does, it does not require medical emergency and can be achieved upon regular medical (surgical) appointments.

Painful erections often resulting from Peyronie's disease, characterized by the development of a plaque on the tunica albuginea, which limits the stretching capacity of the penile tissues and results in penile curvature and painful erections (Garaffa et al, 2012). Although the etiology is unknown, the condition could result from a wound-healing disorder with repeated (even mild) penile trauma. As scar tissue develops, penile curvature appears during erection and evolves with inflammation and curvature progression over 6 to 18 months. Following the acute stage, a chronic condition develops which can require surgery depending on the degree of penile curvature and pain during erection (Garaffa et al 2012).

Ejaculation disorders include a variety of conditions ranging from anejaculation, to retrograde, delayed ejaculation, and premature ejaculation. The disorders can also include anorgasmia (ejaculation without climax), or sensory deficits associated with painful or asthenic ejaculations (Porst & Cruz, 2012).

Anejaculation is the inability to ejaculate. It is usually associated with anorgasmia (Porst & Cruz, 2012) and must be differentiated from retrograde ejaculation, in which semen is derived into the bladder (and hence appears to be absent) but where orgasmic sensations are usually preserved (Porst & Cruz, 2012). Retrograde ejaculation is often observed in neurological conditions (eg. spinal cord injury) where the bladder neck is denervated and therefore relaxed, or where the urethral sphincter contracts during ejaculation, forcing the semen into the bladder rather than forward through the meatus. Retrograde ejaculation can also develop following radical prostatectomy (or other prostate surgery) or upon medical treatments (eg. alpha-blockers) relaxing the bladder neck.

Delayed ejaculation is a persistent delay in reaching ejaculation and orgasm despite adequate sexual stimulation (in intensity and duration). While the exact delay for an established diagnosis is not clearly defined, sexually functional men usually ejaculate within 4 min, so that ejaculatory delays above 25 min are usually considered pathological, especially if the individual reports distress (a condition required for the diagnostic) or if he reports ejaculation upon physical exhaustion or genital irritation (Porst & Cruz, 2012).

Premature ejaculation (PE), in contrast to delayed, has been extensively studied in the past few years, in particular using stopwatch techniques to allow precise definition of the time required for a diagnosis. Multicenter studies using stopwatch techniques have shown that the average latency to reach ejaculation once intromission is achieved is 8.5 min (Waldinger et al, 2009). In men with lifelong premature ejaculation, the delay is less than 1 min (independent of circumcision or wearing of a condom), with a range from 1-3 min. Ante portas ejaculation is defined as an extreme PE where ejaculation occurs before intromission can be achieved

(Porst, 2012). In general, PE is among the most commonly observed sexual dysfunctions in men along with erectile dysfunctions (Porst 2012).

Ejaculation without orgasm, also called anhedonic ejaculation, is characterized by the lack of climactic sensations despite the feeling of ejaculation. It can result from neurological conditions where the sensations are impaired or the ejaculation less propulsive and asthenic, or in lower urinary tract disease and prostate infections where the sensations are diminished or the ejaculation painful, or in psychological and psychiatric conditions where the condition and the side effects of medication can alter climactic sensations (eg. antidepressive, antipsychotic medication) (Porst & Cruz, 2012).

In women, hypoactive sexual desire is defined as a diminished or absent sensation of desire, sexual thoughts or fantasies, or as a failure to respond to the partner advances. It is often (but not necessarily) described following menopause, but it can arise from many other conditions including neurological and psychological or psychiatric conditions and their treatment. Sexual aversion is further corresponding to an anxiety or disgust associated with sexual activities or with the thought or anticipation of such sexual activities (Basson et al, 2000). It is most often associated with psychological or psychiatric conditions, which has lead to the suggestion of including it as an anxiety disorder (along with sexual phobias) (Kirana, 2012).

Sexual arousal disorder generally focuses on genital arousal and is defined as the inability to achieve or maintain sufficient genital swelling and/or vaginal lubrication despite adequate stimulation (in type or intensity) (Kirana, 2012). Subjective arousal can be present despite the lack of genital responding, but conversely, psychogenic arousal dysfunction can be the presenting complaint, whith vulvar congestion and vaginal lubrication being adequate.

In contrast to diminished sexual arousal syndromes, sexual arousal disorders can include increased arousal or hypersexual conditions. Persistent genital arousal is defined as an involuntary, intrusive arousal that can last hours or days despite the absence of sexual desire or specific genital stimulation. Female priapism, a rare but described condition, is a persistent erection of the clitoris despite orgasm or cessation of stimulation (Cuzin, 2012). The associated subjective sexual arousal is typically unpleasant in such persistent syndrome.

Sexual pain syndrome includes dyspareunia defined as a persistent or recurring pain during penetration or tentative penetration (Petersen, 2012). Vaginism often accompanies dyspareunia as a result or the origin of it, and is defined as a persistent or repeated difficulty in vaginal penetration despite the desire to do so and whether penetration is attempted with the penis, a finger or an object (eg. speculum, tampons, dilators). It is usually accompanied with anticipation or fear of pain.

Orgasmic disorders cover symptoms such as the absence or a persistent or recurring delay in reaching climax despite adequate sexual stimulation and proper sexual arousal. It can also include a diminished intensity of orgasm. However, because of the variability in the type and intensity of stimulation that have been described in women to reach orgasm, clinical judgment must consider what is reasonably expected for the women's age, sexual experience and description of adequate stimulation, in order to conclude on a diagnosis.

Sexual dysfunctions in men and women therefore cover a wide range of disorders, sometimes sharing similarities, sometimes being specific to one sex. In all cases, the sexual dysfunction can be primary or secondary, generalized or situational. Its clinical assessment requires considering the contributing (risk) factors, which predispose, precipitate or maintain the sexual dysfunction. These factors include the organic or psychiatric conditions that are covered in this book and that can act as predisposing factors to the development of sexual dysfunctions, or contributing to the emergence of the sexual dysfunction, or precipitating factors as a sexual symptom revealing the existence of underlying emerging disease.

This book addresses the various aspects of men and women sexual dysfunctions, including a description of their normal functioning, and a description of the etiologies that can contribute to these sexual dysfunctions, including neurological conditions, prostatic diseases and benign activities such as bicycle riding which can all affect genital neural transmission, as well as disease such as diabetes and depression that can disrupt sexual function. Women's pathologies including urogynecological disorders and aspects of aging are finally addressed along with a discussion on the limitations of some assessment instruments and that on some unit care concerns (eg palliative care) on their limitations to provide adequate support.

REFERENCES

American Psychiatric Association. *Diagnostic and Statistical Manual of Mental Disorders, Text Revision (DSM-IV-TRTM).* 4th ed. Washington, DC: American Psychiatric Association; 2000.

Basson R. The female sexual response: a different model. *J Sex Marital Ther.* 2000;26(1) 51-65. Review.

Cuzin B. Anatomy and physiology of female sexual organs. In Porst J & Reisman Y. *The ESSM Syllabus of Sexual Medicine.*Amsterdam: MEDIX publishers, 2012.

Cuzin B. Female external genital disorders. In Porst J & Reisman Y. *The ESSM Syllabus of Sexual Medicine.*Amsterdam: MEDIX publishers, 2012.

Garaffa J, Porst H, Ralph D. Peyronie's disease. In Porst J & Reisman Y. *The ESSM Syllabus of Sexual Medicine.*Amsterdam: MEDIX publishers, 2012.

Kirana E. Female sexual arousal disorder (FSAD). In Porst J & Reisman Y. *The ESSM Syllabus of Sexual Medicine.*Amsterdam: MEDIX publishers, 2012.

Petersen CD. Female orgasmic disorders. In Porst J & Reisman Y. *The ESSM Syllabus of Sexual Medicine.*Amsterdam: MEDIX publishers, 2012.

Petersen CD. Sexual pain dirsorders. In Porst J & Reisman Y. *The ESSM Syllabus of Sexual Medicine.*Amsterdam: MEDIX publishers, 2012.

Porst H. Erectile dysfunction. In Porst J & Reisman Y. *The ESSM Syllabus of Sexual Medicine.*Amsterdam: MEDIX publishers, 2012.

Porst H & Cruz N. Basic anatomy and physiology of ejaculation, classification of ejaculatory disorders. In Porst J & Reisman Y. *The ESSM Syllabus of Sexual Medicine.* Amsterdam: MEDIX publishers, 2012.

Waldinger MD, McIntosh J, Schweitzer DH. A five-nation survey to assess the distribution of the intrevaginal ejaculatory latency time among the general male population. *J Sex Med* 2009;6:2888-2895.

In: Sexual Dysfunctions
Editor: Frédérique Courtois

Chapter 1

NORMAL SEXUAL FUNCTION IN MEN

Frédérique Courtois[*1], *Kathleen Charvier*[2]
and Nicolas Morel Journel[2]
[1]Université du Québec à Montréal, Sexology Department, Montreal Canada
[2]Hospices civils de Lyon, Saint-Genis Laval, France

ABSTRACT

This chapter describes the basics of normal sexual functioning in men. It begins with a review of the anatomy of the penis, its cavities, envelopes, blood vessels and nerves fibres, and is followed by a description of the physiology and neuropharmacology of the erection process. The chapter follows with a description of the anatomy of the internal reproductive organs, in particular the vas deferens, prostate gland and seminal vesicles involved in the process of ejaculation, the latter being then described according to its dual phases, emission and expulsion. The neurophysiology of ejaculation and the coordination of its events are then explained, along with the neural pathways involved. The neural substrate of climax follows, along with the role of the brain controlling and interpreting the sexual responses. Overall, the chapter's descriptions help understanding the aetiology of various sexual dysfunctions, which will be covered in the other book chapters, and the rationale for treatments also covered throughout the chapters of this book.

Sexual function in men involves a series of responses starting with erection, itself divided into tumescence and rigidity; ejaculation divided into emission and expulsion; and climax. These responses involve an interplay between genital receptors, spinal pathways and brain modulation, all of which explains how various pathological conditions can affect sexual function and how treatments can provide successful options. The following chapter describes the basics of sexual function in men.

---

[*] Corresponding author: Frédérique Courtois. Université du Québec à Montréal. Department of Sexology Department. CP 8888, succ centre ville. Montreal Canada. H3C 3P8. Phone: 1 514 835-6784. Fax: 1 514 987-6787. Email: courtois.frederique@uqam.ca.

THE ANATOMY OF THE PENIS

The penis is composed of three cavities, two corpora cavernosa located dorsally and composing the shaft, and one corpus spongiosum located ventrally, surrounding the urethra and also composing the glans penis (Gruenwald 2012; Netter, 1984).

The two corpora cavernosa are parallel to each other on the dorsal aspect of the penis and separated by a septum, the septum pectiniform, which allows some communication between the two structures. At the basis of the penis, each corpus cavernosum diverges laterally to form a crus, surrounded by a striated muscle, the ischiocavernosus muscle, which contracts during ejaculation and to some extent during erection (see below). At the distal end, the two corpora cavernosa are slightly inserted into the glans penis, a conic and slightly hollow structure (figure 1).

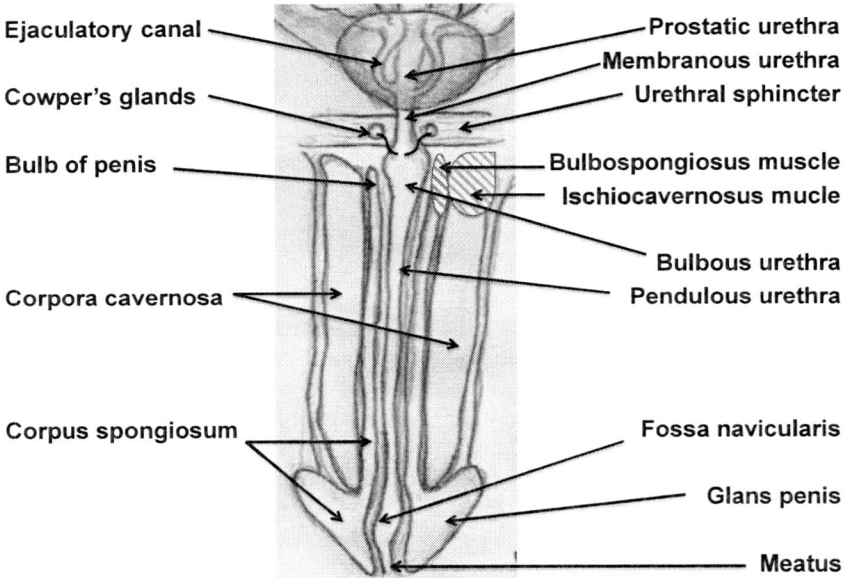

Figure 1. Penile cavities.

The corpus spongiosum surrounds the urethra along the shaft and extends distally to form the glans penis, and proximally to form the bulb of the penis. Underneath the glans penis lie two small odorous glands called Tyson's glands. The smooth surface of the glans penis is delimited by the coronal sulcus, which joins the frenulum on the ventral aspect of the penis. The proximal portion of the corpus spongiosum shows another enlargement, the bulb, surrounded by a penile striated muscle, the bulbospongiosus muscle, which is easily palpated underneath the scrotum and is involved in the ejaculation process, and to some extent in the erection process as well (see further below).

The urethra runs along the corpus spongiosum and is described according to four subdivisions: the prostatic urethra surrounded by the prostate gland and receiving the ejaculatory canals, the membranous urethra at the level of the urethral sphincter, the bulbous urethra at the base of the penis, and the penile or pendulous urethra along the shaft of the penis (Netter, 1984). The urethra terminates with an external opening, the meatus, which is immediately preceded by an enlargement called the fossa navicularis.

Along the shaft of the penis, the roof of the urethra is covered with small openings, called the lagunae of Morgani, connecting with small glands, called the glands of Littré (Netter, 1984), which secrete a mucous substance during erection that alkalinizes the urinary canal and ultimately protects the spermatozoa from the acid environment of the urine during ejaculation. Two other glands, called Cowper's glands, located and embedded within the urethral sphincter, also secrete a mucous substance into the bulbous urethra, which lines the urinary canal and protect the spermatozoa during the expulsion phase of ejaculation.

The penile cavities and the overall penis are surrounded by several membranes (figure 2), starting with the skin or integument, a thin membrane deprived of fat, and extending over the glans penis, where it folds to compose the prepuce or foreskin (Netter, 1984). Underneath the skin lies the dartos composed of smooth muscles fibres and covered on its internal layer by Colle's fascia. Between the two run the arteries and veins irrigating the penile skin. Underneath Colle's fascia lies Buck's fascia, which provides a strong, fibrous envelope surrounding and holding the three penile cavities together, and passing a membrane separating the two corpora cavernosa dorsally and the corpus spongiosum ventrally. Immediately beneath Buck's fascia, and surrounding each penile cavity individually, is the tunica albuginea, a thick membrane composed of connective tissue and a few elastic fibres. Each tunica albuginea surrounds the penile cavities individually. It is composed of a superficial and an internal layer, the latter giving off membranes of fibrous, elastic and smooth muscle fibres that penetrate the penile cavities and provide the trabeculae subdividing the penile cavities in many compartments responsible for their sponge-like appearance (Netter, 1984). In the normal state of detumescence, the smooth muscles of the trabeculae are under tonic contraction, which prevents the vascular congestion of the penis. Upon tumescence, the smooth muscles relax, allowing erection (see later).

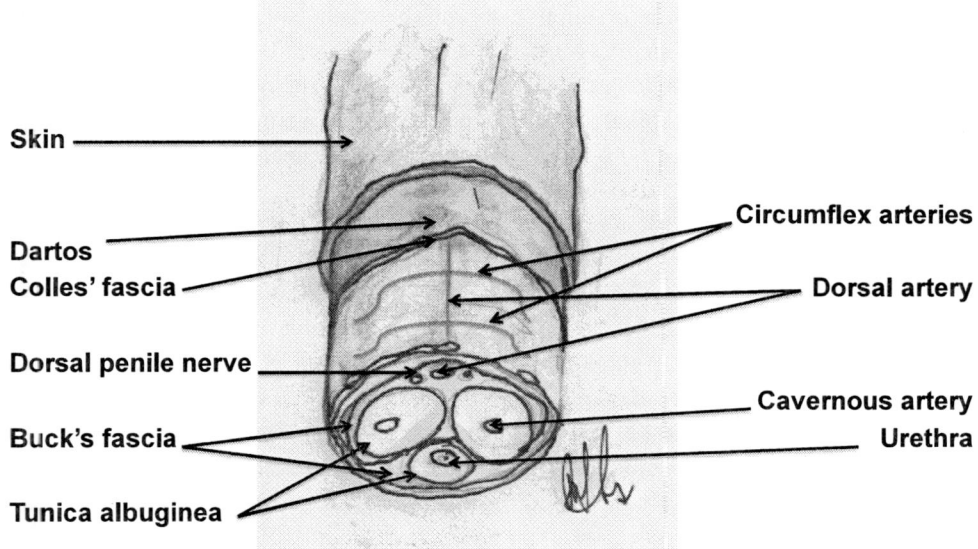

Figure 2. Penile envelopes and neurovascular bundle.

Between Buck's fascia and the tunica albuginea travel the blood vessels and nerve fibres that are responsible for erection (figure 2). Three major arteries are responsible for this process: the dorsal penile artery, the cavernous artery, and the bulbourethral artery (Gruenwald, 2012; Porst & Sharlip, 2006). Each originates from a subdivision of the internal pudendal artery running through Alcock's canal in the pelvis. The dorsal penile artery runs along the shaft of the penis and travels up to the glans penis where it subdivides into numerous terminal branches that irrigate the glans penis. Along its longitudinal course over the penile shaft, the dorsal penile artery gives off regular branches, called the circumflex arteries, which penetrate the corpora cavernosa laterally. The two cavernous arteries, also called the deep arteries of the penis, run along the midline of each corpus cavernosum and subdivide into the helicine arteries, which irrigate the cavernous spaces and trabeculae. The bulbourethral artery irrigates the bulb and continues anteriorly to subdivide into capillaries irrigating the penile cavity around the urethra up to its meatus (Gruenwald, 2012). These three arteries of the penis provide a system that may compensate for any occlusion on one given artery.

The venous drainage of the penis is provided by the veins running parallel to the arteries (Porst & Sharlip, 2006). From the glans penis, five to eight veins drain into the retro-coronal plexus located just beneath the coronal sulcus. The venous drainage of the corpora cavernosa is provided by the emissary veins located within the corpora cavernosa and which drain into the circumflex veins, coursing laterally and draining back into the deep dorsal vein. The deep dorsal vein runs along the penile shaft, but leaves just before the bulb where it shows an upward curve and drains into the peri-prostatic plexus. The proximal cavities of each corpus cavernosum are drained by a deep dorsal vein (also called cavernous vein), which drains into the internal pudendal vein. Venous drainage from the bulb of the corpus spongiosum is provided by the bulbourethral vein, which empties into the bulbous vein, while the body of the corpus spongiosum empties into the bulbourethral and the bulbous veins, themselves draining into the internal pudendal vein (Gruenwals, 2012; Porst & Sharlip 2006).

The nerve fibres mediating erection also run between Buck's fascia and the tunica albuginea on each side of the penile veins and arteries (Netter, 1984). Three types of nerve innervate the penis, the pudendal nerve a somatic component originating from the sacral segments S2, S3, S4 of the spinal cord, the pelvic nerve an autonomic parasympathetic component also originating from the sacral segments of the spinal cord, and the sympathetic nerves originating from the thoracolumbar segments T11, T12, L1, L2 of the spinal cord (figure 3) (Courtois et al 2013; Giuliano, 2011; Giuliano & Rampin 2004; Tajkarimi & Burnett, 2011).

The pudendal nerve comprises a sensory branch called the dorsal penile nerve and a motor branch called the perineal nerve. The dorsal penile nerve is stimulated by the penile receptors mostly located in the glans penis and frenulum, but also in the shaft and penile muscles. The receptors include the free nerve endings, which respond to touch, stretching, vibration, temperature and pain (Tajkarimi & Burnett 2011); the encapsulated Krause-Finger corpuscles located in the subcutaneous penile tissue, and the Pacini and Ruffini corpuscules located in deeper layers of the penis which respond to pressure and vibration (Giuliano & Clément 2005; McMahon et al, 2004; Tajkarimi & Burnett 2011); the mechanoreceptors located in the urethra, the tunica albuginea and the penile cavities which respond to stretch; and the muscles spindles and Golgi tendons located in penile muscles and urethral sphincter and responding to the vascular congestion of the penile cavities and the muscular contractions occurring during erection and ejaculation (Tajkarimi & Burnett 2011)

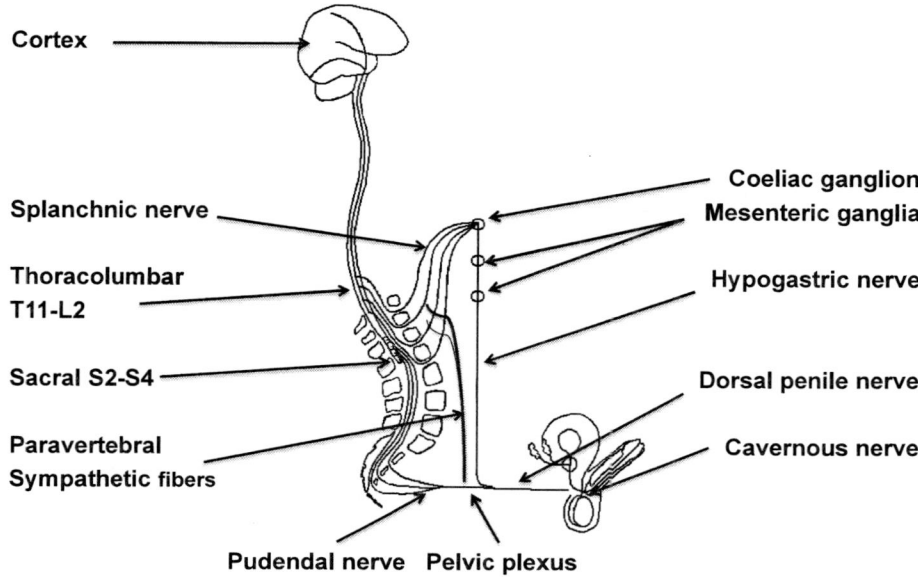

Figure 3. Penis Innervation.

The motor component of the pudendal nerve, namely the perineal nerve, innervates the penile muscles including the bulbospongiosus and the ischiocavernosa muscles, as well as the urethral sphincter. Although a primary motor nerve, the perineal nerve also contains a few sensory fibres originating from the ventral aspect of the penis, and specifically the frenulum.

The autonomic parasympathetic fibres of the penis travel through the pelvic nerve, a preganglionic fibre, travelling across the pelvic plexus and reaching the base of the penis where it connects with the post-ganglionic parasympathetic cavernous nerve responsible for mediating erection.

The autonomic sympathetic fibres originating from the thoracolumbar segments of the spinal cord exit through the pre-ganglionic splanchnic nerves and give off a first contingent running down the sympathetic chain and feeding into the pelvic plexus (where they ultimately synapse with the cavernous nerve described above), and a second contingent synapsing in the coeliac and mesenteric ganglia with the post-ganglionic hypogastric nerve innervating the internal reproductive organs (vas deferens, seminal vesicles, prostate gland) and mediating the emission phase of ejaculation (see below) (Courtois et al 2013; Giuliano 2011; Giuliano & Rampin, 2004).

THE NEUROPHYSIOLOGY OF ERECTION

The neurophysiology of erection, involves both tumescence and rigidity, the first results from the vascular congestion of the penis, and the second from the sporadic contractions of the penile muscles (Karacan et al 1983; 1987; Lavoisier et al 1986; 1988a; 1988b). Overall these responses arise from genital stimulation and/or psychogenic arousal, and involve the interplay between perineal nerves and spinal pathways conveying information from the genitals to the brain, and vice versa (Courtois et al 2012).

Although arising from both genital and psychogenic stimulation, the erection of the penis is primarily a reflex. The reflex receives both excitatory and inhibitory influences from the brain, which modulates the response at the level of the genitals (i.e. facilitating or inhibiting the reflex) and which allows perception of the congestion of the resulting erected penis (Andersson, 2011; Courtois et al 2013; Giuliano 2011; Giuliano & Rampin 2004) (figure 3).

The reflex response mediating penile tumescence is conveyed by the genital receptors that are activated during touch (eg. genital caresses), congestion (stretching of penile tissues), pressure against the glans penis (eg. during penetration), vibration (eg. during rapid thrusting or from the use of a sex toy), or increased temperature (eg., from vasocongestion of the penis), all of which provide genital arousal.

Incoming sensory information from these genital receptors is conveyed through the dorsal penile nerve, for the dorsal aspect of the penis (glans, coronal sulcus) and the distal urethra, and through the sensory fibres of the perineal nerve, for the ventral aspect of the frenulum and bulbar urethra (Courtois et al 2013; Tajkarimi & Burnett 2011). As the dorsal penile nerve and sensory fibres of the perineal nerve reach the base of the penis, they join to become the pudendal nerve, which enters the spinal cord at the level of the S2, S3, S4 sacral segments (Courtois et al 2013; Tajkarimi & Burnett 2011).

In the cord, synapses are made with the parasympathetic pre-ganglionic pelvic nerve, which run through the pelvic plexus to the base of the penis, where it connects with the post-ganglionic parasympathetic cavernous nerve (Courtois et al 2013; Tajkarimi & Burnett 2011). This cavernous nerve is responsible for the simultaneous relaxation of the smooth muscles of the penile trabeculae and the smooth muscle envelop of the penile arteries, resulting in the vasodilation and vasocongestion of the penis during tumescence (Courtois et al 2013; Giuliano 2011; Tajkarimi & Burnett 2011).

The process is mediated by nitric oxide synthase (NOS), which is released by the cavernous nerve (nNOS) and the penile endothelium (eNOS), and activates a series of transformations leading to smooth muscle relaxation and penile tumescence relax (Andersson 2011; de Tejeda et al., 2004 ; Giuliano 2011; Guay 2005 ; Lue 2000). The release of nNOS from the cavernous nerve, particularly upon initiation of sexual arousal, and liberation of eNOS particularly during maintenance of sexual arousal, activate the enzyme guanylyl cyclase (figure 1), which transforms guanosine triphosphate (GTP) into cyclic guanosine monophophase (cGMP) and raises the intracellular concentration of cGMP. This increased concentration of cGMP stimulates a specific protein kinase located in the smooth muscles of the trabeculae and in the penile arteries (Andersson 2011) which triggers changes in the smooth muscle cell, hyperpolarizing them and causing them to relax (de Tejeda et al., 2004 ; Giuliano 2011; Guay 2005 ; Lue 2000). Together, the vasodilation of the penile arteries and the relaxation of the penile trabeculae allow the penile cavities to fill with blood and become congested, resulting in tumescence.

At the same time as the penile cavities fill with blood, parasympathetic stimulation of the cavernous nerve triggers the secretion of the genital accessory glands (Giuliano 2011; Giuliano & Clément, 2005a; 2005b), namely Tyson's glands, Littré's glands, and Cowper's glands. The distal parasympathetic innervation of the cavernous nerve, running to the prostatic plexus, further stimulates the secretion of the prostate gland and the seminal vesicles

(Tajkarimi & Burnett 2011) and is responsible for their congestion during this early phase of sexual arousal (Giuliano 2011; Giuliano & Clément, 2005a; 2005b).

As tumescence develops and blood gradually fills the penile cavities, the sinusoidal spaces of the penis distend and gradually compress the penile dorsal veins and arteries, temporarily occluding them. Entrapment of the blood in this closed system maximizes tumescence, and enhances penile rigidity through the sporadic contractions of the penile muscles (Karacan et al 1983; 1987; Lavoisier et al 1988a; 1988b). As the bulbospongiosus and ischiocavernosa muscles surround the base of each penile cavity - which are now filled with blood -, their sporadic contraction increases the internal penile pressure up to and sometimes even beyond 350mmHg, maximizing rigidity and further congesting the glans penis distally (Karacan et al 1983; 1987; Lavoisier et al 1986; 1988a; 1998b; Claes et al 1996).

This muscular process of erection is mediated by the efferent fibres of the pudendal nerve, namely the perineal nerve, which originates from Onuf's nucleus (1901) in the anterior portion of the sacral spinal cord, and innervates the bulbospongiosum and ischiocavernosa muscles.

The reflex mediation of erection through genital stimulation is also accompanied by psychogenic mediation, arising from arousal produced by sensory feedback from the genitals as well as from brain stimulation including visual, olfactory, and/or auditory stimulation that can be perceived or fantasized, and memories of sexual events that contribute to sexual arousal. In all cases, psychogenic inputs can modulate erection by either 1) feeding into the sacral reflex pathway and enhancing (or inhibiting) its activity, or by 2) running down the spinal cord and reaching the thoracolumbar pathway (Courtois & MacDougall 1993; Giuliano et al 1996; 1997; Root & Bard, 1947), existing the cord through the splanchnic nerves and running down the sympathetic chain to feed into the pelvic plexus of erection (Giuliano et al 1996; 1997; Yaïci et al. 2002).

THE ANATOMY OF THE INTERNAL REPRODUCTIVE ORGANS

The internal reproductive organs, sometimes called the sexual accessory glands, are composed of the vas deferens and their ampullas, the seminal vesicles and the prostate gland (Figure 4) (Netter, 2984).

The ampullas of the vas deferens are reservoirs that store the mature spermatozoa awaiting to be expelled during ejaculation, and providing them with a slightly acid environment, which keeps them immobile before ejaculation. The ampulla is an enlargement of the vas deferens itself, a canal originating from the epididymis and testicles where the spermatozoa are formed. The vas deferens and its ampullas are surrounded by a layer of smooth muscle, which contracts during ejaculation and is responsible for the peristaltic movements moving the spermatozoa up the vas deferens, segment by segment, during each ejaculation.

The seminal vesicles are small glands located under the ampullas of the vas deferens, which are also surrounded by a smooth muscle envelope that contracts during ejaculation. The secretions of the seminal vesicles contain a mixture of fructose that is essential for sperm motility, alkaline fluid that is essential for neutralizing the acid environment of the semen, and fibrinogen, a protein that coagulates the semen, and forms a bolus, which maximizes the expulsion of semen upon ejaculation.

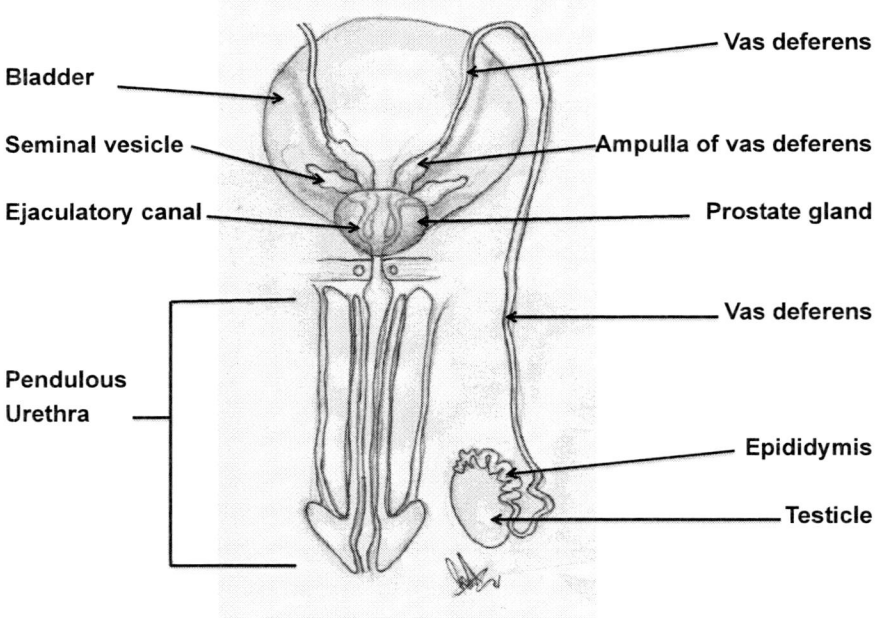

Figure 4. Internal Reproductive Organs in Men.

The secretion of the seminal vesicles composes 60% of the semen. The lateral wall of each seminal vesicle and the lateral wall of each ampulla of the vas deferens join to form the ejaculatory canals, which cross the prostate gland and empty their content in the prostatic urethra.

The prostate gland is a cluster of 30 to 50 small glands collected around the urethra. Located immediately beneath the bladder, the prostate gland is divided into three lobes, a lateral lobe surrounding the urethra and composing the major portion of the prostate, a posterior lobe often involve in prostate cancer and easily accessible (palpable) through the rectum, and a small anterior lobe with an unknown (vestigial) function. The prostate gland has no excretory canal per se and secretes its content directly into the urethra, which explains its role in urinary retention upon prostate hypertrophy or hyperplasia. Prostatic secretions compose 40% of the semen and provide an additional vehicle for the seminal fluid to be expelled during ejaculation. The secretions contain fibrinolysin, an enzyme which liquefies the coagulated semen some 15 to 20 min after ejaculation. This liquefaction liberates the spermatozoa from the ejaculated bolus, allowing them to move up the female's reproductive organs to fertilize the ovum in the fallopian tube (see female chapter).

THE NEUROPHYSIOLOGY OF EJACULATION

The ejaculation process is composed of two phases: emission and expulsion (Courtois et al 2013; Giuliano 2011; Porst 2012; Rampin & Giuliano 2004). The first phase of emission involves the contraction of the smooth muscular envelopes surrounding the internal reproductive organs, namely the vas deferens, the seminal vesicles, and the prostate gland. These smooth muscle contractions stimulate these structures to release of their content into the prostatic urethra, creating the semen. As the semen is contained and trapped between the closed neck of the bladder and the urinary sphincter, it distends the urethral wall and activates its stretch receptors. This initiates the second phase of ejaculation, namely expulsion (McMahon et al 2004; Newman et al 1982). During this phase, the perineal striated muscles, including the bulbospongiosus and ischiocavernosa muscles surrounding the penile cavities, contract and propel the semen out of the urethra.

The neural process mediating the ejaculation process involves an interplay between the sympathetic and somatic nervous system. The coordination of events is most likely controlled by a spinal generator of ejaculation (SGE), identified in animals at the level of the L3-L4 spinal segments (Carro-Juárez et al 2008; Truit & Coolen 2002; Truit et al 2003). While the phase of erection preceding emission is controlled by parasympathetic activity originating from the sacral segments of the spinal cord, emission is mediated by sympathetic activity originating from the thoracolumbar segments T11, T12, L1, L2. Once erection reaches the threshold of ejaculation (i.e., the point at which ejaculation can no longer be controlled), intraspinal connections are established, probably through the SGE, between the sacral and thoracolumbar pathways to initiate emission. Splanchnic nerves originating from the thoracolumbar segments exit the cord and synapse in the coeliac and mesenteric ganglia with the post-ganglionic fibers of the hypogastric nerve (Giuliano 2011; Giuliano & Clément 2005a; 2005b).

As the hypogastric nerve innervates the internal reproductive organs, it stimulates the secretion of the ampulla of the vas deferens, seminal vesicles and prostate gland, resulting in the emission of semen into the prostatic urethra. The resulting emission of seminal fluid distends the urethral wall and activates its stretch receptors, triggering a new reflex with the sacral pathway to provoke in the rhythmic contractions of the perineal muscles surrounding the penile cavities that expel the semen from the urethra.

According to Borgdorff et al (2008), the SGE coordinates the sequence of events from erection to expulsion of the semen, starting with the summation of sensory inputs from the genitals and brain during sexual arousal, followed by activation of the parasympathetic fibers responsible for the internal reproductive organs' secretions, followed by the sympathetic peristaltic contractions of these internal reproductive organs, releasing their contents into the prostatic urethra and culminating in the somatic contractions of the perineal muscles responsible for seminal expulsion (Borgdorff et al, 2008 ; Giuliano 2011).

THE NEUROPHYSIOLOGY OF CLIMAX

Climax usually accompanies ejaculation and is perceived through the powerful contractions of the perineal muscles that characterize the expulsion phase of the process (McMahon et al 2004). It is also perceived through the contribution of autonomic responses that are recorded in men and women upon orgasm and that include hypertension, which can reach levels as high as 160mmHg to 180mmHg, tachycardia, which can reach levels as high as 100 to 180 beats per min (Masters & Johnson 1966; Pollock & Schmidt 1995), and other signs of autonomic activity such as hyperventilation, piloerection, and red skin spots, to name the most common ones (Kaplan, 1974; Levin, 2006; Mah & Binik 2001; 2005; Master & Johnson, 1966; Meston & al., 2004a; 2004b).

These cardiovascular and autonomic responses that characterize orgasm in able bodied men and women are also observed in men with spinal cord injury upon ejaculation (Anderson et al 2007; Courtois et al 2008a; 2008b; Sipski et al 2006; S0ler et al 2011), in a phenomenon called autonomic dysreflexia (Courtois et al 2011; 2013). This phenomenon of autonomic dysreflexia, which occurs in particular upon ejaculation (Courtois et al 2012; Karlsson, 1999; Kavchak-Keyes 2000; Krassioukov, 2004; Silver 2000; Teasellet al 2000), can cause severe hypertension in men with spinal cord injury (Ekland et al, 2008; Elliot & Krassioukov 2005; McBride et al 2003; Thurmbikat & Tophill, 2003). However, in able-bodied men, hypertension at ejaculation reaches high (but rarely dangerous) levels, and returns to baseline very rapidly, that is within 2 min following ejaculation (Courtois et al 2004). The similarity between ejaculation in able-bodied men and men with spinal cord injury has lead Courtois et al (2008a; 2008b; 2011; 2013) to suggest that orgasm is a transient autonomic hyperreflexia normally submitted to immediate supraspinal inhibition. The autonomic hyperreflexia triggered explains the overall climactic response, while the rapid inhibition over blood pressure (and other signs of autonomic activity) explains the transient and pleasurable experience of orgasm in able-bodied men.

The hypothesis of orgasm as an overall autonomic hyperactivity explains the perception of orgasm possible in men even in the absence of ejaculation, for example following radical prostatectomy (Barnas et al 2004; Dubbelman et al 2009 ; Newman et al 1982; Perelman 2008), or in prepuberal boys who experience orgasm before having reached the physiological maturity for ejaculation, as well as able-bodied women who experience orgasm despite the lack of ejaculation (Masters & Johnson 1966; Meston & al., 2004a; 2004b) .

The neurological process ascribed to this process of climax has further been suggested be Courtois et al (2011; 2013) to results from a multisegmental reflex triggered upon emission in men and activating, not only the hypogastric nerve responsible for emission, but the entire sympathetic chain responsible for all other signs of climax. The process begins upon emission in men, where the splanchnic nerves originating from the thoracolumbar segments T11-L2 of the spinal cord synapse, not only with the coeliac and mesenteric ganglia stimulating the hypogastric nerve, but with the entire sympathetic chain innervating the other viscera (heart, lungs, blood vessels and the like) and stimulating the other components of climax, namely hypertension, tachycardia, hyperventilation, smooth muscles and perineal muscles contractions, piloerection, red skin spots and the like (Courtois et al, 2011; 2013).

BRAIN MODULATION AND PERCEPTION OF SEXUAL RESPONSES

The perception of orgasm is necessarily encoded at the brain level, which receive and interpret peripheral activity (genital and extra-genital), and which adds inputs modulating this peripheral activity and interpreting the orgasmic sensations as a joyful, rewarding, pleasant experience (or on the contrary a stressful aversive experience). Studies from functional magnetic resonance imaging (fMRI) and positron emission tomography (PET) show that many brain areas, including the cortex, thalamus, hypothalamus, brainstem and cerebellum are activated upon orgasm in able-bodied men and women (Bianchi-Demicheli & Ortigue

2007; Georgiadis et al;. 2009; Hostege et al 2003) and in women with spinal cord injury (Komisaruk et al 2004; Whipple et al 2002). The studies sometimes make it difficult to differentiate the activity pertaining specifically to sexual desire as opposed to arousal, or to arousal as opposed to climax. Furthermore, while some studies suggest that climax results from, or in, the activation of many brain structures (Bianchi-Demicheli & Ortigue 2007; Hostege et al 2003), others show that the brain literally ceases its activity at the very moment of orgasm (Georgiadis et al 2009), suggesting that the recordings are a function of prior arousal or an after-effect of climax.

Among the structures identified in these fMRI and PET scan studies the medial preoptic area (MPOA) of the hypothalamus and the paraventricular nucleus (PVN), have been found to have excitatory effects on sexual responses, and the paragigantocellularis nucleus (nPGI) in the lower brain stem (more specifically the reticular formation) as having inhibitory effects on the spinal pathways mediating sexual responses (Andersson 2011; Tajkarimi & Burnett 2011). The periacqueductal gray (PAG) in the midbrain has also been found to have inhibitory effects on the nPGI, which removes the inhibition of an inhibitory structure and which results in the expression of sexual responses. Pituitary hormones are further released upon climax, thereby contributing to sexual responses (Georgiadis et al. 2009; Mestin et al., 2004; Pfaus 2009). [195]

At the higher brain level, cortical activity from the sensory and visual cortex have been recorded and would contribute sensory and visual inputs to ejaculation and climax (Bianchi-Demicheli & Ortigue 2007; Georgiadis et al;. 2009; Hostege et al 2003). Recorded activity in the prefrontal, temporal and enthorinal cortex would participate to the hedonic experience of climax and its feeling of satiety (Bianchi-Demicheli & Ortigue 2007; Georgiadis et al;. 2009; Hostege et al 2003). Thalamic areas such as ventroposterior thalamus would contribute to increased visceral perception, while limbic structures including the nucleus accumbens, amygdala and hippocampus, and their reciprocal connections with the ventrotegmental area (VTA) and mesodiencephalic area, would participate to the euphoric and rewarding effect of climax.

In the brainstem, the reticular formation, which receives many inputs from the genitals and viscera (Bianchi-Demicheli & Ortigue 2007; Georgiadis et al;. 2009; Hostege et al 2003) and which regulates cardiovascular and respiratory function (Rampin & Giuliano, 2000) are also expressed during arousal and climax, which is interesting in the context of the autonomic discharge characterizing climax. The cerebellum and its projection to the pontine tegmentum, which have also been found to be light up at climax, similarly participate to cardiovascular arousal and the emotional and motor components of orgasm.

Many structures have therefore been found to be involved in the process of sexual pleasure and climax. The question remains as to whether all of these activities, or which of these activities, actually reflect the effect of climax, as opposed to sexual arousal preceding orgasm, or the after - relaxing and rewarding - effect of climax.

CONCLUSION

The anatomical and neurophysiological substrates of normal sexual responses in men explain how various aetiologies can contribute to sexual dysfunctions, and often explain the rationale for the development of various treatments, both of which are covered throughout the chapters of this book.

ACKNOWLEDGMENTS

The authors wish to thank Thomas Lefebvre (tal.illustrator@gmail.com) for his drawing the figures.

REFERENCES

Anderson KD, Borisoff JF, Johnson RD, Stiens SA, Elliott SL. The impact of spinal cord injury on sexual function: concerns of the general population. *Spinal cord* 2007;45:328-337.

Andersson KE Mechanisms of penile erection and basis for pharmacological treatment of erectile dyfunction. *Pharmacological Reviews* 2011;63(4):811-859.

Barnas JL, Pierpaoli S, Ladd P, Valenzuela R, Aviv N, Parker M, Qaters WB, Flanigan RC, Mulhall JP. The prevalence and nature of orgasmic dysfunction after radical prostatectomy. *BJU Int*, 2004; 94(4):603-5.

Bianchi-Demicheli F & Ortigue S. Toward an understanding of the cerebral substrates of womand's orgasm. *Neuropsychologia,* 2007;45:2645-2659.

Borgdorff AJ, Bernabé J, Denys P, Alexandre L, Giuliano F. Ejaculation elicited by microstimulation of lumbar spinothalamic neurons. *European Urology*, 2008, 54(2), 449-456.

Carro-Juárez M, Rodríguez-Manzo G.The spinal pattern generator for ejaculation. *Brain Res Rev.* 2008;58(1):106-20.

Claes H, Bijnens B, Baert L. The hemodynamic influence of the ischiocavernosus muscles on erectile function. *J. Urol* 1996;156:986-90.

Courtois F, Carrier S, Charvier K, Guertin PA, Morel Journel N. The control of male sexual responses. *Current Pharm Design*, 2013;19.

Courtois FJ, Charvier KF, Leriche A, Vézina, J.-G., Côté, M & Bélanger, M. Blood pressure changes during sexual stimulation, ejaculation and midodrine treatment in spinal cord injured men. *BJU*, 2008b; 101(3); 331-337.

Courtois FJ, Charvier KF, Leriche A, Vézina, J.-G., Côté, M, Raymond D., Jacquemin, G, Fournier C. & Bélanger, M. Perceived physiological and orgasmic sensations at ejaculation in spinal cord injured men. *J. Sex Med*, 2008a, 5(10); 2419-2430.

Courtois, F, Charvier, K., Vézina, J.-G., Morel-Journel N, Carrier S., Jacquemin, G, Côté, I. Assessing and conceptualizing orgasm following a spinal cord injury. *British Journal of Urology,* 2011;108(10):1624-1633.

Courtois F, Geoffrion R, Landry E, Bélanger M. H reflex and physiologic measures of ejaculation in men with spinal cord injury. *Archives of Physical Medicine and Rehabilitation* 2004;85:910-918.

Courtois F, Rodrigue X, Côté I, Boulet M, Vézina J-G, Charvier K, Dahan V. *Sexual function and autonomic dysreflexia in men with spinal cord injuries: How to treat. Spinal cord* 2012:1-9.

Courtois FJ, MacDougall, J.C. & Sach, B.D. Erectile mechanism in paraplegia. *Physiology & Behavior,* 1993;53:721-726.

De Tejada IS, Angulo J, Cellek S, González-Cadavid NF, Heaton J, Pickard R, Simonsen U. Dans Lue TF, Basson R, Rosen R, Giuliano F, Koury S, Montorsi F Eds. *Sexual Medicine: sexual dysfunctions in men and women.* Paris: Editions 21, 2004.

Dubbelman Y, Wildhagen M, Schröder F, Bangma C, Dohle G. Orgasmic dysfunction after open radical prostatectomy: Clinical correlates and prognostic factors. *J. Sex Med* 2009;13.

Ekland MB, Krassioukov AV, McBride KE, Elliott SL. Incidence of autonomic dysreflexia and silent autonomic dysreflexia in men with spinal cord injury undergoing sperm retrieval: implications for clinical practice. *Spinal Cord Med.* 2008;31(1):33-9.

Elliot S, Krassioukov, A. Malignant autonomic dysreflexia in spinal cord injured men. *Spinal Cord* 2005.

Georgiadis JR, Reinders AATS, PaansAMJ, Renken R, Dortekaas R. men versus women on sexual brain function: prominent differnces during tactile genital stimulation, but not during orgasm. *Human Brain Mapping,* 2009, 30:3089-3101.

Giuliano F. Neurophysiology of erection and ejaculation. *J. Sex Med* 2011;8(4):310-315.

Giuliano F, Bernabe J Brown K, Droupy S, Benoit G, Rampin O. Erectile response to hypothalamic stimulation in rats: role of peripheral nerves. *Am. J. Physiol* 1997;273(6):R1990-R1

Giuliano F, Clément P. Physiology of ejaculation: emphasis on serotonergic control. *Eur. Urol* 2005a;48:408-17.

Giuliano F Clément P. Neuroanatomy and physiology of ejaculation. *Annu. Rev. Sex Res* 2005b;16:190-216.

Giuliano F, Rampin O. Neural control of erection. *Phys. Behav* 2004;83:189-201.

Giuliano F, Rampin O, Brown K, Courtois F, Jardin A, Benoit G. Stimulation of the medial preoptic area of the hypothalamus in the rat elicits increases in intracavernous pressure. *Neurosci. Lett* 1996;209(1):1-4.

Gruenwald I. Male genital anatomy and physiology. In Porst J & Reisman Y. *The ESSM Syllabus of Sexual Medicine.* Amsterdam: MEDIX publishers, 2012.

Guay A T. Relation of endothelial cell function to erectile dysfunction : implications for treatment. *American Journal of Cardiology* 2005;96(12)suppl2:52-56.

Hostege G, Georgiadis JR, Paans AMJ, Meiners LC, van der Graaf FHCE, Reinders AATS. Brain activation during male ejaculation. *J. Neuroscience.* 2003, 23(27):9185-9193.

Kaplan HS. *The new sex therapy.* New York, Brunner/Mazel. 1974.

Karlsson AK. Autonomic dysreflexia. *Spinal Cord* 1999;37:383-91.

Karacan I, Aslan C, Hirshkowitz M. Erectile mechanisms in man. *Science.* 1983;220(4601):1080-2.

Karacan I, Hirshkowitz M, Salis PJ, Narter E, Safi MF. Penile blood flow and musculovascular events during sleep-related erections of middle-aged men. *J. Urol.* 1987;138(1):177-81.

Kavchak-Keyes MA. Autonomic hyperreflexia. *Rehabil Nurs* 2000;25(1):31-5.

Komisaruk BR, Whipple B, Crawford A, Liu WC, Kalnin A, & Mosier K. Brain activation during vaginocervical self-stimulation and orgasm in women with complete spinal cord injury: fMRI evidence of mediation by the vagus nerves. *Brain Res.*, 2004 1024(1-2), 77-88.

Krassioukov A. Autonomic dysreflexia in acute spinal cord injury: incidence, mechanisms, and management. *SCI Nursing*, 2004, 21(4), 215-216.

Lavoisier P., Proulx, J., Courtois, F.J., de Carufel, F. & Durand, L.-G. Relationship between perineal muscle contractions, penile tumescence and penile rigidity during nocturnal erections. *Journal of Urology*, 1988a, 139, 176-179.

Lavoisier P., Proulx, J. & Courtois, F.J. Reflex contractions of the ischiocavernosus muscles following electrical and pressure stimulations. *Journal of Urology*, 1988b, 139, 396-399.

Lavoisier P., Courtois, F.J., Barres, F. & Blanchard, M. Correlation between intracavernous pressure and contractions of the ischiocavernosus muscle in man. *Journal of Urology*, 1986, 136, 936-939.

Levin RJ. Vocalised sounds and human sex. Science update. *Sexual Relationship Therapy* 2006;21(1):99-107.

Lue TF. Erectile dysfunction. *N. Engl. J.Med.* 2000 15;342(24):1802-13.

Mah K & Binik YM. The nature of human orgasm: a critical review of major trends. *Clin Psychol Rev.* 2001;21(6):823-56.

Mah K & Binik YM. Are orgasms in the mind or the body ? Psychosocial versus physiological correlates of orgasmic pleasure and satisfaction. *J. Sex Marital Ther* 2005;31(3):187-200.

Masters W.H., & Johnson, V.E. *Human Sexual Response*. Boston, Little Brown. 1966.

McBride F, Quah SP, Scott ME, Dinsmore WW. Tripling of blood pressure by sexual stimulation in a man with spinal cord injury. *J. R Soc Med.* 2003;96:349-50.

McMahon CG, Abdo C, Incrocci L, Perelman M, Rowland D, Studkey B, Waldinger M ChengXin Z. Disorders of orgasm and ejaculation in men. In T Lue, Basson R, Rosen R, Giuliano F, Khoury S, Montorsi F (Eds). Sexual Medicine: Sexual Dysfunctions in Men and Women. *2nd International consultation on Sexual dysfunctions*, Paris: Editions 21, 2004.

Meston CM, Hull E, Levin RJ, Sipski M. Women's orgasm. In T Lue, Basson R, Rosen R, Giuliano F, Khoury S, Montorsi F (Eds). Sexual Medicine: Sexual Dysfunctions in Men and Women. *2nd International consultation on Sexual dysfunctions*, Paris: Editions 21, 2004a.

Meston, C., Levin, R., Sipski, M., Hull, E. & Heiman, J. Women's orgasm, review. *Annual Review of Sex Research*, 2004b, *15,* 173-257.

Netter FH. Reproductive System. *The CIBA Collection of Medical Illustrations* (Vol 2). New York: CIBA Pharmaceutical Company (7th ed), 1984.

Newman HF, Reiss H, Northup JD. Physical basis of emission, ejaculation and orgasm in the male. *Urology* 1982;9(4):341-350.

Onuf B. On the arrangement and function of the cell groups of the sacral region of the spinal cord in man. *Arch Neurol Psychopath* 1901;3:387-412.

Perelman MA Post-prostatectomy orgasmic response. *J. Sex Med*, 2008, 5(1)248-9. Epub 2007 Oct24.

Pollock ML, Schmidt DH. *Heart Disease and Rehabilition*. Champaign, IL: Human Kinetics, 1995;372.

Porst H. & Cruz N. Basic anatomy and physiology of ejaculation, classification of ejaculatory disorders. In Porst J & Reisman Y. *The ESSM Syllabus of Sexual Medicine*. Amsterdam: MEDIX publishers, 2012.

Porst H & Sharlip ID. Anatomy and physiology of erection. In Porst H and Buvat J and the standards committee of the International Society of Sexual Medicine (ISSM). *Standard Practice in Sexual Medicine* . Oxford: Blackwell Publishing: 2006.

Rampin O & Giuliano F. Physiology and pharmacology of ejaculation. *J. Soc Biol.* 2004;198(3):231-6.

Rampin O & Giuliano F. Central control of the cardiovascular and erection systems: possible mechanisms and interactions. *Am. J. Cardiol.* 2000;86(2A):19F-22F.

Rawicki HB, Hill S. Semen retrieval in spinal cord injured men. *Paraplegia* 1991;29(7): 443-6.

Root WS, Bard P. The mediation of feline erection through sympathetic pathways with some remarks on sexual behavior after deaffferentation of the genitalia. *Am. J. Physiol* 1947;151:80-89.

Silver JR. Early autonomic dysreflexia. *Spinal Cord* 2000;38:229-33.

Sipski M, Alexander CJ, Gómez-Marín O. Effects of level and degree of spinal cord injury on male orgasm. *Spinal Cord* 2006;44:798-804.

Soler JM & Previnaire JG. Ejaculatory dysfunction in spinal cord injury men is suggestive of dyssynergic ejaculation. *Eur. J. Phys. Rehabil Med.* 2011;47(4):677-81.

Tajkarimi K & Burnett AL. The role of genital nerve afferents in the physiology of the sexual response and pelvic floor function. *J. Sex Med* 2011;8:1299-1312.

Teasell RW, Arnold MO, Krassioukov A, Delaney GA. Cardiovascular consequences of loss of supraspinal control of the sympathetic nervous system after spinal cord injury. *Arch Phys Med Rehabil* 2000;81:506-16.

Thurmbikat P, Tophill PR. Autonomic dysreflexia. *J. R. Soc. Med* 2003;96(12):618-9.

Truitt WA, Coolen LM. Identification of a potential ejaculation generator in the spinal cord. *Science.* 2002;297(5586):1566-9.

Truitt WA, Shipley MT, Veening JG, Coolen LM. Activation of a subset of lumbar spinothalamic neurons after copulatory behavior in male but not female rats. *J. Neurosci.* 2003;23(1):325-31.

Whipple B & Komisaruk BR. Brain (PETG) responses to vaginal-cervical self-stimulation in women with complete spinal cord injury: preliminary findings. *J. Sex Marital Ther* 2002;28:79-86.

Yaïci ED, Rampin O, Tang Y, Calas A, Jestin A, Leclerc P, Benoit G, Giuliano F. Cathecholaminergic projections on to spinal neurons destined to the pelvis including the penis in rat. *Int. J. Impotence research* 2002;14(3):151-166.

In: Sexual Dysfunctions
Editor: Frédérique Courtois

ISBN: 978-1-62808-765-9
© 2013 Nova Science Publishers, Inc.

Chapter 2

PENIS SIZE AND WOMEN'S SEXUAL SATISFACTION

Roberto Vaz Juliano, Margareth de Mello Ferreira dos Reis,
Renata Gimenez Costa, Ricardo Moreno, Luana Lee, Lívia Job,
Fernanda Gomiero, Ricardo Zagatti, Daniel Amado,
Alexandre Borgheresi, Antonio Carlos Lima Pompeo
*and Marcos Tobias-Machado** *

Section of Urologic Oncology and Andrology, Department of Urology,
ABC Medical School, São Paulo, Brazil

ABSTRACT

The penis is the symbol of masculinity. In many cultures it symbolizes attributes such as strength, intelligence, courage, domination of men over women and possession. For that, many men attribute great importance in its size and seek ways to enlarge it. However, it is not known if the size of the penis in fact matters for the women and her sexual satisfaction. The aim of this chapter is to conduct a literature review to know the average penis size of men and their satisfaction with it, as well as researching the importance given by women to the size of the penis, in length and width, and its relationship on the sexual satisfaction. A systematic review of the literature using the PubMed database was conducted searching penile size and sexual satisfaction as keywords. We found 38 references but only 10 papers reporting women satisfaction were included. In general, the literature suggests that penis size is a factor with less importance to women than personality and external appearance. About 2-5% of women consider penis length very important, 20-30% important and 49-55% consider it unimportant to their satisfaction. On the other hand, one study shows that 90% of women who reported that their partner was average or large were very satisfied with their partner's penis size, compared to 68% who rated their partner as small and who wished their partner had a larger penis. Another study reported that 1 in 3 women are more conditioned to orgasm if their partner's penis is larger than average. There are few and superficial studies that

---

* Corresponding author: Marcos Tobias-Machado MD. Head, Section of Urologic Oncology. Section of Andrology, Department of Urology. ABC Medical School. São Paulo, Brazil. Tel: +55 11 9932-9944. Email: tobias-machado@uol.com.br

address the influence of the size of the penis in female sexual satisfaction in a scientific manner. Results are contradictory and the question is not fully understood. The challenges of this survey are encompasses other confounding factors as social, cultural, psychological and others that can influence women sexual satisfaction. The importance of penile augmentation surgery was not defined. A deeper study on this subject considering different populations may help many men to improve couple sexual satisfaction.

INTRODUCTION

According to Masters and Johnson, "the bigger the penis, more efficient is the man in his coital connection". The size of the male sexual organ, both in the flaccid state as erect, has been considered by many cultures to be able to reflect the sexual bravery of the male [1].

Penis size is a hot topic that generates discussion. Many men tend to seek medical advice because of the dissatisfaction with the size of his penis. However, in most cases, the size of the penis is normal. [2] For example, a survey held with 123 young Korean military showed that some of them underestimates the length of their own penis [3].

The aim of this study is to conduct a literature review to know the average penis size of men and their satisfaction with it as well as researching the importance given by the women to the size of the penis, in length and width, and its relationship on the sexual satisfaction.

METHODS

A systematic review of the literature using the PubMed database was conducted searching penile size and sexual satisfaction as keywords. We found 38 references but only 10 papers that report women satisfaction were included. We try to describe the length variation of penile in different ethnic populations and correlate to information regarding women's satisfaction related to penile dimensions.

RESULTS

The average penis length varies from one country to another. In Italy, the average length of the penis in the erect form is 12.5 cm, in Netherlands the average is of 15.2 cm and in Brazil that average is of 14.3 ± 2cm. [4, 5, 6] The length of the flaccid penis in maximum traction (CRTmax.) was the measure used in a cross-sectional study in Brazil, which correlates the length of the erect penis. When evaluating the CTRmax. of 2,010 children aged 0 to 18 years, the average score for boys aged 18 years (n = 84, of which 71 were in stage 5 of Tanner sexual maturation) was 14.5 cm. Micropenis was considered for this age values under 10.5 cm. [7] The true micropenis is due to hormonal abnormality in the tenth-second week of pregnancy. It is defined by an abnormal size with normal internal genitalia and that can be perceived in the childhood. To be considered a micropenis, the person should be 2.5 standard deviations below the mean for age and must not have other abnormalities [8, 9].

However, studies show that many men are seeking ways to enlarge their penis without having properly a micropenis driven by the thought that they might have a penis too small

[12] The great importance given to the penis is due to its symbol of masculinity. "In many cultures it symbolized attributes such as strength, intelligence, courage, domination of men over women and possession, a symbol of love and be loved" [10].

The big question would be if women attribute so much importance to penis size as men do. Or how much the size influences on female sexual satisfaction? Literature suggests that penis size is among the factor with minor importance to women, far behind personality and external appearance [3,8,11].

However, a Dutch study that evaluated 170 questionnaires of sexually active women concluded that 20% considered penis length important and 55% considered it unimportant. Besides 22% of women found the length of the penis totally unimportant and only 0.6% found it very important. Opinions about the girth of the penis were very similar: 31% found girth important, 2% found it very important and 49% found girth unimportant [5].

In a study conducted in California, USA, views about penis size were assessed in an Internet survey of 52,031 heterosexual men and women. Most men (66%) rated their penis as average, 22% as large, and 12% as small. Also in the study, most women rated their partner's penis size as average (67%), some women viewed their partner's penis size as large (27%), and few women perceived their partner's penis size as small (6%). Turning to satisfaction, most women (84%) were satisfied with their partner's penis size, only 14% wanted their partner to be larger, and 2% wanted their partner to be smaller [11].

Whereas 85% of women were satisfied with their partner's penis size, only 55% of men were satisfied with their penis size, 45% wanted to be larger, and 0.2% wanted to be smaller. Many patients also worry that their romantic partner may not be satisfied with their penis size [13]. These concerns are mostly representations of problems related to anxiety and/or other clinical problems such as erectile dysfunction [3].

For women as for men, there was an association between ratings of penis size and satisfaction with penis size. The vast majority of women who reported that their partner was average or large were very satisfied with their partner's penis size (86% and 94%, respectively). In contrast, the majority of women (68%) who rated their partner as small wished their partner had a larger penis [11].

In another study, with 1,000 Czech women the authors found that female orgasm is strongly associated with the sexual education that vagina is important in orgasm. Approximately 33% of women said they are more conditioned to orgasm if their partner's penis is larger than average, considering the idea that a larger penis stimulates a broader area and thus increase the chances of orgasm [12].

Therefore, the physiological sexual response is also visually stimulated leading women to achieve the state of climax more easily. However, women surveyed reported that there was no preference about penis size [12].

CONCLUSION

After reviewing the literature, we concluded that there are few studies that address the influence of penis size in female sexual satisfaction in a scientific manner. Results are contradictory and this question is not fully understood. The great challenges of this surveys are encompasses other confounding factors as social, cultural, psychological and others that can influence women sexual satisfaction. The importance of penile augmentation surgery was not defined. A deeper study on this subject considering different populations may help many men to improve sexual satisfaction, as they place great importance on the size.

REFERENCES

[1]   Masters W, Jonhson V. *A resposta sexual humana*. São Paulo: Roca; 1984.

[2]   Van Driel MF, Schultz WC, Van de Wiel HB, Mensink HJ. Surgical lengthening of the penis. *Br. J. Urol.* 1998;82(1):81-5.

[3]   Son H, Lee H, Huh JS, Kim SW, Paick JS. Studies on self-esteem of penile size in young Korean military men. *Asian J. Androl.* 2003;5(3):185-9.

[4]   Ponchietti R, Mondaini N, Bonafè M, Di Loro F, Biscioni S, Masieri L. Penile length and circumference: a study on 3,300 young Italian males. *Eur. Urol.* 2001;39(2):183-6.

[5]   Francken AB, van de Wiel HB, van Driel MF, Weijmar Schultz WC. What importance do women attribute to the size of the penis? *Eur. Urol.* 2002;42(5):426-31.

[6]   Ros CT, Teloken C, Sogari PR, et al. Estudo da dimensao peniana em ereçao farmaco-induzida [Study of penile dimension on pharmacological erections]. *J. Bras Urol.* 1993;19(3):130-2.

[7]   Gabrich PN, Vasconcelos JSP, Damião R, Silva EA. Avaliação das medidas do comprimento peniano de crianças e adolescentes [Penile anthropometry in Brazilian child and adolescent]. *J. Pediatr (Rio J.).* 2007;83(5):441-6.

[8]   Lee PA, Mazur T, Danish R, et al. Micropenis. I. Criteria, etiologies and classification. *Johns Hopkins Med J.* 1980;146(4):156-63.

[9]   Wiygul J, Palmer LS. Micropenis. *ScientificWorldJournal.* 2011;11:1462-9.

[10]   Talalaj J, Talalaj S. *The strangest human sex, ceremonies and customs*. Melbourne: Hill of Content Pub; 1995.

[11]   Lever J, Frederick DA, Peplau LA. Does size matter? Men's and women's views on penis size across the lifespan. *Psychology of Men & Masculinity.* 2006;7(3):129-43.

[12]   Brody S, Weiss P. Vaginal orgasm is associated with vaginal (not clitoral) sex education, focusing mental attention on vaginal sensations, intercourse duration, and a preference for a longer penis. *J Sex Med.* 2010;7(8):2774-81.

In: Sexual Dysfunctions
Editor: Frédérique Courtois

ISBN: 978-1-62808-765-9
© 2013 Nova Science Publishers, Inc.

Chapter 3

MALE NEUROGENIC SEXUAL DISORDERS: AN OVERVIEW

Rocco Salvatore Calabrò, Angela Marra and Placido Bramanti*
IRCCS Centro Neurolesi "Bonino-Pulejo," Messina, Italy

ABSTRACT

Sexual function in patients with physical or neurological disabilities is often disregarded by healthcare professionals, even though it is a topic of great importance to patients and to those with whom they share significant relationships. Nevertheless, too often physicians believe that sexuality is not as important as the injury or illness that brought the patient to the rehabilitation team. Neurological disorders frequently alter sexual response by changing the process of sexual stimuli to preclude arousal, decreasing or increasing desire, curtailing genital engorgement. Patients with a neurological disease may be challenged in the physical ability to communicate, embrace, stimulate, engage in intercourse, and maintain urinary and bowel continence during sexual activity. Epilepsy, demyelinating disorders, brain and spinal cord injuries, peripheral neuropathy as well as treatments used for these diseases, may often cause erectile and/or ejaculation dysfunctions; moreover, sexual desire is often affected in many neurological disorders. Thus, neurological patients, especially if male and young, may regard their sexual loss as the most devastating aspect, further worsening their quality of life. This chapter is aimed at investigating sexual dysfunctions in men with neurological disorders, exploring the anatomo-physiology of sexual function, the prevalence and main features of the different neurogenic sexual disorders, and highlighting the importance of proper counseling, diagnosis and treatment.

INTRODUCTION

Sexual function in patients with physical or neurological disabilities is often disregarded by healthcare professionals, even though it is a topic of great importance to patients and to

---

* Corresponding author: Rocco Salvatore Calabrò, MD, PhD. IRCCS Centro Neurolesi "Bonino-Pulejo". Messina, Italy. Email: salbro77@tiscali.it.

those with whom they share significant relationships. Too often, physicians believe that sexuality is not as important as the injury or illness that brought the patient to the rehabilitation team. The quality of personal relationships, sexual ones in particular, exert great impact on a patient's self-esteem and support network. The multiple physical, psychological, and emotional changes that may occur after a catastrophic injury, or as a result of a congenital disability or chronic illness, must be addressed not only in the context of the patient, but also of the patient's support system. The issue of sexuality must be addressed during the acute and long-term rehabilitation processes. Sexual function recovery is no less important than any other aspect of functional rehabilitation from a disabling disease or injury. Indeed, people with disabilities are sexual individuals with sexual desire; their concerns require the attention of health care providers [1].

Neuroanatomic and Physiological Basis of Sexual Function

The key brain regions mediating human sexual behavior and modulating genital reflexes have been identified in humans by examining the effect of neurological insult on sexual behavior and through recent functional neuroimaging findings [2].

Six main regions with their complex neuronal connections play a pivotal role in human sexuality:

1)   the *hypothalamus* that mediates neuroendocrine and autonomic aspects of sexual drive and is thought to be responsible for sexual orientation;
2)   the *septal region*, involved in the mediation of orgasm and sexual pleasure;
3)   the *ansa lenticularis* and *pallidus* implicated in sexual drive;
4)   the *frontal lobes*, in particular the prefrontal cortex, involved in the motor components of sexual behavior and the control of sexual response ;
5)   the *parietal lobes*, in particular the paracentral lobule, implicated in genital sensation;
6)   the *temporal lobes*, with particular regard to the *amygdala*, involved in sexual orientation, sexual drive and sexual dysfunctions (i.e. paraphilia) and to the *hippocampus*, responsible for both emotion and memory in relation to the complex cerebral modulation of sexual behavior.

Other important areas such as nucleus paragigantocellularis (nPG1), locus coeruleus (LC), raphe nuclei, periaqueductal gray area are located in the brainstem and intimately connected to the spinal cord and are mainly involved in erection and ejaculation. Moreover insula seems to play an important role in sexual behavior modulating homeostasis and emotions [2, 3].

The human sexual response cycle is a four-stage model of physiological responses during sexual stimulation, proposed for the first time by William H. Masters and Virginia E. Johnson in their book *Human Sexual Response* (1966) and composed of the sequential phases of excitement, plateau, orgasm, and resolution.

The mechanisms underlying *generalized arousal* are complex and involve many cerebral circuits [4]. Regarding ascending pathways, five major neurochemical systems are classically recognized as contributing to the arousal of the forebrain, i.e. those signaled by norepinephrine, dopamine, serotonin, acetylcholine and histamine, while the role of glutamate is less widely recognized. Of special importance to the regulation of CNS arousal are the reticular neurons along the ventral and medial borders of the medullary and pontine reticular formation, that are crucial to the life of the organism as they respond to pain, genital sensation, to CO_2 levels in the blood, to changes in body temperature and cardiovascular functions. Other important axons descend from the paraventricular nucleus and from the preoptic area of the hypothalamus affecting all the arousal aspects. A neurobehavioral and multifaceted model of neural mechanisms for sexual arousal has been proposed which includes a cognitive, an emotional, a motivational, and an autonomic component.

Cerebral areas which have been found to be linked to the cognitive mechanism include the "attentive" network relaying in orbitofrontal cortex and the superior parietal lobules, motor imagery in inferior parietal lobules, while the motivational component would be stored in the caudal part of the anterior cingulate cortex, related to motor preparation processes; finally, the autonomic mechanism would involve the hypothalamus, insula, and the rostral part of the anterior cingulate cortex [5].

Erection is a neurovascular event characterized by the tumescence of the cavernous bodies that relies upon integration of neural and humoral mechanisms at various levels of the nervous system. It requires the participation of autonomic and somatic nerves, i.e. sacral parasympathetic (pelvic), thoracolumbar sympathetic (hypogastric and lumbar chain) and somatic (pudendal) nerves, and the integration of numerous spinal (L1-L2 and S2-S4) and supraspinal sites, with regard to Hypothalamic and limbic pathways.

Ejaculation is a complex and still poorly understood neurological mechanism, at both spinal and cerebral levels as it is closely associated with orgasm, which refers to the ejaculation extragenital responses and the subjective pleasurable feelings.

Physiologically ejaculation consists of two phases: emission, which is characterized by the secretion from epithelial cells and the accessory sex glands of seminal fluids, excreted and stored in the proximal urethra, is mainly a sympathetic reflex (T10-L3) and expulsion, whereas expulsion is a mixed spinal circuit with parasympathetic afferents, a parasympathetic and somatic spinal centre (Onuf's nucleus) and somatic efferents.

Orgasm refers to the subjective experience of pleasure associated with those somatic phenomena occurring during ejaculation such as the rhythmic contractions of the genital and reproductive organs, cardiovascular and respiratory changes and the release of sexual tension. This subjective sensation could be the consequence of both sympathetic and parasympathetic cerebral tension-release processes occurring together. It is important to underline that ejaculation and orgasm can be dissociated in men as the possibility of ejaculation without orgasm (anesthetic ejaculation) has been documented and orgasm can occur without ejaculation ("nonsexual orgasm").

Considering the complex interplays between several CNS regions in determining sexual function, it is clear that many neurotransmitters and hormones are also involved.

Among them, serotonin (5HT) and dopamine are to be considered of particular importance, taking also into account their receptors' potential role as psychoactive drug target [6]. .

Generally speaking, 5-HT has an inhibitory effect on male sexual function. Antidepressants of the selective serotonin reuptake inhibitor class (SSRI) impair ejaculatory/orgasmic function and frequently inhibit erectile function and sexual interest as well. Interestingly, experimental lesions of a major source of 5-HT to spinal cord, the nPG1, disinhibit the urethrogenital reflex (a model of sexual climax) and reflexive erections and penile anteroflexions, confirming the potential inhibitory role of serotonin on sexuality.

The role of dopamine in human sexuality is not completely understood yet and most of our knowledge comes from animal models. Dopamine in the striatum disinhibits pathways through which the cortex elicits movements: this neurotransmitter is released during copulation, but not during precopulatory exposure to a receptive female, suggesting that striatal dopamine is important for motoric aspect of copulation, but not for sexual motivation. Indeed, the mesolimbic system is critical for appetitive behavior and reinforcement; in fact, it is activated before and during a variety of motivated behaviors, including eating, drinking, copulating and drug-self administration. Furthermore, dopamine in the MPOA facilitates male sexual behavior in many species, suggesting that it plays a central role in this process.

Sexual Dysfunction in Neurological Disorders

Stroke could soon be the most common cause of death worldwide. Indeed, it is currently the second leading cause of death in the Western world, ranking after heart disease and before cancer, and causes 10% of deaths worldwide. The most difficult aspect of having a stroke is living with the disability caused by this condition. Stroke is associated with high morbidity rates, meaning that many patients experience both physical and mental disability following the event.

Various studies have shown a significant decrease in sexual satisfaction after cerebrovascular accidents (CVA) [7,8]. In men affected by stroke, a decline in libido and poor or tailed erection and ejaculation are frequently observed. Indeed, the reported prevalence of post-stroke diminished libido varies from 17% to 42%. Korpelainen et al. [9] showed a significant decline in libido, sexual arousal and satisfaction with sexual life in both male and female stroke patients, but the frequency of patients who ceased having sexual intercourse was lower (28% at 2 months and 14% at 6 months) than in the previous studies. The same authors demonstrated that sexual dysfunction (SD) was strictly related to the presence of sensory hemisyndrome, with changes in the frequency of intercourse were related to the degree of cutaneous sensibility impairments and levels of independence in activities of daily living, but not with the degree of motor impairment.

The cause of SD is often multifactorial with a complex interplay between psychological and organic factors. In fact, sexual problems seem to be related to various factors, like the general attitude toward sexuality, an incipient depression with anxiety after the CVA or prior medical conditions such as hypertension, diabetes mellitus, or the use of specific drugs [10].

Some authors have postulated a relationship between the location of the lesion and sexual change, since sexual disorders appear to be more frequent when the right hemisphere is involved.

Epilepsy (from the Ancient Greek επιληψία *epilēpsía*) is a common chronic neurological disorder characterized by recurrent unprovoked seizures. These seizures are transient signs and/or symptoms of abnormal, excessive or synchronous neuronal activity potentially involving all the brain areas.

Sexual health is one of the most important aspects of quality of life (QoL), and it is often impaired in epileptic patients. Sexual disorders associated with epilepsy can be directly related to seizures (ictal), or unrelated in time to seizures occurrence (interictal). Seizures may also be provoked by "normal" sexual activity. Epilepsy has been described in association with self-mutilation, transvestitism, sadomasochism, exhibitionism and fetishism and these sexual disorders may be resolved with the cessation of attacks through medical or surgical treatment. Hypersexuality, i.e. excessive sexual activity which produces no lasting relief or satisfaction has been occasionally reported. However, the most common SD in epileptic patients is hyposexuality, defined as "a global reduction in sexual interest, awareness and activity".

Gastaut [12] was the first author to underline the association between sexual dysfunction and epilepsy. In his uncontrolled study, he found a global hyposexuality in over two-thirds of patients with temporal lobe epilepsy. Since then many studies have been performed in epileptic men with regard to partial epilepsy, showing rates of sexual dysfunction from 22% to 67%.

The dysfunction most often mentioned includes reduced potency, decreased desire and impaired sexual performance even if it has been suggested that epilepsy interferes specifically with physiological function while sexual desire remains unaffected (12).

There has not been a consensus regarding the prevalence of erectile dysfunction (ED), which varies within particular epileptic patients with a frequency as low as 3% in outpatients to as high as 58% in patients evaluated for epilepsy surgery [14]. Moreover, epileptic men have been found to have an increased risk of ED of up to 57% compared to 3-9% in the general population.

Despite sexual disorders are common in people with epilepsy, the etiology remains still unknown but it is likely to be multifactorial involving neurological, iatrogenic, endocrine psychiatric and psychosocial factors.

In particular, both seizures and antiepileptic drugs can affect the hypothalamic-pituitary-gonadal male axis causing changes in hormones and sexuality.

Liver enzyme-inducing AEDs, that is, phenobarbital, phenytoin, and carbamazepine, can cause SD by decreasing bioactive testosterone, accelerating sexual hormone metabolism, and stimulating sexual hormone binding globulin production. On the other hand, valproate, a liver enzyme-inhibiting drug, seems to increase estrogen levels, perhaps by suppressing enzymatic metabolism of estradiol. New AEDs are thought to cause sexual disorders through complex and poorly understood mechanisms, involving a possible imbalance in CNS neurotrasmitter concentrations, with regard to dopamine/serotonin rate [16].

Multiple sclerosis (MS) is a common inflammatory disorder of the central nervous system affecting about 2.5 million people around the world. MS represents the most common cause of neurological disability among young adults.

Historically, clinical studies have reported a prevalence of SD in male patients with MS ranging from 7% to 91% [17,18]. More recent studies have confirmed a high prevalence of SD in men, ranging from 45% to 70% [19]. SD prevalence is significantly higher in MS patients than in the general population. In a large case-control study [9], male patients with MS experienced decreased libido, ED and ejaculatory dysfunction with a higher frequency than patients with other chronic diseases or healthy controls.

In recent years, a comprehensive conceptual model of SD in MS has been developed, categorizing SD in three general components: primary, secondary and tertiary SD. The primary SD is directly due to MS-related neurologic deficits affecting the sexual response. Men complain of altered genital sensation, decreased libido, ejaculation and orgasmic dysfunction and, most commonly, erectile dysfunction (ED). The secondary SD is attributed to MS-related physical impairments and symptoms that affect indirectly the sexual response, including spasticity and contractures, fatigue, bladder dysfunction and cognitive symptoms. Furthermore, adverse effects of MS medications are frequently causes of secondary SD. The tertiary SD is caused by the psychological, social and cultural issues of having a chronic disabling disease that affects sexual functioning.

Spinal cord injury. Despite advances in the field of medicine, injury to the spinal cord remains a devastating problem. Spinal cord Injury (SCI) often results in permanent neurological deficit and, depending on the level of injury, may leave the patient severely disabled. SCI has a dramatic emotional impact on the patient and his family and represents a high burden to society. Moreover, patients with SCI have a poor quality of life, often worsened by the presence of SD, which is really dramatic especially at a young age [20].

According to the International Standards for Neurological Classification, SCI can be classified as *tetraplegia* (quadriplegia) if it involves a cervical spinal segment or *paraplegia* if it involves a thoracic, lumbar, or sacral spinal segment. SCI is further identified as being *complete* (absence of all motor or sensory functions at the lowest sacral level) or *incomplete* (at least some preservation of motor or sensory functions below the level of the injury, including the lowest sacral level).

Complete SCI is a *functional* transection of the spinal cord in which electrical impulses of sensory information going up to the brain, as well as motor information coming down from the brain, are disrupted.

Studies on war veterans identified spinal reflex and psychogenic pathways for erection and showed that level and completeness of spinal cord damage determine the extent to which erectile and ejaculatory capacity is affected. Indeed, the impact on sexual functioning depends on the degree of injury and its location on the spinal cord [21, 22]

After SCI involving specific spinal centre, male patients may present erection, ejaculation and fertility dysfunction [23-25].

Erectile dysfunction is one of the main male SD following SCI, especially in lower complete lesions. Reflexogenic erection is induced by cutaneous or mucous membrane stimulation from areas below the level of the lesion, thus requiring an intact reflex arc, including S2 - 4. Psychogenic erection is induced by psychic stimulation: visual, auditory, olfactory, as well as dreams, memories, and fantasies: in men with SCI below L2 it is believed that this kind of erection occurs via the thoracolumbar sympathetic outflow. Mixed erection may occur when the level of the lesion is below L2 and above S2, but the erectile response may differ individually regarding the duration and quality of the erection.

Damage to the cauda equina is likely to affect both the anterior and posterior sacral pathways that contain somatic and parasympathetic fibers, thus determining both loss of perineal sensation and sexual response and loss of voluntary control of the anal and uretra sphincters and leading to ED.

In addition to having ED problems, ejaculatory function may be compromised in SCI because of an impairment in the coordinated neurologic impulses between the sympathetic, parasympathetic and somatic nervous systems [21]. Men with incomplete SCI are more likely to achieve simultaneous orgasm than men with any other patterns of SCI, although a number of men with SCI achieve orgasm without ejaculation [26].

Male infertility associated with SCI occurs from a combination of erectile dysfunction and ejaculatory failure. In the acute phase of SCI, semen quality is normal (6-12 days post-injury) but in the following weeks, sperm motility and viability declines [25].

Other factors that contribute to infertility include frequent urinary tract infections, impaired scrotal thermoregulation and retrograde ejaculation.

Neurodegenerative disorders. Alzheimer disease (AD), a neurodegenerative disease predominantly affecting associative brain regions such as medial temporal, posterior cingulate, lateral temporal, parietal and frontal cortices, is clinically characterized by a progressive decline in memory and higher cognitive functions. AD patients are mainly impaired in controlled cognitive processes such as explicit memory recall, and they frequently rely on familiarity-based processes, allowing them to perform routine (automatic) activities.

AD is the most common form of dementia affecting about 5% of 65 years older and 20% of 85 years older people, and followed by vascular dementia and Lewy body disease.

Although general population has historically held vague assumptions and myths concerning sexual issues and practices of the older people, several studies have highlighted how they experience sexual interest and activity [28].

The most frequent sexual disorder in AD-patients is hypersexuality or inappropriate sexual behaviour [29, 30]. Many authors refer to these altered behaviors using the following two definitions: (1) overt acts associated with increased libido; (2) persistent, uninhibited, sexual behaviors directed at oneself or other people. Sexual altered behaviors are often verbal and/or physical acts with sexual meaning or intent. Patients could present with increased libido, change in orientation, sexual comments, excessive hugging/kissing, preoccupation with sex, masturbation in public, grabbing at the genitals and/or breasts of other residents or staff, sexual hallucinations, delusions of spousal infidelity, attempting to seduce other residents or staff, chasing other residents for sexual purposes, exposing one's genitals in public, and disrobing in public. Indeed, some behaviors are thought to be inappropriate because they are performed publicly. Moreover, even when inappropriate sexual behavior is not so bouncy, it can be profoundly disruptive to caregivers and other residents in assisted living and skilled nursing facilities [30, 31].

Parkinson's Diseases (PD) involves motor system, mental, cognitive and autonomic functions, and is clinically characterized by motor and non-motor impairment. Among the latter, the SD are frequent, impairing QoL and welfare, but are often overlooked for various reasons, including: reluctance of patients in dealing with sexual problems, lack of awareness about the possible relationship between PD and SD, omission of sexual anamnesis.

SD in PD can result from alterations in motor, mental or cognitive disease-specific functions and involve both the desire and sexual arousal. Indeed, alterations in arousal are believed to be related to the interference of motor impairments and other non motor disorders on sexual activity (sialorrhea, seborrhea, bradykinesia, akinesia, etc.). Motor disorders of PD (bradykinesia, rigidity, tremor, immobility in bed, difficulty in movements of the fingers and hands) can alter the physical contact between partners and make sexual intercourse very difficult, leading the patient to have a more passive role with the sexual partners and to require a patient with a more active role [35]. Some events such as sweating, drooling, disorders of posture, and tremor make patients less attractive, while hypomimia could be interpreted by the partner as a lack of feeling or desire. Loss of libido with a related ED are the most frequently reported SD in Parkinsonisms [36-38]. Finally, several drugs can cause either hyposexuality or hypersexuality. For example, libido seems to rise after dopaminergic therapy: L-Dopa in 8% of patients is used to restore sexual activity and in 1% of patients induces hypersexuality; the dopamine agonists may induce hypersexuality in 3% of patients, and apomorphine and ropinirole probably have an effect on stimulation of D2 receptors of preoptic area with an increase of oxytocin at the lumbosacral spinal level, which cause erectogenic stimuli [39-40].

Traumatic brain injury. Sexual impairment is a commonly described consequence of traumatic brain injury (TBI) [41]. Indeed, many authors believe that sexual dysfunction is "more often the rule than the exception" . A brain trauma could involve all those brain regions activated during a normal sexual response. Nevertheless, sexual impairment in injured people seems to be related both to a direct effect of trauma on sexual pathway and to a situational change in the patient's mood, the latter contributing to higher rates of SD after brain trauma (about 36-54%). Sexual dysfunctions after TBI are more reported in men than in women, and mostly in severe rather than minor trauma [42-43].

Physiopathology and type of sexual disorders of post TBI patients are closely dependent on the damaged brain area, although poor attention has been paid on understanding the specific nature or the impact of SD in these individuals. The most reported sexual dysfunctions in men after TBI are ED and disorders of desire, mainly when anterior brain regions are damaged [43].

Erectile Dysfunction is considered to be due either to post TBI depression or to damage of the hypothalamic-pituitary axis. Indeed, although many authors reported that head injured males experience ED when associated to depression, it has recently been found how erectile problems are often accompanied by signs and symptoms of cerebral damage and impaired libido. Since anterior brain regions are associated with emotional and behavioral impairment, prefrontal and lobar lesions might more frequently generate hyposexuality rather than hypersexuality. The latter is often reported as an intensified sexual experience after brain injury, an inappropriate sexual attention towards others, or a kind of sexual exhibitionism leading to sexually deviant criminal activities (i.e. rape or pedophilia) [43, 44]. Injury of pituitary gland is a frequent complication of head trauma and it is associated with high mortality rate during the acute phase. Serious and life-threatening adrenal crisis due to adrenocorticotropic deficiencies following TBI is widely highlighted in many clinical studies. The prevalence of endocrine dysfunction after TBI, due to anterior pituitary lesions, ranges from 15% to 68%. Both anterior and posterior parts of the gland could be damaged. Hemorrhage, necrosis and fibrosis in the context of pituitary gland are common complications of TBI. Moreover, they are often associated with hypothalamopituitary impairment of the chronic TBI phase [45].

Lesions of the anterior part of pituitary gland is associated with altered sexual desire related to Luteinizing Hormone (LH), Follicle-Stimulating Hormone (FSH), Prolactin (PRL) and Growth Hormone (GH) alterations.

Klùver-Bucy Syndrome (KBS) is one of the most common temporo-limbic syndromes caused by a bilateral damage of anterior temporal lobes. KBS is quite frequent in post TBI patients due to the injury of temporal and orbitofrontal areas with the bone of middle and anterior cranial fossae [46].

In 1939 Klùver and Bucy bilaterally removed the anterior temporal lobes in primates and noted six different neuropsychiatric symptoms, i.e. "Psychic blindness", hypersexuality, altered emotional behavior, hyperorality, "hypermetamorphosis" and memory deficit, related to limbic cortex and amygdala involvement. They termed psychic blindness as the inability of animals to recognize emotional significance of the object, while they used hypermetamorphosis to indicate the tendency to react to every visual stimulus especially with the mouth. Indeed, their animals became tame with an excessive and sometimes life-threatening oral exploration of the environment.

In humans, KBS is rare and described as typical in the post-traumatic remission phase and associated with favorable prognosis in the outcome of traumatic disturbances of consciousness in survivors of head trauma [47].

Diagnostic Work-up

Diagnostic assessment of sexual disorders in male patients consists of three phases: anamnesis, physical examination and instrumental investigation [48, 49].

Anamnesis or medical history is the key element of clinical approach. It leads to the identification of risk factors (personal habits including smoking, alcohol intake and use of psychoactive drugs, endocrino-metabolic diseases, psychological and/or social stressors) in order to look into either the organic or psychological pathogenesis of the sexual dysfunction, and acts as a guide for further diagnostic evaluation.

A psychological screening for depression and anxiety disorders should always be performed, using validated scales such as Hamilton Rating Scale for Depression and Anxiety, to rule out the possible psychological/psychiatric causes in determining SD.

Medication history plays an important role since there are many drugs commonly used in neurological patients, i.e., antidepressants, neuroleptics, sedatives, β-blockers, diuretics, which may lead to sexual side effects.

Although SD is common in male patients with neurological disorders, its quantification is limited by the paucity of validated, user-friendly scales. Sexual functioning may be easily measured by using the Arizona Sexual Experience Scale (ASEX), a brief five-item scale designed to assess the core elements of sexual function (i.e., drive, arousal, penile erection/vaginal lubrication, ability to reach orgasm, and satisfaction with orgasm), or by the IIEF, a standardized and validated 15-item self-evaluation scale that provides pre–post treatment clinic evaluations of erectile function, orgasmic function, sexual desire, satisfaction in sexual intercourse, and general satisfaction.

General, neurological and urogenital examination is necessary to point out medical comorbidities. Indeed, ED can be the first clinical sign of an unknown and untreated cardiovascular disease, so an accurate evaluation of the heart and of the main arteries should be done in selected individuals.

A full endocrine and metabolic workup, including serum levels of testosterone and thyroidal function, may be of some help in some cases.

The instrumental investigation is built up to confirm the suspicion made by history and physical examination and, typically, used to evaluate erectile function and capacity since the other aspects of normal male sexual response are better assessed by a psychological approach and better diagnosed using DSM-IV and ICD-10.

It is well known that some erectile episodes are present during REM sleep. The neural mechanism of this sleep related erection (SRE) remains largely unknown, although the involvement of several structures of the brainstem, acting directly on the spinal center of the erection, or on the hypothalamic (preoptic area), and other diencephalic structures was hypothesized. The screening of SRE through Nocturnal Penile Tumescence REM sleep Monitoring (NPTRM) is widespread used to differentiate the psychogenic ED from the organic one [50]. When NPTRM is inconclusive a penile colour duplex ultrasound (PCDU) should be requested to investigate abnormalities or disease of penile vessels leading to ED and strengthening the suspicion of a psychogenic etiology of ED. While basal PCDU can show arterial or venous abnormalities of the penis, a dynamic PCDU, with intracavernous injection test, studies the hemodynamic changes occurring during pharmacological erection [51]. In patients affected by neurological disease and suffering of ED and/or ejaculatory disorders, a diagnosis of involvement of neural and muscular structures related to sexual function may be strengthened, refined and documented by neurophysiological testing [52]. The Dorsal Penile Nerve Conduction gives information about the speed of sensitive nervous conduction through an orthodromic sensitive nerve conduction performed by distending the penis and applying two electrodes to the extremities. The bulbocavernosus reflex is the neurophysiological correlate of the elicited bulbocavernosus reflex during the neurological examination, often requested when the response to physical stimuli is not clear; it is performed in men by stimulation of the dorsal penile nerve and detecting the response in the pelvic floor muscle through the aid of concentric single fiber needle Electromyography (EMG). The pudendal-SEP evaluates the speed of conduction to cortex of stimuli applied at peripheral level with a percutaneous bipolar electrode placed on the penile shaft. giving information whether the site of the lesion is peripheral or central.

Other helpful neurophysiological tests include the Pelvic Floor muscle EMG, the Sympathetic Skin Response and the CardioVascular Reflex Tests.

Finally, *Penile Angiography, Cavernosometry and Cavernosography are* three diagnostic tools that are considered as third level investigations and used to better evaluate arterial and venous pathologies. They are performed only when PCDU exam is unconclusive to refine the diagnosis of a vascular and especially in young subjects candidate for surgical repair.

Treatment

Significant advances in the understanding of the physiology and pathophysiology of male sexual function, and in methods of its investigation and treatment, have been attained during the past decades. Since SD are very common in male affected by neurological diseases, it is mandatory that neurologists are aware of sexual problems and of their treatment in order to improve patient's quality of life. *Oral pharmacotherapy* is currently the mainstay of treatment for ED [53]. Although a number of oral prescription drugs may have the potential to be used to treat impotence, most of these drugs act centrally, they are not so effective in this regard and have a number of side effects. Significant advances in the pharmacologic treatment of ED have occurred in recent years, most notably after the introduction of sildenafil, the first oral selective phosphodiesterase type 5 (PDE5) inhibitor, in 1998. Sildenafil quickly gained acceptance by the medical community and the public because of its broad efficacy for different types of ED and its ease of use [54]. Two PDE5 inhibitors, Vardenafil and Tadalafil, have since joined sildenafil to compete in the ED market [55]. Common adverse events with all three PDE5i include headache, flushing, nasal congestion and dyspepsia. Specific drug-related adverse effects include visual disturbance, mainly for sildenafil and Vardenafil, and myalgia/back pain, mainly for Tadalafil. However, these adverse events are generally mild, self-limited after long-term use and not associated with treatment discontinuation. Lastly, the possible relationship between non-arteritic anterior ischemic optic neuropathy (NAION) and

PDE5i use has raised important questions; nevertheless, to date, there is no epidemiological evidence that the incidence of NAION is higher in patients receiving PDE5i [54].

Of particular recent interest has been the utilization of PDE5i as routinely dose medication. Based on existing animal data, it has been hypothesized that administration of daily PDE5i may help to prevent apoptosis in the corporal sinusoids, preserve smooth muscle content, and reduce collagen accumulation in a variety of disease states. Therefore, routine dose PDE5i has been investigated as means for long-term modulation and treatment of ED (typically ED related to cavernous nerve or corporal tissue damage), stuttering ischemic priapism, and some lower urinary tract symptoms.

Injectable and intraurethral agents were relegated to second line therapy after the appearance of the effective oral PDE5i. However, the local delivery of medication (i.e. PGE1 and papaverine) remains useful as in about 25-30% of ED patients PDE5i are ineffective.

About 40% of patients with ED have evidence of abnormal arterial flow, only partly involving aortoiliac carrefour, since most men with major vessel disease rarely present with impotence. Conversely, the majority of vascular ED patients have pathological changes in the small vessels of the penis and, generally, *revascularization* for such smaller arteries is challenging with long-term patients' dissatisfaction and complications including pain, altered sensation, shortening of penile length and glans hyperemia. Also the long-term success rate of *penile vein ligation* is poor. *Penile prosthesis* offers a valid therapeutic alternative for patients who fail vasoactive drugs and vacuum-constrictive devices and who are not candidates for vascular reconstruction procedures [56].

Since *premature ejaculation* (PE) is mostly due to a psychogenic etiology, *psychosexual treatment* is considered the mainstay with high rates of success. Nevertheless, it has been shown that the failure of psychosexual-behavioral therapy, such as the stop-start technique and the start-stop-squeeze by Master and Johnson, may be related to the pooled patients with different PE categories, age groups, anxiety level, sexual experience and somatic vulnerabilities (i.e. urologic and neurogenic hypersensitivities), investigated in many of the studies [57-58].

Since the most common etiology of *anorgasmia* is the intake of psychotropic agents, regaining of the orgasmic sensation may be achieved with discontinuation and/or substitution of the incinting drug. In cases of anejaculation, vibratory stimulation may be helpful, but intact dorsal penile nerves are necessary for the ejaculatory response. If the aim is to retrieve sperm for assisted fertilization, electroejaculation is preferred [58].

Ejaculatory pain represents a component of sexual dysfunction that has received little attention in the literature so far. Postorgasmic pain is associated with prostatitis, chronic pelvic pain syndrome, benign prostatic hyperplasia, ejaculatory duct obstruction, prostate radiation, and radical prostatectomy. The treatment options vary from self-care to medication with alpha-blockers such as tamsulosin, antidepressants such as amitriptilyne, antiepileptics, antinflammatory agents and muscle relaxants, and even surgical procedures such as pudendal nerve decompression [58].

Priapism may be a side effect of intracorporeal injection and, less frequently, can be associated with systemic drug intake such as phenotiazine and trazodone. Mild cases may be treated with oral intake of α-receptor agonists such as pseudoephedrine. More severe cases of priapism lasting for more than 4 h usually require corporeal aspiration and irrigation with a solution of heparin and epinephrine. Occasionally, prolonged priapism (of more than 24-36 h duration) requires surgical placement of an arterio-venous shunt, which will cause a venous leakage and a possible failure of response to future vasoactive drugs.

CONCLUSION

Sexuality is one of the most complex aspects of human life. Sexual expression is dependent on functioning anatomical and physiological systems, which are influenced by cognitive and emotional processes. To assess and treat problems in this area requires knowledge of those factors influencing both the dynamics of the relationship and the physical and psychological aspects of sexual functioning. Neurological disease and trauma have long been recognized as causing sexual dysfunction, through complex and multifaceted mechanisms.

Nevertheless, practicing neurologists have not traditionally paid much attention to SD in their patients, partly because therapeutic possibilities were scant. With emerging awareness of the primary importance of quality of life as the most important indicator of good patient management, and with the advent of more effective treatment of SD, ignoring this very important dimension of life is no longer acceptable.

REFERENCES

[1]   Rees PM, Fowler CJ, Maas CP. Sexual function in men and women with neurological disorders. *Lance Neurologyt.* 2007;369:512-25.

[2]   Baird AD, Wilson SJ, Bladin PF, Saling MM, Reutens DC. Neurological control of human sexual behaviour: insights from lesion studies. *J. Neurol Neurosurg Psychiatry.* 2007;78:1042-9.

[3]   McKenna K. The brain is the master organ in sexual function: central nervous system control of male and female sexual function. *Int J. Impot Res.* 1999;11 Suppl 1:S48-55.

[4]   Pfaus JG. Pathways of sexual desire. *J. Sex Med.* 2009; 6:1506-33.

[5]   Meston CM, Frohlich PF. The neurobiology of sexual function. *Arch Gen Psychiatry.* 2000 ;57:1012-30.

[6]   Hull EM, Muschamp JW, Sato S. Dopamine and serotonin: influences on male sexual behavior. *Physiol Behav.* 2004; 83:291-307.

[7]   Tamam Y, Tamam L, Akil E, Yasan A, Tamam B. Post-stroke sexual functioning in first stroke patients. *Eur. J. Neurol.* 2008;15:660-6.

[8]   Giaquinto S, Buzzelli S, Di Francesco L, Nolfe G Evaluation of sexual changes after stroke. *J. Clin. Psychiatry.* 2003;64:302-7.

[9]   Korpelainen JT, Nieminen P, Myllylä VV. Sexual functioning among stroke patients and their spouses. *Stroke.* 1999;30:715-9.

[10]   Calabrò RS, Gervasi G, Bramanti P. Male sexual disorders following stroke: an overview. *Int J. Neurosci.* 2011;121:598-604.

[11]   Calabrò RS, Marino S, Bramanti P. Sexual and reproductive dysfunction associated with antiepileptic drug use in men with epilepsy. *Expert Rev Neurother.* 2011;11:887-95.

[12] Gastaut H and Collomb H. Etude du comportement sexual chez les epileptiques psychomotors. *Annales Medico-Psychologiques*. 1954; 112: 657-659.

[13] Morrell MJ, Sperling MR, Stecker M, Dichter MA. Sexual dysfunction in partial epilepsy: a deficit in physiologic sexual arousal. *Neurology*. 1994;44:243-7.

[14] Smaldone M, Sukkarieh T, Reda A, Khan A. Epilepsy and erectile dysfunction: a review. *Seizure*. 2004;13: 453-9.

[15] Calabrò RS. Erectile dysfunction and epilepsy: what is the link? *J. Sex Med.* 2013;10:615-6.

[16] Calabrò RS. Sexual disorders related to new antiepileptic drugs: a need for more studies! *Epilepsy Behav*. 2011;20:734-5.

[17] McCabe, MP. Exacerbation of symptoms among people with multiple sclerosis: impact on sexuality and relationships over time. *Arch Sex Behav*, 2004, 33, 593-601.

[18] Zorzon, M; Zivadinov, R; Monti Bragadin, L, et al. Sexual dysfunction in multiple sclerosis: a 2-year follow-up study. *J. Neurol. Sci*, 2001, 187, 1-5.

[19] Demirkiran, M; Sarica, Y; Uguz, S; Yerdelen, D; Aslan, K. Multiple sclerosis patients with and without sexual dysfunction: are there any differences? *Mult. Scler*. 2006, 12, 209-14.

[20] Dikaios S. If not the disability, then what? Barriers to reclaiming sexuality following spinal cord injury. *Sex Disabil* 2006,24:101-11.

[21] Jonson RD. Descending pathway modulationg the spinal circuitry for ejaculation: effects of chronic spinal cord Injury. *Prog Brain Res*. 2006;152:415-26.

[22] Sipski ML. Sexual functioning in the spinal cord Injured. Int J Import Res 1998;10 (suppl 2): S1 28-30, (discussion: S 1 38- 40).

[23] Deforge D, Blackmer J, Garritty C, et al. male erectile dysfunction following spinal cord injury: a systematic review. *Spinal Cord*. 2006;44;465-73.

[24] Ricciardi R, Szabo CM, Poullos AY. Sexuality and Spinal cord injury. Nursing *Clinics of North America*. 2007;42:675-684.

[25] Brown DJ, Hill ST, Baker HW. Male fertility and sexual function after spinal cord Injury. *Prog Brain Res*. 2006;152:427-39.

[26] Allard J, Truitt WA, McKenna KE, et al. Spinal cord control of ejaculaton. *World J. Urol*. 2005;23:119-26.

[27] Anderson KD, Borisoff JF, Johnson RD, Stiens SA, Elliot SL. Long term effects of spinal cord injury on sexual function in men: implications of neuroplasticity. *Spinal Cord* 2007; 45:338-348.

[28] Bouman WP, Arcelus J & Benbow SM. Nottingham study of sexuality & ageing. Attitudes regarding sexuality and older people: a review of the literature. *Sexual and Relationship Therapy* 2006: 21, 149–161.

[29] Higgins A, Barker P, Begley CM. Hypersexuality and dementia: Dealing with inappropriate sexual expression. *BrJ Nurs*. 2004-2005;13:1330-1334.

[30] Kuhn DR, Greiner D, Arseneau L. Addressing hypersexuality in Alzheimer's disease. *J Gerontol Nurs*. 1998;24: 44-50.

[31] Archibald CA. Sexuality, dementia and residential care: managers report and response. *Health and Social in the Community,* 1998, 6, 95–101.

[32] Holmes D, Reingold J & Teresi J. Sexual expression and dementia. Views of caregivers: a pilot study. *International Journal of Geriatric Psychiatry*. 1997; 12, 695–701.

[33] Lyketsos CG, Steinberg M, Tschanz JT, Norton MC, Steffens DC, Breitner JC. Mental and behavioral disturbances in dementia: findings from Cache County Study on Memory and Aging. *Am J Psychiatry.* 2000;157:708-714.

[34] Black B, Muralee S, Tampi RR. Inappropriate Sexual Behaviors in Dementia. *J Geriatr Psychiatry Neurol.* 2005; 18:155-162.

[35] Friedman JH, Brown RG, Comella C, Garber CE, Krupp LB, Lou JS, Marsh L, Nail L, Shulman L, Taylor CB; Working Group on Fatigue in Parkinson's Disease. Fatigue in Parkinson's disease: a review. *Mov Disord.* 2007; 22:297-308.

[36] Meco G, Rubino A, Caravona N, Valente M. Sexual dysfunction in Parkinson's disease. *Parkinsonism Relat Disord.* 2008;14:451-6.

[37] Papatsoris AG, Deliveliotis C, Singer C, Papapetropoulos S. Erectile dysfunction in Parkinson's disease. *Urology.* 2006 Mar;67(3):447-51.

[38] Kummer A, Cardoso F, Teixeira AL. Loss of libido in Parkinson's disease. *J Sex Med.* 2009;6:1024-31.

[39] Vogel HP, Schiffter R. Hypersexuality-a complication of dopaminergic therapy in Parkinson's disease. *Pharmacopsychiatrica.* 1983;16:107-10.

[40] Bronner G. Sexual problems in Parkinson's disease: the multidimensional nature of the problem and of the intervention. *J Neurol Sci.* 2011 15;310(1-2):139-43.

[41] Sandel ME, Williams KS, Dellapietra L, Derogatis LR. Sexual functioning following traumatic brain injury. *Brain Inj.* 1996;10:719-28.

[42] Miller BL, Cummings JL, McIntyre H, Ebers G, Grode M. Hypersexuality or altered sexual preference following brain injury. *J. Neurol Neurosurg Psychiatry.* 1986;49:867-73.

[43] Hibbard MR, Gordon WA, Flanagan S, Haddad L, Labinsky E. Sexual dysfunction after traumatic brain injury. *NeuroRehabilitation.* 2000;15:107-20.

[44] Simpson G, Blaszczynski A, Hodgkinson A. Sex offending as a psychosocial sequela of traumatic brain injury. *J Head Trauma Rehabil.* 1999;14:567-80.

[45] Lieberman SA, Oberoi AL, Gilkison CR, Masel BE, Urban RJ. Prevalence of neuroendocrine dysfunction in patients recovering from traumatic brain injury. *J. Clin Endocrinol Metab.* 2001;86:2752-6.

[46] Carroll BT, Goforth HW, Carroll LA. Anatomic basis of kluver-bucy syndrome. *J. Neuropsychiatry Clin Neurosci.* 1999;11(1):116.

[47] Formisano R, Saltuari L, Gerstenbrand F. Presence of kluver-bucy syndrome as a positive prognostic feature for the remission of traumatic prolonged disturbances of consciousness. *Acta Neurol Scand.* 1995;91:54-7.

[48] Kandeel FR, Koussa VK, Swerdloff RS. Male sexual function and its disorders: physiology, pathophysiology, clinical investigation, and treatment. *Endocrine Reviews.* 2001;22:342-88.

[49] Lundberg PO, Ertekin C, Ghezzi A, Swash M, Vodusek D. Neurosexology. Guidelines for Neurologists. European Federation of Neurological Societies Task Force on Neurosexology. *European Journal of Neurology* 2001, 8 (suppl 3):2-24.

[50] Schmidt MH, Schmidt HS. Sleep-related erections: neural mechanisms and clinical significance. *Current Neurology and Neuroscience Reports.* 2004;4:170-8.

[51] Meuleman EJ, Diemont WL. Investigation of erectile dysfunction. Diagnostic testing for vascular factors in erectile dysfunction. *Urologic Clinics of North America.* 1995;22:803-19.

[52] Diemont WL, Meuleman EJ. Neurological testing in erectile dysfunction. *Journal of Andrology*. 1997;18:345-50.

[53] Calabrò RS, Polimeni G, Bramanti P. Current and future therapies of erectile dysfunction in neurological disorders. *Recent Pat CNS Drug Discov*. 2011;6(1):48-64.

[54] Francis SH, Corbin JD. Sildenafil: efficacy, safety, tolerability and mechanism of action in treating erectile dysfunction. *Expert Opin Drug Metab Toxicol*. 2005;1:283-93.

[55] Feifer A, Carrier S. Pharmacotherapy for erectile dysfunction. Expert Opin Investig Drugs. 2008;17(5):679-90.

[56] Hatzimouratidis K, Hatzichristou DG. Looking to the future for erectile dysfunction therapies. *Drugs*. 2008;68:231-50.

[57] McMahon CG. Dapoxetine for premature ejaculation. *Expert Opin Pharmacother*. 2010;11:1741-52.

[58] Calabrò RS, Polimeni G, Ciurleo R, Casella C, Bramanti P. Neurogenic ejaculatory disorders: focus on current and future treatments. *Recent Pat CNS Drug Discov*. 2011;6(3):205-21.

In: Sexual Dysfunctions
Editor: Frédérique Courtois

ISBN: 978-1-62808-765-9
© 2013 Nova Science Publishers, Inc.

Chapter 4

SEXUAL DYSFUNCTION, QUALITY OF LIFE AND PSYCHOLOGICAL IMPACT OF SPINAL CORD INJURY ON MEN

Ana I. Cobo-Cuenca[*,1], *Miguel Vírseda-Chamorro*[2], *Juan Pedro Serrano-Selva*[1], *Antonio Sampietro-Crespo*[3], *Manuel Esteban-Fuertes*[2] *and Noelia Martín-Espinosa*[1]

[1]University of Castilla la Mancha (UCLM), Spain
[2]Paraplegics' National Hospital, Public Health Service of Castilla-La Mancha, Spain
[3]Hospital Virgen de la Salud, Public Health Service of Castilla la Mancha, Spain

ABSTRACT

This chapter is based on a cross-sectional correlational study. The objectives were to assess the quality of life of 85 men with traumatic spinal cord injury and sexual dysfunction. To assess the coping strategies, depression, anxiety and levels of self-esteem observed in men with chronic spinal cord injury and sexual dysfunction. The setting was the National Hospital of Paraplegics, Toledo, Spain. The methods included the Fugl-Meyer Life Satisfaction Questionnaire Scale (LISAT-8), The Hospital Anxiety and Depression Scale (HADS), The COPE and Rosenberg's Self-esteem Scale were all used for data collection. The results showed that 17.5% of the participants showed signs of depression, 38.7% showed signs of anxiety and 34% showed a lower-moderate level of self-esteem. The coping strategies that were most frequently used by the participants were "personal growth", "acceptance", "positive reinterpretation" and "planning and active coping". The participants reported a high general quality of life (QOL) and a high satisfaction with their quality of life but reported that their satisfaction with their sexual lives was only acceptable. There were significant correlations between general quality of life, emotional-sexual life QOL and social and economic QOL. The QOL, the coping strategies, the self-esteem and the anxiety and depression levels also correlate significantly among themselves.

* Corresponding author: Ana I Cobo-Cuenca PhD. University of Castilla la Mancha (UCLM). Departamento de enfermeria y fisioterapia de Toledo. Campus Tecnológico "Fábrica de Armas" Av. Carlos III. Toledo, Spain. Tel.: 902 204 100 / Fax: 902 204 130. Email: anaisabel.cobo@uclm.es.

In conclusion, men with spinal cord injury and sexual dysfunction achieve to adapt to their situation, being important the relationship between the type of strategies used with the quality of life and mood (depression). Sexuality and employment status are the areas where they get less satisfaction

INTRODUCTION

Spinal cord injury (SCI) is defined as the pathological process produced by any etiology that affects the spinal cord, potentially altering sensory or autonomous motor functions below the level of the injury [1].

The cause of spinal cord injuries may be traumatic (car accidents, falls, sporting injuries...), or the result of birth defects (spine bifid, myelomeningocele) or medical problems (herniated discs, vascular pathologies, or infections). The etiology of most spinal injuries is traumatic [2]

Spinal cord injuries can be classified according to the degree and extent of the injury. The degree depends on the segment that is most distal from the spinal cord and that is neurologically intact. In this sense, we can distinguish two types of injuries: tetraplegic (C1-C8) and paraplegic (from T1 onwards). Depending on where the injury is, it may be classified as cervical, thoracic, lumbar, sacral/conus terminalis and cauda equina lesions.

The extent of the spinal cord injuries is established using the ASIA (American Spinal Injury Association) scale. The injury may be complete or incomplete. If it is complete, it will cause a loss of sensory and motor function below the level of the injury, whereas if it is incomplete, the motor or sensory function is partially preserved at a perilesional level. ASIA distinguishes five types of injuries (A, B, C, D, E) according to the neurological impact of the injury (see table 1).

Table 1. ASIA scale of neurological affectation

Complete injury A	Absence of motor and sensory functions
Incomplete injury B	Incomplete injury complete motor sensory, sensory preservation below the level of the injury, with an absence of motor function.
Incomplete injury C	Incomplete non-functional sensory-motor injury (more than half of the key muscles beneath the level of the injury score below 3).
Incomplete injury D	Incomplete functional sensory-motor injury (more than half of the key muscles beneath the level of the injury score above 3).
Normal E	Normal sensory and motor function

Incomplete spinal cord injuries can be divided into five different groups: Centromedular syndrome, cruciate paralysis, Brown-Séquard syndrome, or spinal hemisection, anterior spinal syndrome and conus medullaris and cauda equine [2].

It is estimated that the incidence of traumatic spinal cord injury in developed countries ranges from 12.1 and 57.8 new cases per million in habitants. The male to female ratio is between 3:1 and 4:1. The most frequent etiology is traumatic: Car accidents (35-53.8%) and falls (22.6-37%). Between 37-55.6% of these injuries are complete [3] 39-62% of which are tetraplegic and the remaining 42.2-56% paraplegic [4]

In Spain, the estimated number of spinal cord injuries is 16-25 cases per million in habitants per year. The most frequent age group is 16-40 years of age. Of the affected individuals, three quarters (3/4) are males and 70% of the injuries are traumatic. Tetraplegia is more common than paraplegia [2]

In the last few years, advances in the medical field have lengthened the life expectancy of individuals suffering from spinal cord injuries. In addition, these medical advances have increased the chances of survival at the moment of injury, as well as in other extreme cases.

The consequences of a spinal cord injury (physical, functional, psychological, familial, social...) are dramatic and require significant coping strategies.

Coping strategies are formed by a combination of personal characteristics and environmental pressures and are fundamental to the evolution and recovery of spinal cord injuries (SCIs) [4,5]. Psychological adaptation is better predicted by coping strategies than by variables such as age, spinal cord injury level, severity of the spinal cord injury or time elapsed since injury [6, 7]

Various studies have concluded that the most frequent coping strategies are those described as "adaptive, such as acceptance, positive reinterpretation and personal growth. The least frequent strategies were described as "maladaptive," and included behavioral disengagement, denial, and drug and alcohol abuse [4-7]. These coping strategies remained constant for up to 10 years after the lesion [8].

One study of adults who had suffered an SCI at age 18 or younger concluded that more than 90% of the participants in the study relied on positive reinterpretation and active coping.[9] The least frequent coping strategies were the negative strategies: behavioral disengagement and drug and alcohol use.

A higher prevalence of depression and anxiety disorders has been found among people suffering from SCIs, ranging from 20%-48. [9-11] Neither depression nor anxiety are related to the degree of the injury, severity or functional independence, and individuals vary extensively in terms of these factors [8, 9].

High anxiety and depression scores are associated with coping strategies such as behavioral disengagement, drug and alcohol use ideation and denial [8]. Generally, people who possess SCIs have a lower quality of life (QOL) than people without SCIs. [12, 13]

A lower QOL exists for individuals who experience urinary infections [13] urinary and/or intestinal dysfunction, motor dysfunction, pain, pressure ulcers and sexual dysfunction [12]

Males with spinal cord injuries can experience problems with sexual performance that lead to changes in the sexual conduct of the patient [14-17]. The degree of sexual dysfunction depends on the extent of the injury, the level of the injury, and the period of time that has transcurred since the spinal cord injury itself [16, 17, 18,19].

The following types of sexual dysfunction tend to occur in males suffering from spinal cord injuries: a decrease in sex drive, erectile dysfunction (ED), non-ejaculation or retrograde ejaculation, anorgasmia, and in some cases, dyspareunia or intracoital pain [15, 17, 19, 20].

The type of erection depends on the extent of the spinal cord injury (SCI). Males with C1 to T9 spinal cord injuries experience reflex erections. Males with cauda equina injuries maintain the ability to have psychogenic erections, and paraplegic patients, with less than L2 and more than S2 spinal cord injuries, maintain both types of erections. However, their sexual performance is abnormal because there is no cortical integration of both types of erections, because the spinal canals have been disrupted. In most cases, patients are not able to maintain an adequate erection [14, 15, 16].

Recent studies have shown that between 25 and 89.5% of males suffering from SCI require treatment to be able to maintain an adequate erection [16-22]. The most frequently used erection treatments are pharmaceutical treatments, intracavernosal injections, penile prosthesis, and vacuum system with penile rings (see table 2) [18, 21]. The most successful of these treatments in terms of achieving a successful erection are pharmaceutical treatments and intracavernosal injections [18, 21, 23, 24]. Individuals that used vacuum system with penile rings tended to be less satisfied with the result [18, 25].

Table 2. Treatment of erectile dysfunction in patients suffering from spinal cord injury

General measures
Abstention from toxic substances, alcohol, and tobacco

Sexual therapy

Mechanical therapy:
Vacuum systems.
Constrictor penile rings.

Oral therapy:
Sildenafil.
Vardenafil

Hormonal treatment

Intercavernous and intraurethral treatment
Prostaglandine E1.
Alprostadil.
MUSE

Surgical therapy:
Penile prosthesis.

In studies of individuals with sexual dysfunction and without spinal cord injury (SCI) reported having worse QOL and having worse self-esteem than those without sexual dysfunction [26, 27]

There are various studies that evaluate the intense emotional impact of erectile dysfunction (ED) on males suffering from this condition. It is associated with depression, anxiety, and a loss of self-esteem [31, 32, 33].

Sexual relations are considered very important for people who possess SCIs, independent of their age and partner status [34]

Sexual performance is recognized as an area that has not been sufficiently addressed. Individuals with SCIs reported dissatisfaction with their sex life [35, 36].

Few studies have investigated the relationship between quality of life, coping strategies, self-esteem and sexuality in individuals with spinal cord injury and how they relate specifically to sexual dysfunction.

For this reason, the objectives of this study are: 1) To understand the different types of sexual dysfunction that can be experienced by males suffering from chronic spinal cord injuries; 2) To assess the quality of life of men who possess SCI and who report having experienced sexual dysfunction (SD); 3) To identify the coping strategies that are most frequently used by these men; 4) To assess their current affective states of mind (anxiety and depression) and their levels of self-esteem; 5) To assess the relationship between quality of life, coping strategies, and levels of anxiety, depression and self-esteem in men suffering from spinal cord injury (SCIs) and sexual dysfunction.

MATERIALS AND METHODS

Design and Participants

A cross-sectional study was carried out at the National Hospital of Paraplegics in Toledo (Spain).

The sample of our study of 85 men with spinal cord injury (SCI) and sexual dysfunction (SD) is a representative sample from the Urology Unit of the National Hospital of Paraplegics (HNP) during the data collection period (January 2009- December 2012), of all individuals who met the criteria of the study.

The study inclusion criteria were as follows: a) males between 18 and 55 years, b) who were suffering from chronic spinal cord injury, the onset of which began more than one year ago and c) from C6 level injury to the cauda equina.

Calculation of sample size: A minimum sample size of 50 patients is required to extrapolate a reliable value from the HADS test for the sample population suffering from SCI and erectile dysfunction (estimating an average measurement error of 4 points, a 5% alpha error and a statistical power of 80%) [9].

Procedures

The participants in the study are males suffering from chronic spinal cord injuries who attend the National Hospital for Paraplegics of Toledo for annual check-ups.

All of the patients in the Urology unit who met the inclusion criteria of this study were invited to participate. The objective and voluntary character of the study was explained to them. In addition, anonymity and protection of privacy was assured to the patient in accordance with applicable legislation.

Individual interviews with patients, lasting between 30-45 minutes, were conducted at the Urology unit. Firstly, the patient was asked a series of socio-demographic questions (age, civil status, level of education, employment status....) clinic information (level and extent of injury, etiology of the injury, consumption of substances, alcohol, tobacco, previous pathologies...). Lastly, the participants were asked to respond to various auto-administered questionnaires. Patients who had difficulties writing or understanding the material were assisted by the researcher.

Measures

- The Fugl-Meyer Life Satisfaction Questionnaire (LISAT-8) [26] is self-administered and contains 8 items, each of which contains 6 answer options. Either a total General Life Satisfaction score can be calculated or the items can be grouped into three categories: Satisfaction with Social Life, Sexual Life and Economic Life. This scale has shown acceptable psychometric properties, ROC curve analysis showed cutoff point >= 15 with a sensitivity of 81.7% (95% confidence intervals: 80.5–82.9), a specificity of 79.2% (77.5–80.8) and Kappa agreement coefficients were 0.60 (LISAT-8 vs. International Index erectile Function (IIEF)).

- The COPE[38] scale assesses dispositional and situational coping in stressful situations. This questionnaire contains 60 items, each of which contains 4 answer options. This scale has shown an adequate internal consistency (Cronbach's α 0.6-0.93) and a test-retest reliability of over 0.5 in studies of people who possess SCIs [5, 6, 7]. This scale was validated for a Spanish population and employed in this study [39]. The situational format was employed, where the patient has to answer questions according to the following instructions: describe a stressful event that occurred in the last few months in relation to an aspect of their sexuality, explaining where the event took place, who it involved, why it was important, and how the patient responded to the situation. After doing so, the patient had to respond to the 60 items.

- The Hospital Anxiety and Depression Scale (HADS) [40] detect anxiety and depressive disorders in a non-psychiatric hospital environment. This questionnaire contains 14 items, each of which contains 4 answer options. This scale has shown an internal consistency of 0.86 for HADS-A and 0.85 for HADS-D and a test-retest reliability of greater than 0.85 based on a study of 963 adults with SCI [11]. It is translated and validated for a Spanish sample [41]. A score is considered normal if it is between 0 and 7, whereas a score of 8-10 indicates anxiety and a score of 11-21 indicates depression.

- The Rosenberg Self-Esteem Scale (RSES), designed by Rosenberg in 1965. This scale is used for evaluating overall self-esteem. This scale has shown an adequate internal consistency (Cronbach's α 0.87) and a test-retest reliability of over C.8 in studies of Spanish people[42]. This questionnaire comprises 10 items, each of which contains 4 answer options.

- The Sexual Health Evaluation Scale (VASS), [43], which is designed to assess sexual health. It records information on symptoms of sexual dysfunction such as 1) disorders of sexual desire (DSD): a decrease or absence of sexual fantasies or a desire sexual. 2) Erectile dysfunction (ED): persistent or reoccurring inability to obtain or maintain an erection until the end of the sexual act. 3) Ejaculation disorders: Difficulty ejaculating during intercourse and anorgasmia. 4) Dyspareunia (Dis): Pain before, during, or after intercourse.

Ethics

All procedures were approved by the institution's Human Ethics Research Committee. In addition, all patients signed an informed consent form in which they consented to participate in the study.

Data Analysis

Data analysis was conducted using the statistical program for the social sciences SPSS version 19. First, a descriptive analysis of participant characteristics was performed. Afterwards, the Kolmogorov-Smirnov (K-S) comparison was used to verify the normal distribution of the quantitative variable data. The following statistical tests were used to determine the relationship between the variables: Chi-square (χ^2), Student's t-test, ANOVA with Scheffés post-hoc comparison, Pearson's correlation coefficient and Rho´Spearman correlation coefficients.

RESULTS

The Sociodemographic Characteristics of the Participants

Table 3 presents the main characteristics of the sample. The pathological history of the group is shown in table 4.

Types of Sexual Dysfunction (VASS)

Out of the 85 males that participated in the study, 9.4% suffered from disorders of sexual desire (DSD). 84.7% experienced difficulty maintaining an adequate erection for sexual activity (ED). 70.6% reported experiencing difficulties ejaculating during intercourse as well as anorgasmia. Only two individuals (2.4%) reported experiencing pain or discomfort during intercourse.

Quality of Life: The Fugl-Meyer Life Satisfaction Checklist (LISAT-8)

Table 5 presents the Life Satisfaction scores obtained from the sample, including general life (total QOL), sexual life satisfaction, economic satisfaction and social satisfaction.

Table 3. Social demographic and clinical characteristics (n= 85)

	N (85)	Mean	Standard Deviation
Age		35.61	8.13
Age at lesion		26.45	8.72
Duration of Disability		9.11	6.4
		Number (Percentage)	
Neurological Level:			
• Cervical (C6)		16(18.8%)	
• Thoracic (T1-T12)		46(54.2%)	
• Lumbers		23(27%)	
Neurological classification:			
• ASIA* A		59(69.4%)	
• ASIA B, C, D		26(30.6%)	
Educational Level:			
• Primary School.		25(29.41%)	
• Secondary School		42(49.42%)	
• University		18(21.17%)	
Marital Status:			
• Single		24(28.2%)	
• Single with partner		25(29.4%)	
• Married and Stable partner		36(42.4%)	

*ASIA: American Spinal Injury Association.

Table 4. Pathological history

Medical history	Frequency	Percentage
Heart disease	7	8.2
HTA	4	4.7
Hipercholesterol	11	12.9
Respiratory	2	2.4
Diabetes	2	2.4
Prostate disease	0	0
Tumors disease	0	0
Depression	2	2.4

Table 5. Total and dimension scores of Life Checklist in patients with SCI and standard deviation

	Range	Mean	Standard Deviation	
QUALITY OF SOCIAL LIFE	12-24	20.16	2.804	(20-24) very good
QUALITY OF SEXUAL LIFE	2-12	7.62	2.766	(8-6) acceptable
QUALITY OF FINANCIAL LIFE	2-12	7.71	2.68	(8-6) acceptable
QUALITY OF LIFE TOTAL	6-48	34.27	8.032	(32-40)good

The results showed that the sexual satisfaction of single men without a regular partner was significantly less than that of both single men who had a regular partner (ANOVA =-3.32, p = 0.002) and married men or men who lived with a partner. (ANOVA = -0.380, p = 0.000).

Younger SCI patients reported higher satisfaction with their economic situations (r Pearson = -0.319, p =0.033) and lower satisfaction with their sexual lives (r Pearson= 0.303, p = 0.043).

There were significant correlations between general quality of life (QOL), emotional-sexual life QOL, social QOL and economic QOL and anxiety, depression and self-esteem (Table 6).

Table 6. Product-moment Pearson's Correlation coefficients with LISAT 8, self-esteem, depression and anxiety

	QOL total	QOL sexual	QOL social	QOL Financial	Self-esteem	Depression	Anxiety
QOL total	1						
QOL sexual	.621* .000	1					
QOL Social	.420* .004	.163 .284	1				
QOL financial	.359* .015	-.024 .875	.292 .052	1			
Self-esteem	.403* .006	.184 .226	.628* .000	.207 .173	1		
Depression	-186 .220	-.191 .208	-406* .006	-.270 .072	-.433* .003	1	
Anxiety	.074 .629	.063 .681	-.279 .064	-.188 .216	-.499* .002	.642* .000	1

*P<.005; QOL: Life Satisfaction Checklist.

There were no significant relationships between QOL and SCI etiology, SCI grade, length of time living with SCI and educational level.

Coping Strategies: COPE

The most frequently used strategies were "personal growth", "acceptance", "positive reinterpretation", "planning", "active coping" and "search of social support". The least frequently used strategies were "alcohol/drug use ideation", "suppression of competing activities" and "denial". Table 7 shows the distribution of the coping strategies that were used.

No significant differences were observed between the various strategies in terms of their relationships with lesion type, SCI etiology, or lesion grade. Additionally, the participants' living environments, educational levels, and clinical histories had no effect on the coping strategies employed by patients.

Table 7. Distribution of the coping strategies most used

COPE		
	Mean	Standard Desviation
Personal Growth	3.1	.45
Acceptance	2.78	.73
Positive reinterpretation	2.71	.65
Planning	2.4	.51
Instrumental social Support	2.3	.67
Active coping	2.24	.67
Restraint	2.05	.64
Behavioral disengagement	1.95	.63
Focusing on/Venting of emotions	1.89	.63
Humour	1.87	.84
Religion	1.56	.81
Mental disengagement	1.53	.53
Denial	1.4	.49
Suppression of competing activities	1.28	.55
Alcohol/drug use ideation	1.24	.39

Hospital Anxiety and Depression Scale

HADS scale scores of eight or greater are considered to be indicative of depression or anxiety. 17.5 % of the sample was obtained scores above a clinical cutoff in depression, and 38.7% in anxiety.

There were no significant relationships observed between anxiety and depression and SCI grade level, SCI level, SCI etiology, age at the time of the spinal cord injury, time elapsed since injury, current age of the patient, or current environment, marital status or educational level of the patient.

Self-Esteem: Rosenberg Self-Esteem Scale

Of the total sample, 64.9% reported high-normal self-esteem (scores> 29), 19.9% reported average self-esteem (29-26) and 15.1% reported low self-esteem (<26).

Coping Strategies and Anxiety, Depression and Self-Esteem

There were significant relationships between higher levels of the depression and the anxiety and each of the following: the use of the "suppression of competing activities", "focusing on/Venting of emotions", "behavioral disengagement" and "mental disengagement" strategies. (See table 8)

Lower self-esteem was associated with the "suppression of competing activities" and "focusing on/venting of emotions".

"Acceptance" and "positive reinterpretation" coping strategies were positively correlated with higher levels of self-esteem.

Coping Strategies and Quality of Life

Positive reinterpretation" and "acceptance" coping strategies were positively correlated with a higher degree of satisfaction with social life.

Strategies of "suppression of competing activities" and "focusing on/Venting of emotions" were correlated with a lower satisfaction with social life (which included family, friends and leisure) and a lower general QOL.

Greater reliance on "focusing on/Venting of emotions activities" and "behavioral disengagement" was correlated with less satisfaction with sexual life (Table 8).

DISCUSSION

As previous studies have demonstrated, erectile dysfunction (ED) was the most common type of sexual dysfunction observed in our sample [16-20, 24, 25]. Erectile dysfunction in males with spinal cord injury can be explained by purely neurological causes. In erection there are two neurological channels: Reflex erection, which involves the sacral reflex arc (S2-S4) and which responds to tactile stimuli, and psychogenic erection, which occurs in the sympathetic spinal trunk (T10-L2), which responds to psychic, visual and auditory stimuli [20]

70.6% of the sample experienced ejaculation disorders, the second primary cause of sexual dysfunction. In the Phelps study [43], the percentage of males with SCIs who reported ejaculation failure and anorgasmia was the highest, exceeding the percentage of patients with ED. In the Lauman study, [44] which has a sample without SCI, this disorder is the third most frequent after DSD and ED.

Ejaculation and orgasm are regulated by a series of neurological spinal and cerebral channels. The afferent arm consists of sensory stimuli from the glans and genitals, which circulate through the spinothalamic bundles until reaching the brain. The efferent arm circulates sympathetic and pudenda motor impulses [45].

Ejaculation disorders are far more frequent in males suffering from SCI than in populations without SCI [17]. In various studies on individuals with spinal cord injuries, ejaculation only occurs in 30- 45% of cases [17, 43, 46]. This is a result of the fact that ejaculation is a multi-segmentary centralized reflex in which spinal channels play an important role. In patients suffering from spinal injuries, disruptions in their ability to ejaculate depend on the degree of the injury and the type of nerve systems that are affected.

Table 8. Pearson's Correlation coefficients with coping and QOL

	QOL social life	QOL Sex life	QOL total	Anxiety	Depr	Self-steem	SCA	Venting of emotions	Accept	PR	BD	MD
QOL social	1											
QOL Sexual	.156	1										
QOL total	.561*	.636*	1									
Anxiety	-.303*	.007	-.154	1								
Depression	-.416*	-.29*	-.41*	.586*	1							
Self-Steem	.613*	.110	.406*	-.473*	-.43*	1						
Suppression of competing activities (SCA)	-.398*	-.178	-.29*	.361*	.432*	-.477*	1					
Venting of emotions	-.461*	-.101	-.37*	.421*	.439*	-.602*	.445*	1				
Acceptance	.406*	-.046	.57	-.190	-.247	.333*	-.25	-.298*	1			
Positive reinterpretation (PR)	.138	-.075	-.012	-.114	-.29*	.274*	-.09	-.121	.331*	1		
Behavioral disengagement (BD)	-.109	-.27*	-.209	.276*	.348	-.180	.225	.394*	.072	-.11	1	
Mental disengagement (MD)	-.186	-.150	-.250	.362*	.420*	-.197	.307	.445*	-.030	.042	.387*	1

*P<.005; QOL: Life Satisfaction Checklist.

The other objective of this study was to study the relationship between quality of life, coping strategies, and levels of anxiety, depression and self-esteem in men suffering from spinal cord injuries (SCIs) and sexual dysfunction. Individuals with SCIs can learn to adapt adequately and achieve good quality of life [5, 6] Participants in this study reported that they had a "good" general quality of life and a "very good" social life.

Participants reported less satisfaction ("acceptable") with their sex life and their financial and employment situation. These results coincide with the results of a study conducted by Kennedy et al. that investigated 350 people with spinal cord injury from different European countries (United Kingdom, Germany, Switzerland and Austria) [36].

SCI etiology, length of spinal cord injury, SCI grade, and educational level do not affect quality of life.

It was observed that patients, who were younger, both at the time of the study and at the time of the SCI, reported more satisfaction with their financial situation and less satisfaction with their sex lives.

Men, who had a regular partner, whether single or married, reported greater satisfaction with their sex lives than those who did not have a regular partner [35]. Social and economic satisfaction was also related to general quality of life, but to a lesser extent than sexual satisfaction [27, 28, 35, 36, 37]. The results showed that younger men were less satisfied with their sex life than older men, possibly because they did not have a regular partner. It is logical to assume that sexuality carries special importance during this phase of life and affects QOL in other respects.

In the current study, the most frequent coping strategies were "personal growth", "acceptance", "positive reinterpretation", "planning", "active coping" and "social support instrumental". Consistent with results from previous studies, the least frequent coping strategies were "drug/alcohol use ideation", "suppression of competing activities" and "denial" [8, 10]. The use of these strategies was not related to the type of neurological lesion, the SCI etiology or lesion grade, patient educational level, or clinical history [5, 8].

Men who were younger at the time of spinal cord injury relied on "personal growth" and "positive reinterpretation" strategies more frequently than men who were older at the time of injury [10].

The use of "positive reinterpretation" and "acceptance" strategies was associated with greater social life and general life satisfaction. These strategies are considered "adaptive"; therefore, their use improves QOL.

Despite a lower reported sexual QOL ("acceptable"), the participants reported a high general QOL. This high QOL indicates that the participants are likely to focus on improving other aspects of their general life to compensate for reduced satisfaction in the sexual sphere.

Higher anxiety scores are associated with higher depression scores and lower self-esteem.

Neither depression nor anxiety was related to the level, degree or etiology of the injury or to the educational level or marital status of the patient [8, 9, 11, 12]

Moreover, men with spinal cord injury and sexual dysfunction managed to adapt to their situation. In this sense, the relationship between coping strategies and quality of life and mood (depression) is important. Sexuality and employment status are the areas in which patients experienced the least satisfaction.

After spinal cord injury, individuals can choose to be sexually active or not. As health professionals, it is our role to ensure that they receive accurate information about sexuality and the emotional support that is necessary to make that decision.

It would also be appropriate to provide sexual education and information on health and rehabilitation professionals to ensure that professionals feel comfortable speaking to SCI patients about sexual issues. The Consortium for Spinal Cord Medicine has offered to review the literature and gather the latest information regarding sexuality and reproductive health after spinal cord injuries [22]

Patients' partners should be included in future studies to offer better information on the sex lives of the patients as well as their partners.

ACKNOWLEDGMENTS

We would like to thank the male patients with SCI who participated in this study for their contributions. This study received a FISCAM grant in the 2009 Assembly of Regional Aid for Health Investigation for Standard Projects. Record: PI-2009/62.

REFERENCES

[1]   Wyndaele, M., & Windaele, J.J.(2006) Incidence, prevalence and epidemiology of spinal cord injury: what learns a worldwide literature survey? *Spinal Cord,* 44, 523-9.

[2]   Esclarín, A. (2010). Lesión medular: Enfoque multidisciplinario. (1ª ed). Madrid: Editorial Médica Panamericana.

[3]   Chiu, W.T., Lin, H.C., Lam, C., Chu, S.F., Chiang, Y.H., & Tsai, S.H. (2010) Review Paper: Epidemiology of Traumatic Spinal Cord Injury: Comparisons Between Developed and Developing Countries. *Asia Pac J Public Health*, 22(1),9-18.

[4]   Van den Berg, M., Castellote, J.M., Mahillo-Fernandez, I., & Pedro-Cuesta, J. (2010) Incidence of Spinal Cord Injury Worldwide: A Systematic Review. *Neuroepidemiology,* 34(3), 184-192.

[5]   Chevalier, Z., Kennedy, P., & Sherlock, O. (2009) Spinal cord injury, coping and psychological adjustment: a literature review. *Spinal Cord*, 47,. 778-782.

[6]   Kennedy, P., Duff, J., Evans, M., & Beedie, A. (2003) Coping effectiveness training reduces depression and anxiety following traumatic spinal cord injuries. *Br. J. Clin. Psychol,* 27, 239–246.

[7]   Kennedy, P., Evans, M., & Sandhu, N. (2009). Psychological adjustment to spinal cord injury: the contribution of coping, hope and cognitive appraisals. *Psych of Health Me,* 14,. 17-33.

[8]   Kennedy, P., Marsh, N., Lowe, R., Grey, N., Short, E., & Rogers, B. (2000) A longitudinal analysis of psychological impact and coping strategies following spinal cord injury. *Brit. J. Health Psych*, 5, 157–172.

[9]   Pollard, C., & Kennedy, P. (2007) A longitudinal analysis of emotional impact, coping strategies and posttraumatic growth following spinal cord injury: a ten year review. *Brit. J. Health Psych*, 12, 347-362.

[10]   Anderson, C.J., Vogel, L., Chan, M., & Betz, R. (2008). Coping with spinal cord injury: strategies used by adults who sustained their injuries as children or adolescents. *J. Spinal Cord Med*, 3, 290–296.

[11] Dryden, D.M, Saunders, L.D., Rowe, B.H., May, L.A., Yiannakoulias, N., Svenson, L.W., Schopflocher, D.P., & Voaklander, D.C. (2006) Depression following traumatic cord injury. *Neuroepidemiology,* 25, 55-61.

[12] Woolrich, R.A., Kennedy, P., & Tasiemski, T. (2006) A preliminary psychometric evaluation of the Hospital Anxiety and Depression Scale (HADS) in 963 people living with spinal cord injury. *Psych Health Med*, 11, 80-90.

[13] Lidal, I.B., Veenstra, M., Hjeltnes, N., & Biering-Sorensen, F. (2008) Health-related quality of life in persons with long-standing spinal cord injury. *Spinal Cord*, 46, 710-5.

[14] Haran, M.J, Lee, B., King, M.T., Marial, O., & Stockler, M. (2008) Health status rated with the Medical Outcomes Study 36-Item Short-Form Health Survey after spinal cord injury. *Arch. Phys Med. Rehab*, 86, 2290-5

[15] Salinas, J., Martín, C., & Vírseda, M. (2003). Tipos de disfunción eréctil neurógena: Lesión medular traumática. In J.J. Salinas (Ed.) Bases neurológicas de la erección Disfunción eréctil neurógena. (1ª ed. pp 165-178). Madrid: Gráficas Santher.

[16] Courtois, F.J, Goulet, M.C., Charvier, K.F., & Leriche, A. (1999). Posttraumatic erectile potential of spinal cord injured men: how physiologic recordings supplement subjective reports. *Arch. Phys Med Rehabil*, 80(10), 1268-72.

[17] Virseda-Chamorro, M., Salinas-Casado, J., Lopez-Garcia-Moreno, A.M., Cobo-Cuenca, A.I., & Esteban-Fuertes, M. (2013). Sexual Dysfunction in men with spinal cord injury: a case-control study. *International Journal of Impotence Research*. doi:10.1038/ijir.2013.1

[18] Cobo-Cuenca, A.I., & col. (2012). Calidad de vida del varón con lesión medular traumática y disfunción sexual. *Enfermería Clínica*, 22(4),205-208.

[19] Biering-Sorensen, I., Bolling Hansen, M.D., & Biering-Sorensen, M.D.(2012) Sexual function in a traumatic spinal cord injured population 15-45 years after injury. *J. Rehabil. Med*, 44.

[20] Biering-Sorensen, F., & Sùnksen, J. (2001). Sexual function in spinal cord lesioned men. *Spinal Cord*, 39, 455-470.

[21] Giuliano, F., Sánchez-Ramos, A., Löchner-Ernst, D., Del Popolo, G., Cruz, N., Leriche, A., Lombardi, G., Reichert, S., Dhal, P., Elion-Mboussa, A., & Casariego, J. (2007) Efficacy and Safety of Tadalafil in men with erectile dysfunction following spinal cord injury. *Arch Neurol*, 64(11), 1584-92.

[22] Consortium for Spinal Cord Medecine. (2010). Sexuality and reproductive health ind adults with spinal cord injury: A clinical practice Guideline for Health-Care professionals. *J. Spinal Cord Med.*, 33 (3), 281-336.

[23] Sánchez Ramos, A., Vidal, J., & Jáuregui, M.L. (2001). Efficacy, safety and predictive factors or therapeutic success with sildenafil for erectile dysfunction in patient with different spinal cord injuries. *Spinal Cord*, 39, 637-643.

[24] Anderson, K.D., Borisoff, J.F., Johnson, R.D., Stiens, S.A., & Elliott, S.L. (2007). Long-term effects of spinal cord injury on sexual function in men: implications for neuroplasticity. *Spinal Cord*, 45, 338–348.

[25] Deforge, D., Blackmer, J., Garritty, C., Yazdi, F., Cronin, V., Barrowman, N., & cols. (2006). Male erectile dysfunction following spinal cord injury: a systematic review. *Spinal Cord,* 44, 465–473.

[26] Lloyd, E.E., Toth, L.L., & Perkash, I. (1989). Vacuum tumescence: an option for spinal cord injured ma les with erectile dysfunction. *SCI Nurs,* 6, 25–28.

[27] Moncada, I., Micheltorena, C.F., Martínez-Sánchez, E.M., & Rejas, J. (2008). Evaluation of the psychometrics properties of the LISAT-8 checklist as a screening tool erectile dysfunction. *J. Sex Med.*, 5, 83-91.

[28] Moncada, .I, Martínez-Jabaloyas, .J.M., Rodríguez-Vela, L., Gutiérrez, P.R., Giuliano, F., & Koskimaki, J. (2009). Emotional changes in men treated with sildenafil citrate for erectile dysfunction: a double blind, placebo-controlled clinical trial. *J. Sex Med.*, 6, 3469-77.

[29] Kantor, J., Bilker, W.B., & Glasser, D. B. (2002). Prevalence of erectile dysfunction and active depression: an analytic cross-sectional study of general medical patients. *American Journal Epidemiology*, 156(11), 1035-42.

[30] Makhlouf, A., Kparker, A., & Craig, S. (2007). Depresión y disfunción eréctil. *Clínicas Urológicas de Norteamérica*, 34(4), 565-574.

[31] Rosen, R.C., Fisher, W.A., & Eardley, I. (2004). Men´s attitudes to Life Events and Sexuality (MALES) study: I Prevalence of erectile dysfunction and related health concerns in the general population. *Current Medical Research & Opinion*, 20(5), 607-17.

[32] Althof, S.E., O´Leary, M.P., Cappelleri, J.C., Glina, S., King, R., Tseng, J., & Bowler. J. (2006) Self- Esteem, confidence and relationship in men treated with Sildenafil Citrate for erectile dysfunction. *Jounal of General Internal Medicine*, 21(10), 1069-1074.

[33] Martín-Morales, A., Mejide, F., García, J. I., Regadera, L., & Manero, M. (2005). Repercusiones psicológicas de la disfunción eréctil sobre la autoestima y autoconfianza. *Actas Urológicas Españolas*, 28(5), 493-498.

[34] Delgado, J. A., Blázquez, J., Silmi, A., & Martínez, E. (2008) Factores determinantes de la satisfacción del paciente con el tratamiento para la disfunción eréctil. *Actas Urológicas Españolas*, 32(19), 995-1003.

[35] Lombardi, G., Macchiarella, A., Cecconi, F., Aito, S. & del Popolo, G. (2008). Sexual life of males over 50 years of age with spinal cord lesions of at least 20 years. *Spinal Cord,* 46(10), 679-83.

[36] Kennedy, P., Lude, P., & Taylor, N. (2006). Quality of life, social participation, appraisals and coping post spinal cord injury: A review of four community samples. *Spinal cord*, 44,99-105.

[37] Kennedy, P., Sherlock, O., McClelland, M., Short, D., Royle, J., & Wilson, C. (2010) A multi-center study of the community needs of people with spinal cord injuries: the first 18 months. *Spinal Cord,* 48,15-20.

[38] Carver, Ch. S., Scheier, M.F., & Weintraub, J. (1989) Assessing coping strategies: A theoretically based approach. *J. Pers Soc Psychol*, 56(2), 267-283.

[39] Crespo, M.L., & Cruzado, J.A. (1997). La evaluación del afrontamiento: adaptación española del cuestionario COPE con una muestra de estudiantes universitarios. *Análisis y Modificación de Conducta*, 23(92), 797-283.

[40] Zigmon, A.S, & Snaith, R. P.(1983) The Hospital Anxiety and Depression Scale. *Act Psych Scand*, 67, 361-370.

[41] Caro, I. & Ibañez, E. (1992).La escala hospitalaria de ansiedad y depresión. *Boletín de Psicología,* 36, 44-69.

[42] Vázquez, J., Jiménez, R., & Vázquez, R. (2004). Escala de autoestima de Rosenberg. *Apuntes de Psicología,* 2(22), 247-255.

[43] Tomás R, Tárraga López PJ, Álvarez MC, Cerdán Oliver M, Celada Rodríguez A, Solera Albero. Disfunciones sexuales en Atención Primaria. *MGF*. 2007;92:13---23.

[44] Phelps, J., Albo, M., Dunn, K., & Joseph, A. (2001). Spinal cord injury and sexuality in married or partnered men: activities, function, needs, and predictors of sexual adjustment. *Arch. Sex Behav*, 30(6),591-602.

[45] Laumann, E.O., & Waite, L.J. (2008) Sexual dysfunction among older adults: prevalence and risk factors from a nationally representative U.S. probability sample of men and women 57-85 years of age. *J. Sex Med*, 5(10), 2300-11.

[46] Motofei, I.G., & Rowland, D.L. (2005) Neurophysiology of the ejaculatory process: developing perspectives. BJU Int, 96(9), 1333-8.

[47] Slot, O., Drewes, A., Andreasen, A., & Olsson, A. (1989) Erectile and ejaculatory function of males with spinal cord injury. *Int. Disabil Stud*,11(2), 75-7.

In: Sexual Dysfunctions
Editor: Frédérique Courtois

ISBN: 978-1-62808-765-9
© 2013 Nova Science Publishers, Inc.

Chapter 5

SEXUAL DYSFUNCTION AFTER RADICAL PROSTATECTOMY: RELATED FACTORS AND TREATMENT

Marcos Tobias-Machado[*], *Ricardo Moreno, Renata Gimenez Costa, Fernanda Ramos, Luana Lee, Lívia Job, Margareth de Mello Ferreira dos Reis, Roberto Vaz Juliano and Antonio Carlos Lima Pompeo*
Sections of Urologic Oncology and Andrology, Department of Urology,
ABC Medical School, São Paulo, Brazil

ABSTRACT

Prostate Cancer (PC) is the most common cancer worldwide in men. Radical prostatectomy (RP) is the standard curative treatment for localized PC. However, a significant number of patients may have sexual disorders after surgery with impact on the quality of life of the couple. The objective of this chapter is to review the literature on the impact of sexual dysfunctions (erectile, ejaculatory and psychological aspects) in the individual submitted to RP in association with the surgical technique used. A systematic review of the literature using the PubMed database was conducted. The keywords selected were *prostate cancer, sexual dysfunction, erectile dysfunction, ejaculatory dysfunction, psychological aspects, radical prostatectomy*, and *prophylaxis*. There were 1,062 articles found. There were seventy selected due to the higher level of scientific evidence, which were subdivided into fifty-two about erectile dysfunction, six on ejaculatory dysfunction and twelve on psychological aspects. The rate of Erectile Dysfunction (ED) after RP varies from 10-90% with influences of pre-, intra- and postoperative parameters. The main preoperative factors related to lower recovery of erectile function after RP are any grade of previous ED, patient age older than sixty years and non-preservation of neurovascular bundles. Patients aged between 40 and 45 years

---

[*] Corresponding author: Marcos Tobias-Machado MD, Head, Section of Urologic Oncology, Section of Andrology, Department of Urology, ABC Medical School, São Paulo, Brazil.Tel +55 11 9932-9944; Email: tobias-machado@uol.com.br

have an index of erectile function recovery greater than 80 percent. Among the intraoperative factors, it is agreed that high experience of the surgeon and hospital volume of procedures are protective factors against postoperative ED. There is some influence on urinary control and decreased sexual performance. Some studies suggest that perineal exercises can reduce the recovery time to total continence. Moreover, it is extremely important to preserve urinary sphincter and prostate neurovascular bundle, especially parasympathetic fibers of pelvic plexus. From these fibers originate the cavernous nerves that are responsible for vasodilatation and increased blood flow during erection. In this way, the basic principles of preserving these nervous structures have been well-described: minimum traction, athermic dissection and proper handling of surgical plans (independent of the technique used) in addition to selecting the correct patient. Another relevant intraoperative factor concerns the surgical techniques used for RP: retropubic, laparoscopic or robotic-assisted. New data emerging from systematic review suggests that lower rates and faster recovery from ED are found after robotic surgery compared to the other techniques. In the postoperative period, some authors discuss the use of pro-erectile therapies to aid better erectile recovery. The therapies more often described are the phosphodiesterase inhibitor – type 5 (PDE5), intracavernous injections and penile pumps. There is no consensus on which of these therapies is best. Studies evaluating ejaculatory or orgasmic function post-RP are scarce, but when reported, quality of life can be significantly affected. Pre- and post- operative patients psychological aspects, especially the interest in maintaining sexual function, are important issues related to couple satisfaction after surgery. This psychological impact is frequent in the short term, but less significant in long-term follow-up after surgery. Considering the potential benefits, there is little scientific evidence suggesting that psychological intervention can improve couple's adjustment. Most patients undergoing RP will exhibit any changes in sexual function after surgery. Factors related to patient and disease characteristics, surgeon expertise and technique utilized are extremely important to the functional outcome. Therefore, further studies involving several less-studied aspects are necessary. Multidisciplinary teams with physicians, physiotherapists and psychologists can be important to offer better recovery of sexual function to the patient and his partner.

INTRODUCTION

Prostate Cancer (PC) is the sixth most common type of cancer worldwide and the most common among men, representing 10 percent of total cancer. In the United States it is the most commonly diagnosed after skin cancer and the second leading cause of death from cancer [1]. According to the National Cancer Institute at the National Institutes of Health it was estimated that in United States in 2012 there were 241,740 new cases of PC with 28,170 deaths.

The incidence of PC is around six times higher in developed countries compared to developing countries. There are two main factors that can explain the increased incidence of PC: the increase of life expectancy and the use of Prostate-Specific Antigen (PSA) screening to detect this malignancy.

Radical prostatectomy (RP) is the standard curative treatment for localized PC since Walsh and Donker [2] described the anatomic nerve-sparing technique for Retropubic Radical Prostatectomy (RRP) in 1982. Due to significant postoperative morbidity found in this technique, ten years later Schuessler [3] described the minimally invasive surgical approach to managing PC. Because of the learning curve of Laparoscopic Radical Prostatectomy

(LRP), the use of this technique suffered significant repulsion at the beginning when comparing the results with those of RRP. Subsequently however, with larger LRP series reporting the advantages of this approach, the LRP had increased application in clinical practice by urologic surgeons [4-6].

The introduction of Robot-Assisted Radical Prostatectomy (RARP), Da Vinci platform (Intuitive Surgical Inc., Sunnyvale, CA, USA), again revolutionized the management of clinically localized PC. This minimally invasive technique has some peculiarities compared to RRP and LPR, and approximately ten years after its introduction RARP is now standardized [7, 8]. Independent of the technique used, the objective of RP is complete excision of the prostate providing cancer control while maintaining some fundamental functions such as urinary continence and sexual potency. Presently, RARP has supplanted RRP as the most common surgical approach for RP in United States. Moreover 72.3 percent of RARP were performed at teaching institutions compared with 60.7 percent of RRP [9].

Currently large series, systematic reviews and meta-analysis comparing the three techniques are the main scientific means of establishing different morbidity data. In recent years the number of papers published by high-volume centers about RARP has increased [10].

MATERIAL AND METHODS

A systematic review of the literature using PubMed and CancerLit databases was conducted. The keywords selected were *prostate cancer, sexual dysfunction, erectile dysfunction, ejaculatory dysfunction, psychological aspects, radical prostatectomy, treatment* and *prophylaxis*. All of these keywords are found in the Medical Subject Headings database, which represents the controlled vocabulary used for indexing articles for MEDLIN E and PubMed.

The articles with the highest levels of evidence were selected to compose this review. 1,062 articles were found. Seventy were selected due to the higher levels of scientific evidence, which were subdivided into fifty-two on erectile dysfunction, six ejaculatory dysfunction and twelve on psychological aspects.

The lack of randomized studies comparing the three surgical approaches means that no consensus exists about definitions to describe Positive Surgical Margins (PSM), recurrence, urinary continence, sexual function and others factors about PC. In this scientific scenario the results between series can differ when certain morbidity factors are studied, especially if the study involved few patients or contains the learning curve bias for each procedure [11]. Nevertheless many comparisons can be performed and some conclusions formed.

ERECTILE DYSFUNCTION

Definitions

Probably the most difficult morbidity to compare after RP is potency, besides the fact that preservation of erectile function after surgery remains the greatest challenge for most urologists. This issue involves a broad list of associated factors including age, preoperative potency, use of medications, intraoperative nerve-sparing, stability of the relationship and general partner influence. In these conditions there are an important number of articles about pathophysiology of postoperative erectile dysfunction (ED) and the related prophylaxis and treatment [12]. There is no consensus about potency definition: capability to achieve a spontaneous erection, ability to maintain an erection, an affirmative answer to "Were erections adequate for penetration?" or "Were the erections satisfactory?" are some examples used to define potency. Most studies use IIEF, but some use telephone or personal interviews. Generally only age factor was considered in the majority of the studies, while other factors such as partner relationship were not commonly mentioned [13].

Anatomical Considerations

The cavernous nerves are responsible for erections because of corpora cavernosa innervations. The cavernous nerves form the Neurovascular-Bundle (NVB) localized in the prostate posterolateral margin bilaterally and between the endopelvic fascia (visceral layer) and prostatic fascia. Due to its location, adjacent to the seminal vesicles on the anterolateral wall of the rectum, this structure may be damaged during RP with consequent interference of potency and sexual function after RP. Indeed, patients with both NVB preserved are more likely to have an earlier recovery of erectile function after surgery, so that the volume on neural tissue preserved has a linear association with the quality of erection [14, 15]. Rabbani et al were the first to describe the association between the volume of preserved neural tissue and postoperative erectile function [16].

However, the curse of NVB is linked to more possible anatomical varieties. Tewari et al, for example, described small nerve fibers ramifying in the prostatic and Denonvillier fascia outside the main bundle of NVB [17]. Eichelberg *et al* demonstrated that some nerves can be observed along the ventral circumference of the prostatic capsule [18].

However, despite this data, the total function of all of the nerve fibers along the periprostatic space is not well understood and some authors have proposed modification of the standard nerve-sparing approach aimed at maximizing nerve fiber preservation [19]. Montorsi et al suggested a high anterior incision of the levator and prostatic fascia, which would allow a better plane between prostatic fascia and prostatic capsule (an intrafascial approach). This condition may enable laterally displacing neural structures between the two fasciae and preservation of ventral nerve fibers [20]. Masterson et al, on the other hand, in a non-randomized retrospective study, reported a technique where the NVB was mobilized completely off the prostate apex over the seminal vesicles. With this, the six-month erectile function recovery rate was higher in patients who were submitted to the modified technique compared with patients submitted to standard nerve-sparing approach (67 percent versus 45 percent, respectively, p = 0.01) [21].

There is a consensus that cavernous nerves preservation is key to erectile function recovery after RP. In addition, it is believed that adequate oxygenation is necessary to maintain the erectile tissue integrity. With this, the other anatomical structure involved in this issue is the Accessory Pudendal Artery (APA), also controversial in the literature, which proves the fact that this artery also has an understood function in ED pathophysiolgy.[19] Despite no relationship between vascular system (especially APA) preserving and ED after

RP having been formerly reported [22], a recent literature review was conducted to determinate the available evidence supporting vascular insufficiency as an important contributor to ED after RP [23]. This study stated that in the Urological Community it is appropriate to create the concept of artery-sparing RP. Nevertheless, the authors concluded that the greatest difficulty is to decide which arteries should be preserved and which may be sacrificed.

On the other hand, a prospective study analyzed two hundred potent patients who underwent RARP with a cautery-free technique, analyzing the prevalence of APA. Eighty patients (40 percent) had APA, all APAs were sacrificed and there was no association with having APA and normal or abnormal sexual function. Probably minimizing the age bias, a subgroup of age sixty-five years or less (n=58) was created. Thirty-nine patients had no APA and nineteen had a sacrificed APA. In this group 91 percent (n=53) were potent at the twenty-four months follow-up. Despite not having achieved a statistically significant data (p=0.530), 95 percent (n=19) of patients with sacrificed APA were potent and 90 percent (n=35) without APA [24]. However, larger functional studies will be needed to shed further light on this issue.

Novara et al related that being over age sixty was an independent risk predictor of postoperative ED (OR: 2.828; CI 95 percent; 1.591 – 5.027) [25], as well as Shikanov et al. (OR: 0.92; p < 0.0001) [26] and Kowalczyk et al (OR: 0.94; CI 95 percent; 0.89 – 0.98) [27].

The Influence of Patient Characteristics

The RP with anatomic nerve-sparing approach is considered for patients who have clinically localized PC, classified as clinical T1 or T2, as regards the best candidates for this treatment. So an accurate patient selection is fundamental, especially for patients who have PSA of less than 10 ng/mL and a Gleason sum less than or equal to 7 [28]. Agarwal et al analyzed a large series with more than 3,000 patients and demonstrated that PSA was an independent predictor of complications of any grade, whereas age, Gleason score, presence of hyperlipidemia were associated with surgical complications of any grade [29].

Several trials have reported the best postoperative potency rates in the younger patients, perhaps because of a better preoperative erectile function found in young patients, as well as an increased interest in sexual recovery [14]. A study reported rates of erectile function recovery as high as 92 percent for patients aged forty-forty-nine years [15]. The comparison between patient and partner ages is also important. Descazeaud et al. showed a better recovery of erectile function rate with a difference in couple age as great as twenty years compared with patients who were the same age as their partners (90 percent versus 25 percent, p < 0.001) [30].

When the issue is postoperative erectile function, one condition is very important: the preoperative patient potency or erectile function. Regardless of the surgical technique used, patients submitted to RP that report some degree of ED or who already use Phosphodiesterase Type 5 Inhibitor (PDE5-I) before procedure, are more likely to develop severe ED after RP [31]. Because of this it is very important to apply the International Index of Erectile Function (IIEF) at the first urological consultation [32].

Finally, in compiling the preoperative factors list, any conditions that have an impact on penile hemodynamic may be associated with a higher rate of postoperative ED. Thus, a concomitant diagnosis of some co-morbidity such as Diabetes Mellitus, Hypertension, Hypercholesterolemia, history of Ischemic Heart Disease or Smoking should be taken as a potential negative predictive factor for potency before and after RP, especially Diabetes Mellitus [31].

Comparing Three Surgical Approaches (Retropubic, Laparoscopic and Robotic) Considering Factors Related to Sexual Activity

Urinary Continence

Urinary incontinence is an important factor associated with erectile dysfunction or unsatisfactory sexual relationships and influences a global quality of life. Evaluation of urinary continence after RP is another controversial subject, probably due to the lack of validated institutional questionnaires to evaluate this postoperative co-morbidity. Another limitation is the availability of short- and long-term follow-up in the investigations, so that the heterogeneous follow-up and the different data make the studies' comparison hard. While a review described a virtually equal continence rate between the three approaches [13], the literature is controversial. In general, it is believed that age, BMI, LUTS and prostate volume are relevant factors influencing urinary continence recovery [33]. Although different values were used to determine a large prostate, 70-80 cm^3 could be correlated with a significant risk of urinary incontinence after RARP [34, 35]. On the other hand, Huang et al. analyzed 951 RARP for Benign Prostatic Hyperplasia and showed that prostate size did not affect PSM, urinary continence or sexual function [25].

A non-randomized comparative study related an earlier continence recovery in patients submitted to RARP compared to RRP. After a prospective comparison, this study described a shorter time to continence urinary recovery in the RARP group (44 days *versus* 160 days, p less than 0.05) [36]. Other studies report a similar time to recovery for this function at the first year of follow-up, but there is no statistical significance [37, 38]. Ficarra et al described in a cumulative analysis similar continence rates after RRP and LPR, but considering the learning curve, the recovery of continence is better after RRP. Due the heterogeneity of the studies the author considered it impossible to compare RARP and RRP [39]. In turn, a paper by Touijer et al. reported a statistically significant difference in favor of RRP [40].

Recently, a systematic review and meta-analysis by Ficarra et al. reported an absolute risk of urinary incontinence (twelve months after surgery) of 11.3 percent for RRP (n=105/923) and 7.5 percent for RARP (n=38/509), with an absolute risk reduction of 3.8 percent. The cumulative analysis showed a statistically significant advantage favoring RARP (OR: 1.53; CI 95 percent; 1.04 – 2.25; p = 0.03). Comparing LRP and RARP, the absolute risk of urinary incontinence was 9.6 percent after LRP (n=29/302) and 5 percent after RARP (n=22/436), with an absolute risk reduction of 4.6 percent. The cumulative analysis showed a statistically significant advantage in favor of RARP (OR: 2.39; CI 95 percent; 1.29 – 4.45; p = 0.006) [33].

Sexual Potency

Possibly, despite the anatomical varieties of NVB, RARP may prevent an injury in this structure, because of the peculiarities of the Da Vinci Surgical System, especially the three-dimensional magnified view, which can offer a better condition for a precise dissection of the neurovascular bundle.

Tewari et al. showed an earlier return of erections in patients submitted to RARP than compared to RRP. Half of the patients submitted to RARP recovered the erectile function at an average follow-up of 180 days, in contrast to after 440 days of follow-up with RRP. RARP has also a quicker return to intercourse in comparison to RRP (50 percent at 340 days versus 50 percent at 700 days) [36].

A matched-pair analysis related similar potential rates between RARP and RRP at one year of follow-up but without statistical significance (p = 0.081) [38].

A recent systematic review and meta-analysis demonstrated a prevalence of ED after RRP of 47.8 percent (n=403/843) and 24.2 percent after RARP (n=183/756). The cumulative analysis showed a statistically significant advantage favoring RARP (OR: 2.84; CI 95 percent; 1.48 − 5.43; p = 0.002), with an absolute risk reduction for ED of 23.6 percent. Nevertheless, a comparison between LRP and RARP demonstrated no statistically significance difference (OR: 1.89; CI 95 percent; 0.70 − 5.05; p=0.21) [41].

Postoperative Management and Recovery of ED

Urologists should not worry about patient erectile function only during surgery, since nowadays an important number of trials have demonstrated higher rates of erectile function recovery after RP in patients using any drug already established for the ED treatment. The pathophysiology principle that induced the use of these drugs in the postoperative stage of RP is greater corporeal blood filling and consequent increase of penile oxygenation and decreased penile fibrosis.

Schwartz et al analyzed a cohort of twenty-one patients with localized PC who underwent RP. All of these patients were potent before surgery and were submitted to RP at the same institution. The patients subsequently received Sildenafil at a dose of either 50 mg or 100 mg (Group 1 or 2, respectively) every other night for six months. The patients first took the drug on the day of catheter removal. The twenty-one patients underwent percutaneous penile biopsy both pre- and postoperatively (six months after surgery). In Group 1 there was no statistically significant difference in the average intracavernal smooth muscle contents before and after RP (51.5 percent *versus* 52.6 percent, respectively). On the other hand, Group 2 patients presented a significant increase in the average smooth muscle contents after RP (42.8 percent *versus* 56.8 percent, p < 0,05). These results reinforce the idea of increasing the corporeal blood filling in treating ED, including after RP. They also reinforce the application of sexual pharmacologic prophylaxis after surgery [49], especially because the increased blood flow can prevent the natural steps occurs when there is low penile flow: penile hypoxia, muscle apoptosis, fibrosis, venous occlusion and subsequent difficult to correct ED.

The advent of oral PDE5-I in the ED treatment has revolutionized the management of erectile dysfunction and this is the first line for a majority of patients. The disadvantage is that there is no increment in the 2-year rate of potency compared to placebo, and immediate recovery is not frequently obtained, but it is faster than to patients without treatment.

There are other options for ED treatment after RP. The most utilized is intracorporeal injections of Alprostadil, especially early after surgery for couples that ask for more effective and quicker recovery to sexual intercourse [42, 43]. As with oral medications, the rate of potency after two years is not improved with intracavernous injections but faster recovery is obtained by strong patients.

ORGASMIC DYSFUNCTION

General Considerations

Among the many possible changes caused by radical prostatectomy, such as urinary dysfunction, erectile dysfunction and relationship issues with the partner, there is also a concern with orgasm and ejaculation, which are both still neglected.

Orgasm is a neurophysiologic phenomenon that stimulates bulbocavernous muscles to contract and often coincides with ejaculation [44].

Very few studies evaluate ejaculatory function after RP. Some of them state that both orgasmic and ejaculatory dysfunction are commonly mentioned as undesirable side effects among men that underwent this type of surgery, with some rating it as severe.

A recent a European urological journal article associates the reduced quality of orgasm after RP to the loss of sensation of the prostate and seminal vesicle contractions, and absence of the emission of semen which contributes to the feeling of orgasm, and which are all removed at RP. Another explanation would be psychological processes after the procedure [45].

Incidence

In one study, post-RP orgasm was measured in twenty men, ages averaging sixty-five years old, through interviews and questionnaires associated to a written account of their sexual life. Eighteen questionnaires and seventeen written accounts were returned by the patients.

The results showed that none of the patients were capable of sustaining maximum erection but five of them thought of their erection as sufficient for sexual intercourse. Moreover nine of the patients claimed using intracavernous self-injection therapy and fourteen of them reported reduced libido levels.

Among the fourteen patients that still referred to the presence of orgasm, seven pointed to lower sensation rates and four of them reported no alteration when comparing their sexual life prior to and after surgery. Nine out of fourteen patients noted urinary loss during orgasm, of which five considered it as an impeditive to having any kind of intimate relationship with their partners [46].

A Spanish study reviewed cases of 152 men who underwent RP over the period of one year, ages averaging 64.4 years. Of those, 31.6 percent (42 out of 152) exhibited erectile dysfunction prior to radical prostatectomy.

The evaluation included semi-structured questionnaires and personal interviews that indicated that 91.6 percent of the patients had stable partners, 96.4 percent presented some level of post operatory erectile dysfunction, 44.4 percent were capable of sustaining sexual intercourse, 23.3 percent only practiced masturbation and 32.3 percent did not have any kind of sexual relation.

Concerning orgasmic function, 92.1 percent of patients retained sensation close to normal, 5.2 percent claimed an "abnormal" orgasmic experience, 2.6 percent refer to absence of orgasm and 15.7 percent mentioned urinary loss during orgasm [44].

Climaturia

Yet another study, focused on climacturia, found that the incidence of urinary incontinence during post-RP orgasm reaches 20 percent. The research, through telephonic conversations, surveyed 119 patients, with ages averaging fifty-nine years. Most of them (87 percent) reported discrete urinary loss and 62 percent found it always associated with orgasm. Only 13 percent of them perceived it as an obstacle to their sexual life [47].

Orgasm Associated Urinary Incontinence (OAUI) has been reported in the *European Urological Review*. Between 45 and 93 percent of men suffer from OAUI following RP. Various mechanisms were suggested, the most widely accepted being the one indicating that the dysfunctional bladder neck, that allows bladder contractions during orgasm, may result in urine being ejaculated [45].

Choi et al and Lee et al reported that daytime continence is not associated with climacturia, suggesting that a separate mechanism seems to be responsible [48, 49].

Concordance between Genders

In an American study, from Duke University, North Carolina, the intimate relationship of couples was studied by means of semi-structured questionnaires sent after RP to both patients and their partners. The answers showed concordance between genders as to what extent the surgery affected the couple's life.

Two hundred and forty six men who submitted to radical prostatectomy between 2002 and 2007, and were being monitored for at least twenty-eight months after the procedure, received these questionnaires. The patient ages averaged sixty-two years (between forty-eight and seventy-five), and answered questions concerning libido, sexual foreplay, erection, orgasm, ejaculation and psychological impact of the RP.

Among all couples, just 11.4 percent (28 out of 246) sent the questionnaires back. The answers indicated that 40 percent of them reported being satisfied with their sexual interest (82 percent of concordance), 43 percent of men reported urinary loss during orgasm, and most of them considered that a symptom of great importance.

Ejaculation dysfunction was noted by 96 percent of man (96 percent concordance), and most of them report its absence. Moreover, orgasmic dysfunction was perceived by 86 percent of the patients but only by 36 percent of their partners.

The present study is of great importance showing that men and woman may have different opinions about the same physiologic phenomenon caused by the definitive treatment of prostate cancer. However, these results should be carefully taken into account since that just 14 percent of the questionnaires were returned, and they were not fully structured to evaluate all possible sexual dysfunctions caused by the RP.

Nevertheless this study is relevant because it evaluates the intimate universe of couples that underwent radical prostatectomy and allows a more comprehensive care of both patient and partner during post-RP [50].

PSYCHOLOGICAL ASPECTS THAT IMPACT SEXUAL FUNCTION

The impact of radical prostatectomy (RP) in patient quality of life is the subject of several studies. However, few studies are prospective, with small groups being studied using different questionnaires as well as forms of impact assessment.

Among the possible complications of PR, sexual and urinary dysfunctions have greater impairment in prostatectomy patient quality of life [51, 52]. In addition to these factors, insomnia, anxiety, fatigue and depression are also common among this population [53, 54, 55, 56]. For this reason, during the postoperative follow-up, the physician should look for possible signs of psychological disorders [57].

Studies indicate that sexual desire diminishes with age, being important in 75 to 84 percent among men at the fifth decade of life and 48 to 59 percent at the sixth decade, however each case should be individualized. The patients should be informed of the risks of PR because they are uniquely capable of analyzing the effects of the surgery in their quality of life [58]. Apart from the patient, his partner should also participate in the entire process of diagnosis and choice of treatment [59]. The psychological stress of spouses is often times greater than that of patients, mainly due to concerns related to treatment, possible physical limitations, pain and the diagnosis of cancer itself [60, 61].

The recovery of sexual function depends on several factors such as surgical technique, neurovascular preservation, age and comorbidities of the patient, as well as sexual potency prior to surgery. It also depends on the guidance received by the couple and the psychological preparation for the return to sexual activity, for fear of impotence occurring leads couples to avoid se xual contact after PR [58]. Guidance as to the possibility of erectile dysfunction, treatment for this complication and the recovery time are key to the acceptance of this condition and the stimulus for attempts to return to sexual activity.

Urinary dysfunctions, incontinence among them, may cause greater losses in quality of life than sexual function, since they influence the patient's everyday and social life, sleep and self-esteem [59, 62].

Many studies have evaluated the effects of different surgical techniques on the prostatectomy patient's quality of life. A prospective study followed patients for five years post-PR and post-radiotherapy and concluded that the second group had a poorer quality of life in many aspects compared to the first, but had fewer sexual and urinary symptoms [63]. This is because the effects of PR are immediate in the postoperative period and tend to improve gradually, since radiotherapy presents complications at a later stage. The post-radiotherapy group is more likely to develop psychological disorders [57].

The rate of post-PR impotence is significantly higher than after radiotherapy, 76 percent and 45 percent respectively. However there is a statistically significant interaction between treatment and age regarding bother with sexual function. Patients younger than 60 years of age who reported impotence and loss of quality of life after PR account for 59.4 percent and post-radiotherapy, 25.3 percent. In the group over 60 years there was no difference. Also there are indications of improvement of this complication in young patients in the second year post-PR, while post-radiotherapy patients reported worsening later [64].

Approximately 90 percent of patients report improvement in all aspects of quality of life, including physical, social and health-related, within five months after treatment, except for urinary and sexual dysfunction [58].

The study in relation to the psychological aspects and impact on quality of life is complex. The use of different sexual function questionnaires complicates comparison and analysis of results, as they do not measure erectile function objectively or physiologically. Therefore it is difficult to differentiate between psychological and physiological causes of sexual dysfunction in prostatectomy patients. As for urinary function, there is no questionnaire considered standard and validated for either monitoring or scientific research, although there are several medical exams that the patient can undergo since a common test like urinalysis, blood test and bladder diary to specialized tests like postvoid residual measurement, pelvic ultrasound, stress test, urodynamic test, cystogram and cystoscopy.

Despite the limitations and the difficulty of comparing studies on this topic, it is concluded that the proper orientation for the couple significantly influences the maintenance of quality of life of patients after treatment. It is important to emphasize the risks of impotence and urinary incontinence and the treatments for these complications. The presence of spouses in consultations is also important, since they are directly and indirectly affected by the diagnosis and the possible dysfunctions after treatment [58, 59, 62-64].

CONCLUSION

Most patients undergoing RP will exhibit any changes in sexual function after surgery. Factors related to patient and disease characteristics, surgeon expertise and technique utilized are extremely important to the functional outcome.

Nowadays orgasmic dysfunction has been put aside when compared to erectile dysfunction, but all studies analyzed in this article have suggested repeatedly that orgasmic dysfunction can be as impeditive to a satisfactory sexual life as any other sexual dysfunction.

Since the prevalence of sexual dysfunctions other than ED after RP is substantial, it is important to address the entirety of these aspects during patient counseling. Therapy and prevention of post-RP sexual dysfunction should ideally be individual and cover all facets of sexuality.

Therefore, further studies are necessary involving several aspects still under studied. Multidisciplinary teams of physicians, physiotherapists and psychologists can be important in offering better recovery of sexual functions to the patient and his partner.

Hence, the ideal study design comparing RRP, LPR and RARP would be a randomized trial technique, applying the same clinical approach and methodology for outcomes.

REFERENCES

[1]   Altekruse, S.F., Kosary, C.L., Krapcho, M., et al., eds. *SEER Cancer Statistics Review*, 1975–2007. National Cancer Institute, Bethesda, Md. http://seer.cancer.gov/csr/1975_2007/, based on November 2009 SEER data submission, accessed, 2010.

[2]   Walsh, P.C., Donker, P.J. "Impotence following radical prostatectomy: Insight into etiology and prevention." *Journal of Urology* (1982): 128: 492-497.

[3]   Schuessler, W.W., Schulam, P.G., Clayman, R.V., et al. "Laparoscopic radical prostatectomy: Initial short-term experience." *Urology* (1997): 50: 854-857.

[4]   Guillonneau, B., Vallancien, G. "Laparoscopic radical prostatectomy: The Montsouris xperience." *Journal of Urology* (2000): 163: 418-422.

[5]   Rassweiler, J., Sentker, L., Seemann, O., et al. "Laparoscopic radical prostatectomy with the Heilbronn technique: An analysis of the first 180 cases." *Journal of Urology* (2001): 166: 2101-2108.

[6]   Eden, C.G., Cahill, D., Vass, J.A., et al. "Laparoscopic radical prostatectomy: The initial UK series." *BJU Internacional* (2002): 90: 876-882.

[7]   Binder, J., Kramer, W. "Robotically-assisted laparoscopic radical prostatectomy." *BJU Int* (2001): 87: 408-410.

[8]   Pasticier, G., Rietbergen, J.B., Guillonneau, B., et al. "Robotically assisted laparoscopic radical prostatectomy: Feasibility study in men." *European Urology* (2001): 40: 70-74.

[9]   Trinh, Q.D., Sammona, J., Sun, M., et al. "Perioperative Outcomes of Robot-Assisted Radical Prostatectomy Compared With Open Radical Prostatectomy: Results From the Nationwide Inpatient Sample." *European Urology* (2012): 679-685

[10]   Coelho, R.F., Rocco, B., Patel, M.B., et al. "Retropubic, Laparoscopic na Robot-Assisted Radical Prostatectomy: A critical Review of outcomes reported by high-volume centers." *Journal of Endourology* (2010): 24: 2003-2015.

[11]   Nelson, J.B. "Debate: Open radical prostatectomy vs. laparoscopic vs. robotic." *Urologic Oncology* (2007):25:490–493.

[12]   Briganti, A., Salonia, A., Gallina, A., et al. "Management of erectile dysfunction after radical prostatectomy in 2007." *World Journal of Urology* (2007): 25: 143-148.

[13]   Ferronha, F., Barros, F., Santos, V.V., et al. "Is There Any Evidence of Superiority between Retropubic, Laparoscopic or Robot-Assisted Radical Prostatectomy?" *Internacional Brazilian Journal of Urology* (2011): 37: 146-60

[14]   Ayyathurai, R., Manoharan, M., Nieder, A.M., et al. "Factors affecting erectile function after radical retropubic prostatectomy: results from 1620 consecutive patients." *BJU Internacional* (2008): 101: 833-836.

[15]   Kundu, S.D., Roehl, K.A., Eggener, et al. "Potency, continence and complications in 3,477 consecutive radical retropubic prostatectomies." *Journal of Urology* (2004): 172: 2227-2231.

[16]   Rabbani, F., Stapleton, A.M., Kattan, M.W., et al. "Factors predicting recovery of erections after radical prostatectomy." *Journal of Urology* (2000): 164: 1929-1934.

[17]   Tewari, A., Peabody, J.O., Fischer, M., et al. "An operative and anatomic study to help in nerve sparing during laparoscopic and robotic radical prostatectomy." *European Urology* (2003): 43: 444-454.

[18] Eichelberg, C., Erbersdobler, A., Michl, U., et al. "Nerve distribution along the prostatic capsule." *European Urology* (2007): 51: 105-110.

[19] Briganti, A., Capitanio, U., Chun, F.K.H., et al. "Prediction of Sexual Function After Radical Prostatectomy." *Cancer* (2009): doi: 10.1002/cncr.24349

[20] Montorsi, F., Salonia, A., Suardi, N., et al. "Improving the preservation of the urethral sphincter and neurovascular bundles during open radical retropubic prostatectomy." *European Urology* (2005): 48: 938-945.

[21] Masterson, T.A., Serio, A.M., Mulhall, J.P., et al. "Modified technique for neurovascular bundle preservation during radical prostatectomy: association between technique and recovery of erectile function." *BJU Internacional* (2008): 101: 1217-1222.

[22] Polascik, T.J., Walsh, P.C. "Radical retropubic prostatectomy: the influence of accessory pudendal arteries on the recovery of sexual function." *Journal of Urology* (1995): 154: 150.

[23] Mulhall, J.P., Secin, F.P., Guillonneau, B. "Artery sparing radical prostatectomy – myth or reality?" *Journal of Urology* (2008): 179 (3): 827-31.

[24] Box, G.N., Kaplan, A.G., Rodriguez, E., Jr., et al. "Sacrifice of accessory pudendal arteries in normally potent men during robot-assisted radical prostatectomy does not impact potency." The *Journal of Sexual Medicine* (2010): 7 (1): 298-303.

[25] Novara, G., Ficarra, V., D'Elia, C., et al. "Preoperative criteria to select patients for bilateral nerve-sparing robotic-assisted radical prostatectomy." *The Journal of Sexual Medicine* (2010): 7: 839-45.

[26] Shikanov, S., Desai, V., Razmaria, A., et al. "Robotic radical prostatectomy for elderly patients: probability of achieving continence and potency 1 year after surgery." *Journal of Urology* (2010): 183: 1803-7.

[27] Kowalczyk, K.J., Huang, A.C., Hevelone, N.D., et al. "Stepwise approach for nerve sparing without countertraction during robot-assisted radical prostatectomy: technique and outcomes." *Eur Urol* (2011): 60: 536-47.

[28] Heidenreich, A., Aus, G., Bolla, M., et al. "EAU guidelines on prostate cancer." *European Urology* (2008): 53: 68-80.

[29] Agarwal, P.K., Sammon, J., Bhandari, A., et al. "Safety profile of robotassisted radical prostatectomy: a standardized report of complications in 3317 patients." *European Urology* (2011): 59: 684-98.

[30] Descazeaud, A., Debre, B., Flam, T.A. "Age difference between patient and partner is a predictive factor of potency rate following radical prostatectomy." *Journal of Urology* (2006): 176: 2594-2598.

[31] Montorsi, F., Briganti, A., Salonia, A., et al. "Current and future strategies for preventing and managing erectile dysfunction following radical prostatectomy." *European Urology* (2004): 45: 123-133.

[32] Rosen, R.C., Cappelleri, J.C., Gendrano, N., III. "The International Index of Erectile Function (IIEF): a state-of-the-science review." *Internacional Journal of Impotence Reserch* (2002): 14: 226-244.

[33] Ficarra, V., Novara, G., Rosen, R.C., et al."Systematic Review and Meta-analysis of Studies Reporting Urinary Continence Recovery After Robot-assisted Radical Prostatectomy." *European Urology,* (2012): 62: 405-417.

[34] Boczko, J., Erturk, E., Golijanin, D., et al. "Impact of prostate size in robot-assisted radical prostatectomy." *Journal of Endourology* (2007): 21: 184-8.

[35] Link, B.A., Nelson, R., Josephson, D.Y., et al. "The impact of prostate gland weight in robot assisted laparoscopic radical prostatectomy." *Journal of Urology* (2008): 180: 928-32.

[36] Tewari, A., Srivasatava, A., Menon, M.; Members of the VIP Team. "A prospective comparison of radical retropubic and robot-assisted prostatectomy: Experience in one institution." *BJU Internacional* (2003): 92: 205-210.

[37] Parsons, J.K., Bennett, J.L. "Outcomes of retropubic, laparoscopic, and robotic-assisted prostatectomy." *Urology* (2008): 72: 412-416.

[38] Krambeck, A.E., DiMarco, D.S., Rangel, L.J., et al. "Radical prostatectomy for prostatic adenocarcinoma: A matched comparison of open retropubic and robot-assisted techniques." *BJU Internacional* (2009): 103: 448-453.

[39] Ficarra, V., Novara, G., Artibani, W., et al. "Retropubic, laparoscopic, and robot-assisted radical prostatectomy: A systematic review and cumulative analysis of comparative studies." *European Urology* (2009): 55: 1037-1063.

[40] Touijer, K., Eastham, J.A., Secin, F.P., et al. "Comprehensive prospective comparative analysis of outcomes between open and laparoscopic radical prostatectomy conducted in 2003 to 2005." *Journal of Urology* (2008): 179: 1811-7.

[41] Ficarra, V., Novara, G., Ahlering, T.E., et al. "Systematic Review and Meta-analysis of Studies Reporting Potency Rates After Robot-assisted Radical Prostatectomy." *European Urolpgy* (2012): 62: 418-430.

[42] Montorsi, F., Guazzoni, G., Strambi, L.F., et al. "Recovery of spontaneous erectile function after nerve-sparing radical Retropubic prostatectomy with and without early intracavernous injections of alprostadil: results of a prospective, randomized trial." *Journal of Urology* (1997): 158: 1408-1410.

[43] Montorsi, F., Brock, G., Lee, J., et al. "Effect of nightly versus on-demand vardenafil on recovery of erectile function in men following bilateral nerve-sparing radical prostatectomy." *European Urology* (2008): 54: 924-931.

[44] Martínez-Salamanca Garcia, J.I., Jara Rascón, J.; Moncada Iribarren, I., et al. *Actas Urológicas Españolas* (2004): Nov-Dec 28] (10): 756-760,.

[45] Schmitges, J., Graefen, M.. "Post-operative Sexual Function Following Radical Prostatectomy" *European Urological Review*, (2011): 6 (1): 38-42.

[46] Koemen, M., van Driel, M.F., Schultz, W.C., et al. "Orgasm after radical prostatectomy" *British Journal of Urology* (1996): June 77 (6): 861-4.

[47] Loizaga Iriarte A., Pas Diaz-Romeral, J.L., Arciniega Garcia, J.M., et al. "Climacturia, un síntoma a tener en cuenta tras prostatectomía radical." *Actas Urológicas Españolas* (2007): April 31(4): 345-8.

[48] Choi, J.M., Nelson, C.J., Stasi, J., et al. "Orgasm associatedincontinence (climacturia) following radical pelvic surgery:rates of occurrence and predictors." *Journal of Urology* (2007): 177 (6): 2223-6.

[49] Lee, J., Hersey, K., Lee, C.T., et al. "Climacturia following radical prostatectomy: prevalence and risk factors." *Journal of Urology* (2006): 176 (6, Pt. 1): 2562-5

[50] Tsivian, M., Mayes, J.M., Krupski, T.L., et al. *Internacional Brazilian Journal of Urology* (2009) Vol.35, N.6, Rio de Janeiro Nov.

[51] Eton, D.T., Lepore, S.J. "Prostate cancer and health-related quality of life: a review of the literature." *Psychooncology* 2002; 11: 307-326.

[52] Bacon, C.G., Giovannucci, E., et al. "The association of treatment-related symptoms with quality-of-life outcomes for localized prostate carcinoma patients." *Cancer* 2002; 94: 862-871.

[53] Roth, A.J., Kornblith, A.B., Batel-Copel, L., et al. "Rapid screening for psychologic distress in men with prostate carcinoma." *Cancer* 1998; 82: 1904-1908.

[54] Vordermark, D., Schwab, M., et al. "Chronic fatigue after radiotherapy for carcinoma of the prostate: correlation with anorectal and genitourinary function." *Radiotherapy and Oncology* 2002; 62: 293-297.

[55] Monga, U., Kerrigan, A.J., et al. "Prospective study of fatigue in localized prostate cancer patients undergoing radiotherapy." *Radiation Oncology Investigation* 1999; 7: 178-185.

[56] Savard, J., Morin, C.M. "Insomnia in the context of cancer: a review of a neglected problem." *Journal of Clinical Oncology* 2001; 19: 895-908.

[57] Hervouet, S., Savard, J., et al. Psychological functioning associated with prostate cancer: cross sectional comparison of patients treated withradiotherapy, brachytherapy, or surgery." *Journal of Pain and Symptom Manage* 2005 Nov; 30 (5): 474-84.

[58] Ruth Kirschner-Hermanns, Gerhard Jakse. "Quality of life following radical prostatectomy." *Critical Reviews in Oncology/Hematology* 43 (2002) 141/151.

[59] Evangelos N. Liatsikos, Kostantinos Assimakopoulos, Jens-Uwe Stolzenburg. "Quality of Life after Radical Prostatectomy." *Urologia Internationals.* 2008; 80: 226-230.

[60] Kornblith, A.B., Herr, H.W., et al. "Quality of life of patients with prostate cancer and their spouses." *Cancer* 1994; 73: 2791 /802.

[61] Cliff, A.M., MacDonagh, R.P. "Psychosocial morbitidy in prostate cancer: II. A comparison of patients and partners." *Journal of the British Association of Urological Surgeons*2000; 86: 834/9.

[62] Arai, Y., Okubo, K., et al. "Patient-reported quality of life after radical prostatectomy for prostate cancer". *International Journal of Urology* 1999 Feb; 6 (2): 78-86.

[63] Bacon, C.G., Giovannucci, E., Testa, M., et al. "The impact of cancer treatment on quality of life outcomes for patients with localized prostate cancer." *Journal of Urology* 2001; 166: 1804 /10.

[64] Potosky, A.L., Legler, J., et al. "Health outcomes after prostatectomy or radiotherapy for prostate cancer: results from the prostate outcomes study." *Journal of National Cancer Institute* 2000; 92: 1582/92.

In: Sexual Dysfunctions
Editor: Frédérique Courtois

ISBN: 978-1-62808-765-9
© 2013 Nova Science Publishers, Inc.

Chapter 6

BICYCLE RIDING AS A RISK FACTOR FOR MALE ERECTILE DYSFUNCTION

João Pedro Peralta[1], Ricardo Godinho[1], Carlos Rabaça[2] and Amilcar Sismeiro[3]*

[1] Resident of Urology at the Department of Urology - Portuguese Institute of Oncology, Coimbra, Portugal
[2] Doctor of Urology at the Department of Urology - Portuguese Institute of Oncology, Coimbra, Portugal
[3] Chief Doctor and Head of the Department of Urology - Portuguese Institute of Oncology, Coimbra, Portugal

ABSTRACT

From around the world, people of all ages use a bicycle as a popular means of transportation, recreation, sports and exercise. Bicycle riding is an easy, economic and efficient way to perform aerobic exercise, even for obese, osteoporotic and disabled patients. However, there have been several references to adverse effects of bicycle riding, namely erectile dysfunction. A Pubmed and Medline search for literature related to bicycle riding as a risk factor for erectile dysfunction (ED) was performed. A lot of concern exists about cycling as a risk factor for ED. There seems to be a relationship between cycling and some forms of direct and indirect injuries to the perineum that can lead to vascular and neurogenic dysfunction in men, and consequent development of ED. The most common urogenital symptoms are related to nerve entrapment syndromes, presenting with temporary penile numbness and ED (temporary or permanent). Others include priapism, hematuria, PSA elevation, etc. The data on random studies are scarce but there is a trend for increased awareness of these risk factors. Some preventive maneuvers are advocated, all related to anatomic considerations for the cyclist and the bicycle. Further random studies and standard questionnaires with objective parameters are needed. However, all urologists should be aware of these problems and be alert of some types of urological complaints in their clinical practice regarding cycling.

* Corresponding Author: João Pedro Peralta MD, Department of Urology, Portuguese Institute of Oncology FG EPE, Av. Bissaya Barreto, 3000-075 Coimbra, Coimbra, Portugal. Email: joaopedroperalta@gmail.com

INTRODUCTION

From around the world, people of all ages use a bicycle as a popular means of transportation, recreation, sport and exercise in their everyday practice.

Bicycle riding is an easy, economic and efficient form of aerobic exercise, particularly for obese, osteoporotic and disabled patients.

Nowadays, especially in western countries, cardiovascular diseases are a major cause of death and it is well known from a recently published large study that physical activity reduces the risk of premature cardiovascular death in people with cardiovascular risk factors as well as in inactive individuals without such risk factors [1,2].

It is well known that regular exercise, for a minimum of thirty minutes, three times a week, improves exercise endurance in cardiac chronic patients with stable disease [3].

Nevertheless, several authors describe some negative features of bicycle riding. Most of them, and excluding acute traumatic injuries as part of those, are related to genitourinary and andrological disorders which all urologists should be aware of in their clinical practice [4].

METHODS

A Pubmed and Medline search of the literature related to bicycle riding and erectile dysfunction (ED) was performed. The search yielded about 40 relevant articles on the topic, as well as other related genitourinary issues, which are briefly described (priapism, lower urinary tract symptoms (LUTS), infertility, testis cancer, hematuria and prostate-specific antigen (PSA) changes).

INCIDENCE/EPIDEMIOLOGY

There are several reports which relate ED and bicycle riding to perineal compression syndromes, while only occasional reports are related to other genitourinary disorders. Somer et al., in a study performed in 100 male cyclists with a weekly training exceeding 400 km, reported 61% of complaints of genital numbness and about 24% ED [5].

Likewise, Schwarzer et al. in a sample of 1786 amateur cyclists, reported genital numbness in 58.3-70.3% and 4% of ED. When compared to a matched control group of 155 long distance swimmers, 2% of these complained of ED and none of numbness [6]. Goodson et al. in another study reported penile numbness as a consequence of pudendal neuritis from biking [7].

In a study by Weiss et al. in 1985, 45% of cyclists participating in an 8-day tour of 804,97 km reported penile numbness, with 2% of the patients having had to stop riding temporarily [8].

Most of the participants in the different studies, reported a direct correlation between genital numbness and cycling distance/time [9].

In another population-based epidemiologic study, Marceau et al. surveyed cyclists from the Massachusetts Male Aging Study (MMAS) on 1709 men aged between 40 and 70 years and correlated bicycle riding and ED. When stratified according to riding categories, including recreation, transportation and sport, the study showed that riding more than 3 hours per week was an independent risk factor for men to develop moderate to severe ED, however this did not mean that bicycle riding in general was a risk factor for ED. In the MMAS, in fact, the major risk for ED was seen in men who did not perform exercise [10].

The results from a health hazard evaluation on the members of the Marine Bicycle Patrols from the Long Beach Police Department, in Long Beach, California, showed a 93% incidence of genital numbness and a direct effect on nocturnal penile tumescence (NPT), showing a significant reduction in the duration and quality of nocturnal penile erections when compared to non-bikers. The duration of the nighttime erections was inversely correlated with the average saddle nose pressure and with the duration of riding [11].

There is a great diversity of reported incidences of perineal compression symptoms amongst these studies. This might be due to the studies not being random and match controlled and because multiple variables are often present which may influence the presentation of the reported symptoms, ED and genital numbness. Some of these variables included age, body weight, type of saddle, type of bicycle, duration of training (more than 3 hours seems a consensual limit for weekly training), position during bike riding, and previous erectile function [12, 13].

PATHOPHYSIOLOGY

Male erectile dysfunction resulting from bicycle riding is multifactorial but some theories have been proposed, such as the pudendal nerve entrapment syndrome, caused by the continuous compression and strain on the anatomical pathway located under the pubic arc, but also the vascular occlusion theory [14].

Pudendal Nerve Entrapment Syndrome

The pudendal nerve is a mixed nerve that carries both motor and sensory fibers. It derives from the sacral plexus, originating from roots S2-S4 and transmits somatosensory impulses from the genitalia and perineum, carrying motor efferent fibers to perineal muscles, including the bulbospongiosus and ischiocavernosus muscles, which contribute to the strength and rigidity of penile erection.

On its downward pathway, the nerve crosses the pudendal canal (Alcock's canal) emerging under the pubic arc and innervating the perineum and the genitalia.

The internal pudendal artery, which derives from the anterior trunk of the hypogastric artery, also runs closely to the pudendal nerve in the Alcock's canal, making it vulnerable to the same compression forces on its way down to the genitalia [4, 15].

During bicycle riding, the weight of the body sitting against the saddle generates extreme pressure to the pudendal nerve against the pubic arc. In addition, the nerve can also be stretched as a result of pedaling in a forward leaning position, especially against a narrow, firm saddle with a long nose. This will most likely result in hypoxemia of the nerve and/or neuropraxia, secondary either to nerve ischemia and mechanical pressure [16, 17].

Penile Arterial Insufficiency

Another theory for ED is penile blood insufficiency due to perineal arterial compression. Arterial insufficiency leads to an up-regulation of TGF-B$_1$ expression, which induces collagen and connective tissue synthesis in the corpus cavernosum resulting in fibrosis and decreased smooth muscle content, leading to ED due to a veno-occlusive mechanism. Thus the penile blood flow, and consequently cutaneous penile oxygen content, decrease significantly during cycling and are related to the type of saddle as well as the riding position. The extent of this decrease is worst in the sitting position when compared to a reclining position, but better than a leaning forward position.

Standing up during cycling in turn improves penile blood flow back to normality [18, 19].

Similarly, Broderick et al. reported reduced blood flow after penile PGE1 injection after sitting in a saddle when compared to matched control group not sitting in a saddle [20].

Saddle and Riding Position

Sommer et al. evaluated the effects of seating positions (45-60 vs. 90-degree), saddle size (sport vs. travel) and saddle geometry (uniform flat surface vs. surface with a central hole) on penile oxygen pressure in male cyclists aged 20-37.

Cycling in a reclining position (more than 90 degrees) resulted in 40% better penile oxygenation than cycling in a usual rider's position (45-60 degrees). These results were valid for each saddle type and especially for wider saddles [20].

More recent studies have shown that riding in a sitting position reduces penile oxygenation to a greater extent than a standing position because the penile arteries are compressed against the pubic arc, and because the most likely site of compression is under the pubic symphysis. On the other hand, riding reclining backwards, without compression of the perineum, did not show any difference in penile blood perfusion.

After reviewing reports on saddle types, we realize most authors are consensual regarding the best ergonomic design, suggesting that a wider saddle, with a large groove and without a nose is the most appropriate one. Recently, Jeong et al. showed, using Doppler fluxometry, that the saddle shape can negatively influence penile blood flow, when comparing a wide unpadded with a narrow unpadded saddle [21].

Besides, it is more important for a cyclist, the relationship between the riding position than the saddle type alone.

Bicycle Type

A report from Joseph et al. showed an increased risk of ED among men who cycled in a mountain bicycle compared to a road model. These authors suggested an associated increased risk of ED when the handlebar was higher than the saddle, as it is on mountain bikes. [22]

CLINICAL SYMPTOMS

Genital Numbness

The most common adverse effect of bicycle riding seems to be genital numbness (50-90% of cyclists according to different studies), caused by nerve compression, which arises in the buttocks, scrotum, penis and perineum and is commonly the only symptom. Most of the time it is transient and the site of compression dictates the area of numbness. Numbness is not necessarily synonymous to ED, but ED arising from bicycle riding is usually associated with a history of previous numbness. Hence, numbness may be considered a marker for future ED.

The longer the duration of exposure to perineal compression the greater are the urological complaints. These include perineal numbness/pain and impotence. However, other complaints have been reported, such as orgasmic dysfunction and reduced ejaculation sensitivity.

Likewise, the compression of other urologic structures, like the urethra and the prostate, may cause bladder outlet obstruction symptoms, chronic pelvic pain syndromes and hematuria [23].

Erectile Dysfunction

Another common form of presentation of entrapment syndrome related to bicycle riding is ED (incidence varies between 10-14%).

Ironically, one of the early reports of ED comes from a self-report by a 55 year old physician who described penile numbness and subsequently progressive ED after prolonged daily practice of 20 minutes of vigorous riding exercise. He also reported improvement in penile numbness soon after he had stopped riding, but it took more than one month to completely recover erectile function.

One major study from Marceau et al. reported a 21%, 11% and 17% incidence of ED, respectively, in non-cyclists, moderate cyclists (less than 3 hours per week) and sport cyclists (more than 3 hours per week). After a logistic regression analysis, moderate cyclists still had less ED compared to sport cyclists.

However, this study was underpowered. So even though ED may be an important issue, these conclusions cannot be generalized to the vast majority of sport cyclists because they have a low likelihood of suffering from ED when compared to general population [10].

On the contrary, Taylor et al., in a recent study conducted on the internet, did not show any association between ED and the different cycling variables that were mentioned above [12].

The previously mentioned study on police patrols, showed a decreased quality of NPT tests in the majority of patients, while all of them complained of penile numbness [11].

Lehmann et al. hypothesized that sub-clinical perineal vascular trauma could explain some cases of unexplained ED in young patients, particularly if they were cyclists. In fact, angiograms performed on these patients showed focal lesions in the pudendal and penile arteries along their path through the Alcock´s canal, suggesting a vasculogenic cause for ED [24].

Other Urologic Abnormalities

Aside from genital numbness and ED, other abnormalities in the genitourinary system have been reported, such as priapism, LUTS, infertility, testicular cancer, hematuria and prostate-specific antigen (PSA) changes [25]. A brief summary for some of these reports follows.

There seems to be a link between hematuria and cycling as a result of chronic impact to the perineum, but usually resolves spontaneously [26]. Some cases of high flow priapism have also been reported, suggesting that some form of arterial-venous fistula or shunt, caused by lacerations of the cavernous artery, is the cause of it [27].

Regarding infertility, it has been hypothesized that perineal and testicular blunt trauma, associated with an increased scrotal temperature, and the absence of the usual protective mechanisms to preserve the testes from such environmental aggressions, might be responsible for sperm alterations, namely oligo-teratospermia [28,29].

A controversial question for urologists is the usual indication for stopping bicycle riding a few days before PSA sampling, but there is no proof to the fact that cycling induces clinically significant changes is PSA values. However in older patients with prostate cancer, bicycle riding may have an impact on PSA serum evaluation, so they should be advised about it, and the urologist should also be aware of it.

MANAGEMENT, PREVENTION AND TREATMENT OF THE PUDENDAL COMPRESSION SYNDROME

From a practical point of view, all complaints regarding cycling and the genitourinary system should follow general urological practice and guidelines, and ED is no exception. A correct sexual and medical history, laboratory testing and psychological evaluation should be performed [31]. Eventually Doppler ultrasonography or even dynamic infusion cavernosonometry could be used.

Then, a prevention scheme should be started, comprising several measures to minimize trauma/pressure to the neurovascular bundle of the perineal region. This includes changing the saddle type, the bicycle type and the riding schedule, as well as the riding position at different time intervals during cycling [32,33].

As seen earlier, it can be concluded that mountain bicycles are worse than road models, due to their elevated handlebar, hard tracks and more upright position, which exerts more pressure on the buttocks [34]. From this, we may also conclude that a heavily padded, wide horizontal saddle, with a flexible or absent nose (or a nose saddle that can be faced downward in a 10 degrees position) and a large V-groove shape, is the best option for seating, because it could decrease the pressure exerted on the perineum, which in turn reduces genital numbness and improves penile blood flow [35, 36].

Also, cycling in a reclining position (although not as practical) is better than a sitting position. However, it may be worse, in case the cyclist bends forward (45-60 degrees), putting more pressure on the ischial tuberosities [35]. Likewise, maintaining a slightly flexed leg at the lowest point of rotation on the pedal spin reduces perineal pressure.

An important recommendation, and probably one of the most important ones, is to stand during riding every 10-15 minutes, allowing for the blood to flow freely through the genitalia. Also, frequent time brakes during long distances should be taken [37].

Some *in vivo* as well as *in vitro* studies with phosphodiesterase type 5 inhibitors (PDE-5i) have reported good results in penile rehabilitation following radical prostatectomy. This is because PDE-5i promote penile oxygenation and prevent endothelial dysfunction, which is the main issue behind ED following this procedure. Extrapolating those results along with the ones from a study by Sommer et al., we may conclude that PDE-5i could promote penile oxygenation and prevent vascular damage in long-distance cyclists, making their use a must in these particular circumstances, but special attention must be paid to professional athletes, since PDE-5i may be considered an illicit substance. However, for those who ride for pleasure and recreation and especially in those who have some degree of vascular damage, it could be an asset [38].

CONCLUSION

Although cycling can be a source of genital complaints, with which all urologists may have to deal with sooner or later, parcimony must be used when it comes to conclusions. Bicycle riding is and will continue to be one of the most pleasant and friendly sports, especially for enthusiasts. It should be promoted, particularly in those with cardiovascular risk factors, because it reduces overall mortality, obesity, body fat content and improves glucose status. By reducing these risks cycling also reduces the risk of ED.

However, from a clinical point of view, bicycle riding is also a risk factor for some inconveniences and dangerous accidents, bringing about traumatic injuries that can be life threatening. Moreover, bicycle riding is often a source of transient complaints, which are mostly reported to the genitourinary system. Although usually self-limited, urologists should be aware of them.

After this review, one may conclude that cycling could be a cause of transient or even permanent ED if some preventive maneuvers are not taken and if it is performed in a non-physiologic manner, with adverse features to penile health. These include some types of bicycles and saddles, specific positioning, schedules and duration of riding.

Despite the fact that most urological complaints are transient, one must be aware that continuous aggression to the pudendal nerve during cycling may cause irreversible damage, resulting not only in penile numbness, but also in a permanent form of ED.

The limit between what is healthy, and what is not, regarding cycling, is not yet clearly defined and might not ever be. More random trials have to be made if we are ever to have evidence-based guidelines. Until then, bicycle riding should be regarded as potentially beneficial but with some inherent limitations.

REFERENCES

[1]   Sommer F; Goldstein, I; Korda, JB. Bicycle riding and erectile dysfunction: a review. *J Sex Med* 2010;7:2346-2358.

[2]   Baek S; Lee, SY; Kim, JM; Shin, E; Kam, S; Jung, HC. Bicycle riding: Impact on
        lower urinary tract symptoms and erectile function in healthy men. *Int Neurourol J*
        2011;15:97-101.
[3]   Kiilavuori K, Näveri H, Salmi T, Härkönem M. The effect of physical training on
        skeletal muscle in patients with chronic heart failure. *Eur J Heart Fail* 2000;2:53-63.
[4]   Leibovitch I, Mor Y. The vicious cycling: bicycling related urogenital disorders. *Eur
        Urol* 2005;47:277-287.
[5]   Sommer F; Konig D, Graft C, Schwarzer U, Bertram C, Klotz T, et al. Impotence and
        genital numbness in cyclists. *Int J Sports Med* 2001;22:410-3.
[6]   Schwarzer U, Wiegand W, Bin-Saleh A, Lotzerich H, Kahrmann G, Klotz T, et al.
        Genital numbness and impotence rate in long distance cyclists. J Urol 1999;161:178.
[7]   Goodson JD. Pudendal neuritis from biking. *N Eng J Med* 1981;304:1367-8.
[8]   Weiss BD. Nontraumatic injuries in amateurs long distance bicyclist. *Am J Sports Med*
        1985;13:187-92.
[9]   Andersen KV, Bocim G. Impotence and nerve entrapment in long distance amateur
        cyclist. *Acta Neurol Scand* 1997;95:233-40.
[10]   Marceau L, Kleinman K, Goldstein I, McKinlay J. Does bicycling contribute to the risk
        of erectile dysfunction? Results from the Massachusetts Male Aging Study (MMAS).
        Int J Impot Res 2001;13:298-302.
[11]   Schrader SM, Breitenstein MJ, Clark JC, Lowe BD, Turner TW. Nocturnal penile
        tumescence and rigidity testing in bicycling patrol officers. *J Androl* 2002;23:927-34.
[12]   Schrader SM, Breitenstein MJ, Lowe BD. Cutting off the nose to save the penis. *J Sex
        Med* 2008;5:1932-40.
[13]   Silbert PL, Dunne JW, Edis RH, Stewart-Wynne EG. Bicycle induced pudendal nerve
        pressure neuropathy. *Clin Exp Neurol*, 1991;28:191.
[14]   Taylor JA, Kao TC, Albertsen PC, Shabsigh R. Bicycle riding and its relationship to the
        development of erectile dysfunction. *J Urol* 2004;172:1028-31.
[15]   Oberpenning F, Roth S, Leusmann DB, Van Hahlen H, Hertle L. The Alcock
        syndrome: temporary penile insensitivity due to compression of the pudendal nerve
        within the Alcock canal. *J Urol* 1994;151:423-5.
[16]   Mackinnon SE. Pathophysiology of nerve compression. Hand Clin 2002;18:231-41.
[17]   Nanka O, Sedy J, Jarolim L. Sulcus nervi dorsalis penis: site of origino f Alcock's
        syndrome in bicycle riders? *Med Hypotheses* 2007;69:1040-5.
[18]   Nayal W, Schwarzer U, Klotz T, Heidenreich A, Englemann U. Transcutaneous penile
        oxygen pressure during bicycling. *BJU Int* 199;83:623-5.
[19]   Nehra A, Goldstein I, Pabby A, Nugent M, Huang YH, de las Morenas A, Krane RJ,
        Udelson D, Saenz de Tejada I, Moreland RB. Mechanisms of venous leakage: A
        prospective clinicopathological correlation of corporeal function and structure. *J* Urol
        1996;156:1320-9.
[20]   Broderick, GA. Bicycle seats and penile blood flow: does the type of saddle matter?. *J
        Urol*, suppl.,1999;685:161:178.
[21]   Jeong SJ, Park K, Moon JD, Ryu SB. Bicycle saddle shape affects penile blood flow.
        Int J Impot Res 2002;14:513-7.
[22]   Dettori JR, Koepsell TD, Cummings P, Corman JM. Erectile dysfunction after long-
        distance cycling event: associations with bicycle characteristics. *J Urol* 2004;172:637-
        641.

[23] Doursounian M, Catney-Kiser J, Salimpour P, Adelstein M, Kim C, Goldstein B, et al. Sexual and urinary tract dysfunction in bicyclist. *J Urol* 1998;159(suppl):30.

[24] Lehmann K, Schople W, Hauri D. Subclinical trauma to perineum: a possible etiology of erectile dysfunction in young men. *Eur Urol* 1995;27:306-10.

[25] Kim DG, Kim DW, Park JK. Does bicycle riding impact the development f lower urinary tract symptoms and sexual dysfunction in men? *Korean J Urol* 2011;52:350-354.

[26] Salcedo JR. Huffy-bike hematuria. *N Engl J Med* 1986;315:768.

[27] Montague DK, Jarow J, Broderick GA, Dmochowski RR, Heaton JP, Lue TF, et al. American Urological Association guideline on the management of priapism. *J Urol* 2003;170:1318-24.

[28] Gebreegziabher Y, Marcos E, McKinon W, Rogers G. Sperm characteristics of endurance trained cyclist. *Int J Sports Med* 2004:25;247-51.

[29] Munkelwitz R, Gilbert BR. Are boxer shorts really better? A critical analysis of the role of underware type in male subfertility. *J Urol* 1998;160:1329-33

[30] Luboldt HJ, Peck KD, Oberpenning F, Schmid HP, Semjonow A. Bicycle riding has no impact on total and free prostate-specific antigen serum levels in older men. *J Urol* 1996;156:103-5

[31] Goldstein I, Lurie AL, Lubisich JP. Bicycle riding, perineal trauma and erectile dysfunction: data on solutions. *Curr Urol Rep* 2007;8:491-7.

[32] Lowe BD, Schrader SM, Breitenstein MJ. Effect of bicycle saddle designs on the pressure to the perineum of the bicyclist. *Med Sci Sports Exerc* 2004;36:1055-62.

[33] Munarriz R, Huang V, Uberoi J, Maitland S, Payton T, Goldstein I. Only the nose knows. Penile hemodynamic study of the perineum-saddle interface utilizing saddle/seats with and without nose extensions. *J Sex Med* 2005;2:612-62.

[34] Sommer F, Shwarzer U, Klotz T, Caspers HP, Haup G, Engelmann U. Erectile dysfunction in cyclist. Is there any difference in penile blood flow during cycling in an upright versus reclining position? *Euro Urol* 2001;39:720-3.

[35] Gemmery JM, Nangia AK, Mamourian AC, Reid SK. Digital three-dimensional modeling of the male pelvis and bicycle seats: Impact of rider position and seat design on potencial penile hypoxia and erectile dysfunction. *BJU Int* 2007;99:135-40.

[36] Shwarzer U, Sommer F, Klotz T, Cremmer C, Engelmann U. Cycling and penile oxygen pressure. The type of saddle matters. *Eur Urol* 2002;41:139-43.

[37] Sommer F, König D, Graft C, Schwarzer U, Bertram C, Klotz T, Englemann U. Impotence and genital numbness in cyclists. *Int J Sport Med* 2001;22:410-3.

[38] Sommer F. Cycling and erectile dysfunction (ED): Can sildenafil prevent hypooxygenation of the penis during cycling? Presented at the 100th Annual Meeting of the American Urological Association, May 21-2005, Texas: Abstract 1247.

In: Sexual Dysfunctions
Editor: Frédérique Courtois

ISBN: 978-1-62808-765-9
© 2013 Nova Science Publishers, Inc.

Chapter 7

SEXUAL DYSFUNCTION IN MEN AND WOMEN WITH TYPE 2 DIABETES MELLITUS

Sevilay Hintistan and *Dilek Cilingir*

Karadeniz Technical University, Health Sciences Faculty,
Nursing Department, Trabzon, Turkey

ABSTRACT

Sexuality is a complex phenomenon, which involves not only biological but also psychological and socio-cultural components. Thus, the occurrence of sexual problems in a person's life may be provoked by any or all of these factors. Diabetes mellitus is a systemic disease that is believed to play a principal role in the etiopathogenesis of sexual dysfunction in both men and women. The impact of neurogenic, psychogenic and vascular factors in the pathogenesis of related complications. usually combined, has been cited in a large number of studies. Notwithstanding the similarity between sexual dysfunction in men and women with diabetes as shown in this article, a disparity remains in etiological explanations between male and female sexual dysfunction. The prevalence of female sexual dysfunction and associated risk factors in diabetic women are less clear than in men. Although women with diabetes mellitus are at higher risk of developing sexual dysfunction than those without the disease, study results vary greatly and indicate that SD in these patients is generally linked more to psychological factors rather than organic causes. Sexual problems in women with diabetes primarily include issues related to sexual desire, sexual satisfaction, orgasmic disorder, arousal disorder and lubrication. The prevalence of sexual dysfunction among women with diabetes varies between 20.0% and 80.0%. Sexual problems in men with diabetes include disorders of libido, ejaculatory problems, erectile dysfunction, decreased sexual desire, and intercourse satisfaction. In particular, erectile dysfunction is common in men with diabetes with a prevalence of 20.0% to 85.0%. This chapter attempts to give an overview of sexual dysfunctions in diabetic men and women and its influence on their sexual functioning. The chapter results also aim to add to the present understanding of diabetes and its impact on patients' sexual lives so that more effective clinical guidelines for treatment can be developed.

* Corresponding author: Sevilay Hintistan PhD, Assistant Professor Nursing Department, Pharmacy, Karadeniz Technical University Health Sciences Faculty, Faculty Building, 61080, Trabzon, Turkey. Telephone: 0090 0462 230 04 76; E mail: sevilayhindistan69@yahoo.com

INTRODUCTION

The field of sexuality consists of many dimensions and is a central part of being human. It is influenced by the interaction of biological, psychological, social, economic, political, cultural, ethical, legal, historical, religious, and spiritual factors. The term "sexuality" encompasses numerous and complex aspects of human life, and many elements need to be considered when discussing this topic. These would include male and female characteristic, life span from infancy to old age, physical and emotional needs, love, affection, intimacy, belonging, attitudes, feelings, expression, reproduction, pleasure, cultural and religious influences, self-image, and respect. Sexuality includes a person's sexual knowledge, attitudes, values, and behaviors, as well as anatomy, physiology, and the sexual response cycle. It is integral to marital or romantic relationships and is central to a person's self-concept, self-esteem, and mental and physical health. Since sex is associated with these characteristics, it can be deduced that individuals relate their health status to their sexual activity [64].

As an important part of human life, issues related to sexuality should be an integral part of the challenge to improve the quality of life of diabetic patients. Diabetes is a chronic disease requiring patients to visit health-care providers regularly. Therefore, diabetic patients theoretically have greater access to professional help [38]. Yet current care for DM patients would indicate that although medical professionals understand the importance of sexual health, the reality shows it is often neglected [26]. This article focuses specifically on sexual dysfunction (SD) in men and women with type 2 diabetes, with particular emphasis on information for health care professionals.

1. EPIDEMIOLOGY

Information on the prevalence of SD and diabetes varies widely probably due to the different definitions and the population studied. These differ with respect to the number and selection of participants, cultural background, socioeconomic level, quality of psychosexual relationship and income [51].

1.1. Epidemiology of Sexual Dysfunction in Men with Type 2 Diabetes Mellitus

The research shows that diabetes is an independent risk factor for SD, especially erectile dysfunction (ED) in men. Diabetes has long been considered a major cause of impaired sexual function in men, with prevalence rates of ED approaching 50% in both type 1 and type 2 diabetes [25]. ED is common in men with diabetes with a prevalence of 20% to 85%. Men with diabetes also have a three-fold increased risk for ED compared with those without the disease [2, 38, 43].

1.2. Epidemiology of Sexual Dysfunction in Women with Type 2 Diabetes Mellitus

A few published studies on SD in women with diabetes mellitus (DM) have presented conflicting results. Most studies have shown a higher prevalence of female SD in women with diabetes irrespective of the country of origin [1, 63]. The estimated prevalence varied between 42% and 88% for type 2 DM [15, 49]. In contrast, some studies revealed the presence of objective changes in genital sensation in females with DM with no subjective deleterious effect on sexual functions [6, 24]. Although studies have revealed conflicting results, some general tendencies in predicting sexual dysfunctions in females with DM were observed [49]. The discrepancies in the results of various studies can be explained by the methodological differences in studies as well as the socio-cultural structure and traditional values of the society in which the study was conducted. The prevalence of sexual disorders among diabetic women is reported to range between 20% and 80% [23]. SD is common among sexually active women, with over a third reporting dissatisfaction with overall sexual functioning and up to 40% reporting specific sexual problems [63]. The prevalence of SD in diabetic men approaches 50%, whereas in diabetic women it seems to be slightly lower [26]. However, a recent review of diabetes and female sexuality indicated that diabetes slightly increases the risk of female SD [19].

2. PATHOGENESIS

DM may lead to disruption of normal sexual function in both men and women. The disease process damages the nerves and blood vessels which are essential for normal function of the genital organs [43]. Although both sexes share a similar risk of cardiovascular and neurological complications from diabetes, which presumably may arise from similar pathogenetic mechanisms, the pattern of specific effects of diabetes may differ [25].

2.1. Pathogenesis of Sexual Dysfunction in Men with Type 2 Diabetes Mellitus

The pathophysiology of ED in male diabetes is complex, but probably involves vascular and neurogenic components, together with endothelial dysfunction [16]. A study by Zdravko (2007) supported the hypothesis that diabetic neuropathy is the major pathogenic factor in the complex pathogenesis of diabetic ED [71]. Diabetes causes damage to nerves throughout the body including the penis and ED is a common diabetes complication. The high rate of SD in diabetic patients could stem from damage to small arteries and arterioles, which could impair endothelium-dependent relaxation of the penile smooth muscle. This results in obstruction of optimal blood flow to and from the penis, and thus maintenance of an erection becomes impaired [51].

The pathophysiology of ED in DM is multifactorial, consisting of vascular and neurologic insults. Impaired relaxation of the corpus cavernosal smooth muscle in diabetics occurs in response to neuronal- and endothelial- derived nitric oxide, which may be due to the accumulation of glycosylation products. New evidence has suggested that in addition to problems with the arteries and nerves supplying the penis, men with diabetes may be at increased risk of low testosterone levels. While the precise mechanism of this effect is not entirely clear, in some cases, it may be secondary to a decline in the levels of pituitary hormones responsible for stimulating testicular production of testosterone. Low levels of testosterone may lead to a decline in sexual desire and, directly or indirectly, to ED [43].

2.2. Pathogenesis of Sexual Dysfunction in Women with Type 2 Diabetes Mellitus

Neuropathy, vascular impairment and psychological complaints have been implicated in the pathogenesis of SD among diabetic women [26, 41]. The brain's signal of sexual arousal is transmitted by the autonomic nervous system to the genital erectile tissue in both sexes and to women's submucosal vaginal microvasculature. This neurotransmission to the erectile tissue involves nitric oxide (NO) and other neurotransmitters, and causes relaxation of the smooth muscle surrounding the minute blood spaces (sinusoids) in the clitoris and in the vestibular bulb. It also facilitates the release of NO from the endothelial cells that line the sinusoids. The neurotransmission to the vascular smooth muscle in the vaginal submucosa, which is most likely vasointestinal polypeptide- and NO - mediated, increases the inflow of blood, thereby increasing intracapillary pressure and the transudation of lubricating fluid. This autonomic neurological conduction is most likely inefficient in diabetic patients and can result in less NO in the endothelial cells. Supply arteries may be prematurely stiffened with atheroma, and with time, relative anoxia causes the loss of smooth muscle, further inhibiting the process of engorgement. The engorgement of erectile tissue is clearly of major importance to a man with diabetes but may be less critical to a woman with this disease. Similarly, lubrication may still be "sufficient" even if a decrease in vascular response is documented [5].

3. DIABETES MELLITUS AND SEXUAL DYSFUNCTION

The impact of various illnesses on a person's sexuality is well known, and SD in both male and female patients is very common [73]. In fact, sexual problems may be a warning sign or consequence of a serious underlying illness [64], and for some men SD may be the first sign of diabetes [18]. Current knowledge suggests that DM plays a principle role in the etiopathogenesis of SD in both sexes [23].

Diabetes is known to cause multiple medical, psychological, and sexual problems [19] and can have both direct and indirect effects on sexual functioning. The direct effects are in relation to the vascular changes that occur in diabetes mellitus. Individuals with diabetes mellitus may also experience neurological deficits due to the disease process, which can also affect sexual function [64].

Diabetes affects biological mechanisms that mediate sexual response as well as psychosocial factors, both of which impact broader cognitive and psychological aspects of sexuality. When Type 2 diabetes onset occurs later in life, it may seriously disrupt the stability of a couple and render the relationship less satisfying to the woman and/or her partner [23].

Men and women have very different "sexual programming", and their most common sexual dysfunctions or complaints are not simply physiological equivalents [5].

3.1. Sexual Dysfunction in Men with Type 2 Diabetes Mellitus

SD among diabetic men may include disorders of libido, ejaculatory problems, erectile dysfunction, decreased sexual desire, and intercourse satisfaction [51, 55]. Patients with diabetes have lower libido; men may have lower testosterone levels; and individuals with diabetes may experience decreases in genital sensation and lubrication, which leads to SD and thus affects a person's quality of life [39]. Generally, men have higher levels of spontaneous sexual desire than women, most likely based in part on genetic factors and 10-fold higher testosterone levels compared with women. Men's sexual drive contributes much to the enjoyment of the sexual experience with a partner or alone. For both types of activity, but especially during sexual activity with a partner, a firm and not just tumescent penis is necessary. Thus, the most common male SD is ED [5]. Corona et al. demonstrated that among their ED patients, those with diabetes had a lower prevalence of hypoactive sexual desire than those without diabetes. It suggested that they were more interested in restoring sexual activity than the other ED patients [10].

Still, even non-erectile sexual problems (e.g., low desire, premature ejaculation) often present as erectile failure. The inherent biological vulnerability of the erectile mechanism compounds the requirement of a firm penis. Vascular health, especially the availability of endothelial NO, which is an integral component of the expansion of corporal tissue, commonly decreases with diabetes. Given the perceived mandatory requirement of a firm penis, any physically based deficiency quickly becomes compounded by interpersonal and intrapersonal factors [5].

3.1.1. Erectile Dysfunction

ED, or the persistent inability to attain and maintain an erection adequate for sexual activity, affects many men at some time in their lives [16]. Men with diabetes are more likely to consider their ED to be severe and permanent, compared with men without diabetes. ED is a common complication of diabetes [11], and although it is widespread, the condition often remains undiagnosed and deserves appropriate assessment and proper treatment [35, 73]. Other research findings indicate that the etiology of ED is multifactorial and the management of diabetic ED requires a holistic approach [45].

DM is a major health problem and a leading cause of male ED with an incidence of 500,000 newly-diagnosed Americans each year [39]. It is also one of the most common risk factors associated with ED [16]. A recent report of outcomes of Type 2 diabetes research programs found that of 1460 patients, 34% reported frequent erectile problems and 24% reported occasional problems [31]. In diabetic men, ED severity increases with age, diabetes duration, poor glycemic control, presence of microvascular complications and cardiovascular disease [2]. Therefore, clinicians should take preventive measures to include early screening and treatment in high-risk patients [38].

As with most aspects of diabetes care, routine exercise, careful monitoring of glucose levels, and usage of appropriate therapies to prevent hyperglycemia are key to preventing progression of diabetes-induced sexual problems. Weight management and dietary prudence are also critical in the management of diabetes; research results suggest that weight loss may reverse ED in some men [43].

Factors Affecting Erectile Dysfunction in Men with Type 2 Diabetes Mellitus

One of the most common risk factors associated with ED is diabetes [16], and ED is, in fact, a well-established complication of diabetes [19]. Many factors can contribute to the development of ED, including organic causes (e.g. vascular disease and neurological disease) and psychogenic factors (e.g. anxiety or depression).

1. Age

SD is known to occur in approximately 50% of men with DM prior to age 60 [64]. ED develops at an earlier age in the diabetic population when compared with the general population [11], and its severity increases with age [2]. The prevalence of ED among men with diabetes is 9% in men aged 20-29 years, rising to 95% by 70 years of age [16]. Furthermore, ED has been found to be age dependent and increases with age in diabetic males. ED affects those with diabetes an average 10-15 years earlier than the general population regardless of the insulin dependency status [2]. More than 50% of men with diabetes develop ED within 10 years of diagnosis [16].

Previous reports have shown that diabetic men are at increased risk for SD at an earlier age with an incidence ranging from 20% to 85% [51]. The Giugliano et al. study (2010) with type 2 diabetes male patients found that the rate of ED increased with age. In the Massachusetts Male Aging Study cohort, the annual age-adjusted incidence rate of ED increased with diabetes [31]. Guay's study (2001) reported the occurrence of nearly 36% moderate to severe ED, ranging from 4.6% in young men to 45.5% in older men [34].

2. Diabetes Duration and Severity of Disease

Men with diabetes, whether type 1 or type 2, have a significantly greater prevalence of ED than the general population, and this increases with age, duration, and the severity of disease [34]. ED develops an average of 6.4 ± 4.3 years after the diagnosis of diabetes, and it occurs in approximately half of patients within 10 years after diagnosis [11]. Men with ED and a history of diabetes present with more severe ED compared with men without diabetes [16]. The prevalence of ED in patients with diabetes duration less than 5 years was 60%; the rate for 5-10 years was 68.5%; and for patients with diabetes 10 years or longer the rate was 77.7% [31].

3. Glucometabolic Control

Aside from emotional support, other factors were only weak predictors of HbA1C in men. ED also tended to relate to metabolic control. Men displayed stronger sexual desire, activity, and less satisfaction with their sex life than women. Interestingly, poor glucose control may initiate a vicious cycle leading to ED which could arouse negative emotions, thereby further impairing glucose levels [40]. Additionally, poorly-controlled diabetes may increase the morbidity associated with the treatment of ED in men [43].

4. Diabetes Related Complications

Autonomic neuropathy or cavernosal artery insufficiency, or a combination thereof, are the likely pathophysiologic mechanisms leading to ED in diabetes. Studies of smooth muscle from patients with ED and diabetes have shown the presence of autonomic neuropathy. Biochemical and immunohistochemical evidence suggest diabetes causes a general depletion of neurotransmitter systems and structural damage to the autonomic nerves that control local mechanisms of penile erection. Vasculopathy contributes to diabetic-induced atherosclerosis-associated ED by way of decreased arterial inflow of blood to the lacunar spaces of the corpora cavernosa. Concurrently, alterations occur in the reactivity of the endothelial cells in the lacunar space and corpus cavernosum smooth muscle. The structural modifications induced by diabetes include reduction in smooth muscle content, increased collagen deposition, and thickening of the basal lamina, leading to fibrosis. These combined hemodynamic and structural changes lead to decreased rigidity, a delay in time to maximal erection, and a diminished ability to sustain an erection [31].

5. Obesity

Obesity is associated with a state of chronic oxidative stress and inflammation which impairs endothelial function. This results in SD and lays the groundwork for atherosclerosis. Since atherosclerosis of the arteries supplying genital tissues greatly affects sexual function, it seems rational to assume that conditions predisposing a person to atherosclerosis (diabetes, obesity) might impair sexual function [51]. Weight management and dietary prudence are also critical in the management of diabetes. There is evidence to suggest weight loss may reverse ED in some men [43]. An increase in visceral, central or abdominal adiposity, as measured by waist circumference and possibly weight, can lead to endocrinologic imbalances [51]. A study by Dey et al. indicated that the high prevalence of ED was found to be correlated with obesity [14]. Another study by Bacon et al. determined a positive correlation between body mass index and ED [3].

6. Hyperlipidemia

Hyperlipidemia is one of the risk factors leading to ED in men. Epidemiological studies have found that the decrease in high density lipoprotein (HDL) and elevation of total cholesterol/high density lipoprotein are correlated with ED. Studies have also shown that arterial stenosis and occlusion caused by hyperlipidemia could be attributed to the advanced-stage mechanism of ED induced by hyperlipidemia. Hyperlipidemia may damage a man's erectile function at an early stage by affecting the endothelial cells and smooth muscles of the penis and the peripheral nerves for penile erection [54].

7. Cigarette Smoking

The mechanisms that could explain an association between smoking and diabetes are not known. Experimental findings suggest that smoking causes insulin resistance [53, 72]. This effect could be due to a stimulation of the sympathetic nervous system by nicotine. Indeed, long-term use of nicotine-containing chewing gum was associated with insulin resistance. Other studies also indicate that acute administration of nicotine induces insulin resistance [29, 72]. As to effects on insulin secretion, heavy smoking was not found to affect insulin secretion, whereas an influence on insulin secretion by long-term nicotine use has not yet been investigated [53].

Several studies have linked cigarette smoking to ED [29, 72]. Smokers are 1.5 times more likely to have ED than nonsmokers, and even 2 cigarettes per day may have a detrimental effect on erection [72]. Longitudinal data over a 9-year period from the Massachusetts Male Aging Study showed that the incidence of ED was twice as high among smokers compared with nonsmokers [27]. There is evidence of a beneficial effect of smoking cessation on ED, especially at younger ages [53]. A study conducted by Gades et al. found an association between cigarette smoking and ED [29]. Another study by Bacon et al reported that 1.3 times more ED was seen in smokers than nonsmokers [3].

8. Medication Use

All antihypertensive agents, regardless of composition, have been implicated in causing ED [72]. Although many antihypertensive drugs (diuretics and some beta-blockers) are known to cause ED, renin-angiotensin system inhibitors are often claimed to have fewer debilitating side effects on erectile function [31].

9. Chronic Diseases

Common risk factors associated with ED include heart disease, hypertension and DM. As mentioned earlier, ED in diabetic men may be multifactorial in origin, involving possible vascular, neurological and endocrinological components [2]. It is associated with glycemic control and other classic cardiovascular and neuropathic complications of diabetes; moreover, the prevalence of other cardiovascular risk factors (obesity, hypertension, dyslipidemia) is high, especially in type 2 diabetes. ED is also an independent risk factor and powerful predictor of major cardiovascular events in diabetic patients with known coronary artery disease [25]. ED may also be the presenting symptom for DM and may predict later neurologic sequelae [43]. A number of men with autonomic neuropathy can experience normal erectile function and orgasm but do not ejaculate normally, as verified through urine analysis [73].

Hypertension is a well-known risk factor for ED. The prevalence of ED is significantly greater among men with hypertension than in the general population. Prolonged elevated blood pressure has detrimental effects on the vascular system as a whole, including the penile blood supply. It is now widely accepted that organic ED in a substantial majority of men occurs because of underlying vascular causes, especially atherosclerosis [31]. While the incidence of ED increases with age, this is driven not so much by age but by comorbid conditions associated with aging. Examples include smoking, heart disease, high blood pressure, high cholesterol, and diabetes [43]. In a study conducted on diabetic men by Yalcin et al. the most important risk factor for ED was hypertension (38%) [66]. Moreira et al. reported that ED was seen 2.48 times more in men with hypertension than in those without it [46]. In the Giuliano et al. study, 61% of patients with hypertension, 67% of those with diabetes, and 78% of patients with both hypertension and diabetes reported some degree of ED [31].

10. Self-esteem

ED in men with diabetes causes a decline in their self-esteem. A study by De Bore et al. found the risk of ED in patients with low self-esteem to be 1.25 times higher [12].

11. Psychogenic Factors

ED is a common clinical problem and a serious detriment to quality of life for men and their partners [43]. It is also negatively associated with many aspects of patients' psychological well-being. Therefore, most patients would want their physicians to take the lead in discussing ED [38]. The strong association between SD and impaired quality of life justifies recognition of ED in diabetic patients as a significant public health problem. In this respect, sexual function should be considered an integral part of overall health in diabetic patients [11].

Although psychogenic factors, such as performance distress, can contribute to ED's etiology, ED in diabetic patients is mainly related to organic causes which can include vasculagenic and neurological abnormalities. Furthermore, the occurrence of symptoms of depression, anxiety, panic and forgetfulness are common and may also have a role in ED associated with diabetes [2]. Studies have shown that sexually dysfunctional men had significantly more emotions of sadness, disillusion, and fear, and less pleasure and satisfaction, compared with men without sexual problems [47].

The presence of a normal sexual desire and the inability to physically act on that desire can affect patients' lives in different ways. Problems include disturbed interpersonal relationships, a disrupted sexual life, problems with partners, and increased mental stress. These negative effects make ED a major quality-of-life issue [11], and more effective treatments are needed to improve the lives of both patients and their families [38].

12. Depression

Goldstein and colleagues found a strong relationship between ED and depression; the incidence of depression was more than 2 times higher in people with ED than in those without ED. The same study identified depression at a rate of 2.48 times higher in diabetic subjects under treatment for ED. Depression was found to be more than 7.38 times higher in untreated patients with ED [32]. In particular, patients with ED showed higher levels of frustration and discouragement and a lower acceptance of diabetes, which were, in turn, related to worse metabolic control and higher levels of depressive symptoms [11].

13. Screening ED in Men with Type 2 Diabetes Mellitus

Although some ED patients thought sex was not important, many reasons exist for physicians to screen sexual function. First, ED may be a precursor of other cardiovascular disease. Second, poor glycemic control and unhealthy lifestyle habits, such as smoking, have been associated with ED. In fact, health concerns related to ED may be the impetus for patients to quit smoking or to improve their compliance with DM control measures. ED has also been shown to cause interpersonal relationship problems, increased mental stress, and higher levels of diabetes-specific health distress. Furthermore, a correlation has been found which relates poor psychological adaptation to diabetes with unsatisfactory metabolic control. Therefore, physicians caring for DM patients should not overlook this association and act accordingly [38].

14. Treatment

The treatment of ED in men with diabetes is often considered to be more difficult than that of other patients. Diabetic men with ED tend to be less responsive to treatment, perhaps because the pathogenesis of diabetes-related ED is multifactorial [16]. For example, differences in culture, custom, and socioeconomic status may affect patients' attitudes towards ED treatment [38].

Therapy with oral medication is generally accepted as the optimal first-line treatment for most men with ED, including those with diabetes. The most commonly used oral agents are the phosphodiesterase type 5 (PDE5) inhibitors Sildenafil (Viagra), Tadalafil (Cialis) and Vardenafil (Levitra) [16]. The treatment of ED in general was revolutionized by the availability of Sildenafil, followed by Tadalafil and Vardenafil. The three medications work by a similar pathway. Sexual stimulation provokes the release of NO, leading to increased cellular concentrations of cyclic guanosine monophosphate (cGMP) and subsequent penile smooth muscle relaxation. This process is reversed by the conversion of cGMP to guanosine monophosphate, which is mediated by PDE5- the predominant functional PDE type found in the penis. PDE5i act at this step to maintain elevated levels of cGMP and continued smooth muscle relaxation. Since the release of NO is a neurologically-mediated event, neuropathy (as may occur with diabetes) may blunt the efficacy of PDE5i. This is indeed borne out clinically, as diabetics have a poorer response overall to PDE5i than men with ED due to other causes [43].

Intracavernosal Injection

Intracavernosal alprostadil injection therapy in diabetics was evaluated. In patients for whom injection therapy does not work vacuum erection devices (VED) may be useful. There is a paucity of data specifically evaluating the use of VED in diabetics, and the drop-out rate is quite high, even for patients who are able to achieve a rigid erection with the device. One subset analysis found that despite a good response (i.e. rigid erection) using VED, only 50% of couples found the treatment to be satisfactory. This may be due to the "unnaturalness" of the devices, as well as the fact that they may have several local side effects, including petechiae (small red dots from broken capillaries), a feeling of having a cold penis, and abnormal sensation of ejaculation [43].

Penile Prosthetics

When there is lack of efficacy or dissatisfaction with other modalities, penile prostheses are often the best alternative for ED in diabetics [43].

While PDE5i do not work as well in diabetics as in other populations, they still represent a good first-line treatment. If their use is unsatisfactory, intracorporal injections and an implantable prosthesis are excellent alternatives. Vacuum devices represent another viable alternative, although satisfaction is generally not as high [16, 43].

3.2. Sexual Dysfunction in Women with Type 2 Diabetes Mellitus

Female SD is a common problem worldwide [25]. As SD is considered a taboo topic, sexuality can be overlooked by women and is often neglected by health professionals in patients' assessments [21]. In women, SD is generally a self-reported condition, with a complex pathogenesis (intrapsychic, sociocultural, relational, and organic). Although diabetic women suffer from the same vascular and neurological complications thought to be instrumental in the occurrence of SD in diabetic men, results of sexual functioning of women with diabetes are less conclusive. Furthermore, medical professionals have not yet agreed upon a definition for SD; at this time it is still poorly understood [37]. Consequently, knowledge about SD in diabetic female patients is lacking and needs more research [39]. In spite of limitations, most studies have found a higher prevalence of female SD in diabetic women when compared with nondiabetic women [25].

As mentioned, sexual functioning of women with diabetes has received much less attention in clinical research. However, a recent review on diabetes and female sexuality indicated that diabetes slightly increases the risk of female SD. The most common SD in women with diabetes is decreased sexual arousal with slow and/or inadequate lubrication. These patients may also experience a decreased sexual desire and more pain on sexual intercourse, whereas problems with orgasm are infrequent [19]. Ege et al. revealed that 45% of women had pain during sexual intercourse and this problem was a risk factor for SD [17]. Decreased libido is reported by 30% -50% of women who consult marital and sex therapists and is considered to be the most frequently encountered sexual problem. There may be an initial loss of libido after the diagnosis of diabetes or during a phase of illness, but there is little evidence to suggest that diabetic women have lower libido than nondiabetics. Instead, it is generally psychogenic factors and important physical aspects that affect sexual desire. These include health status, depression (which affects hormonal status), and the use of both prescription and recreational drugs [23].

Sexual problems in women with diabetes primarily present as loss of sexual desire, sexual satisfaction, orgasmic disorder, arousal disorder and lubrication issues [73].

1. Sexual Desire

In contrast to men's sexual desire, women's desire is often perceived as being more responsive than spontaneous, as is reflected in the new American Foundation of Urological Disease consensus definition of female hypoactive sexual desire disorder. It may be triggered by many factors, in addition to conventional sexual stimuli. Women's desire may be expressed more as their need to share physical closeness, intimacy, love, and affection rather than the pure physical pleasure of sexual acts. The need for physical pleasure is, however, commonly accessed once the sexual experience has begun [5]. Doruk and colleagues found that Turkish women with type 2 mellitus had higher rates of sexual desire (82%) than women without diabetes [15].

2. Sexual Satisfaction

Type 2 diabetes has a consistently deleterious effect on both women's sexual behavior and relationships. When compared to controls, diabetic women viewed themselves as less sexually attractive and were generally dissatisfied with their sexual life [23].

SD is a decrease in, or lack of sexual satisfaction. A woman's sexual health can be greatly affected in many ways:

1) Infections and irritation: high blood glucose levels, yeast infections and vaginal irritations [39]. Ozerdogan et al. reported that genital infections in women were

associated with SD [52], and Wallner et al. (2010) found that diabetic women were at greater risk for vaginal infections, particularly yeast candidiasis, which may predispose them to dyspareunia [63]. Other related issues awaiting further detailed studies include the following: Low sexual desire that is associated with high blood sugar levels, interference with sexual response from painful neuropathy, recurrent cystitis, and vaginitis and pain from vulvar vestibulitis syndrome, which is potentially precipitated by Candida Albicans infection [5].

2) Low blood flow, e.g., vascular damage.
3) Medication: tranquilizers, birth control pills, high blood pressure medication; and
4) Menopause: its effects on the body may cause a serious change in the sexual function [39].

A diagnosis of diabetes affects arousal, and decreases genital sensation and lubrication, which may negatively impact women's sexual satisfaction [39].

3. Orgasmic Disorder

Inability to achieve orgasm is related to psychological, organic etiology, or a combination of the two. Erol et al. reported that 49% of diabetic women had difficulty reaching orgasm by sexual stimulation or intercourse, whereas no women in the control group complained of orgasmic disorder. Symptoms which probably contribute to orgasmic dysfunction include decreased libido, low arousability, decreases in vaginal lubrication, sexual desire, and clitoral sensation which occur during the excitement phase of sexual relations. Furthermore, related symptoms in women with SD usually overlap, which means that they combine as presenting complaints [23]. Women with SD experience decreased arousal, desire, and orgasmic capacity because of inadequate stimulation [39].

4. Arousal Disorder

Sexual arousal is difficult to evaluate due to its complexity. Women tend to rate their subjective arousal based on their mental excitement, rather than on an appreciation of genital changes [5]. Doruk and colleagues found that Turkish women with type 2 mellitus had lower rates of arousal than women without diabetes [15]. Neurovascular processes that regulate genital vasocongestion can also become impaired in diabetic patients and are partially responsible for the vaginal discomfort and dyspareunia in diabetic women [23]. Most women are relatively unaware of the state of vasocongestion of the genitalia. They mainly refer to subjective arousal when speaking of sexual arousal. Women's appraisal of sexual stimuli and their context, rather than the conscious appraisal of genital vasocongestion, determines their subjective arousal. Women speak rather infrequently of problems that reflect a lack of engorgement of the clitoris, the vaginal wall, vestibular bulbar tissue or the erectile tissue around the urethra. The vast majority of this erectile tissue is hidden from view in women. Partial rather than full engorgement may not interfere with sexual pleasure from stimulation. Neither a woman nor her partner is likely to be aware that the physiological response is only a partial response [5].

Clitoral response in the arousal phase may also be impaired in DM. Diabetes is well known to cause pathological changes in both the central and peripheral nervous system. Evaluation of the neurogenic components of ED in men by biothesiometry has shown that the penile somatic afferent system is damaged in diabetes [23]. It seems that the somatic sensory system is affected by diabetes and the vagina, labium minora and clitoris are the most deteriorated genital sites in diabetic women. Although sexual difficulties do not always occur, medication can improve blood flow to the clitoris [73]. These changes, and especially the autonomic neuropathy frequently observed in diabetes, result in diminished clitoral sensation. Still, additional objective studies are needed to more fully understand these mechanisms of change [23].

5. Lubrication

Diabetes in women can lead to hardening of the blood vessels of the vaginal wall. Decreased blood flow can affect vaginal lubrication, causing the vagina to be too dry for comfortable intercourse [39]. Sidi et al. indicated that less lubrication was associated with SD in women [59]. Women may complain of insufficient lubrication from vaginal capillaries despite an intact desire for a sexual experience and adequate mental arousal. This situation is usually a reflection of reduced estrogen production in post-menopausal women (estrogen is needed for the process of lubrication, which is, most likely, predominantly vasointestinal polypeptide-mediated) [5]. Previous studies have shown that sexual difficulties are a risk factor for female SD. It is argued that neuropathy, vascular impairment, and psychological complaints are recognized factors in the pathogenesis of female SD in diabetic women [73].

Factors Affecting Sexual Dysfunction in Women with Type 2 Diabetes Mellitus

Studies of SD in women are few and results conflict. Several studies demonstrate a greater prevalence of SD among women with diabetes than women without diabetes, while others do not [63]. Although women with diabetes might be at a greater risk of developing sexual dysfunctions, diabetes-related risk factors for female SD have not been clearly identified. In light of those conflicting results, it is still unclear how diabetes-related parameters might influence sexual functions in females with DM [49].

The impact of several risk factors on female SD also has been investigated [20, 23, 37, 49].

1. Age

Previous studies have found female SD to be associated with age [20, 44]. The incidence of DM for both women and men also increases with age and may be particularly difficult for women as it can intensify the negative effects already associated with aging. For females with DM, ages 45 to 64 and 65 to 79, the rates are 12.5% and 13%, respectively [8]. Epidemiological surveys report a variable prevalence ranging from 19% to 45%, according to age, hormonal status, and focus on single or cumulative disorders. Although discrepancies exist, all studies have concluded that female SD is highly prevalent with an increasing incidence in elderly women [37]. Abu Ali and colleagues found that approximately 60% of Jordanian women with diabetes and older than 50 years of age reported SD. Their study results also showed that diabetic women had lower levels of desire, arousal, lubrication, and orgasm than women without diabetes. However, comparisons adjusting for potential confounders, including marital and menopausal status, were not performed [1].

2. Glucometabolic Control

The prediction of insufficient glucometabolic control as assessed by HbA1C reflected many aspects of the findings. HbA1C was related to the degree of insulin resistance and indicators of insulin resistance, such as abdominal obesity (waist circumference and circulating lipids (triacylglycerol, high density lipoprotein - (HDL) cholesterol) [40]. Inadequate glycemic control and insulin resistance in women with diabetes may cause loss of libido, decreased clitoral sensitivity, orgasm difficulties, dyspareunia and decreased lubrication [70]. Social isolation, reduced sexual desire, insomnia and poor coping strategies were strong predictors of high HbA1C in women [40].

3. Diabetes Related Complications

Studies have identified that vascular and neurogenic changes from the effects of diabetes form the basic pathophysiology of SD in both men and women with diabetes [68, 69]. Most studies suggest that women with diabetes report more sexual dysfunctions than those without the disease and increased diabetes-related complications can intensify the SD problems in patients [73]. It has now become clear that in addition to evaluation of the usual diabetic complications, an assessment of female sexuality in type 2 diabetic women should become routine [25].

Nowosielski et al. (2011) reported that diabetes-related factors have little impact on sexual dysfunctions in women with DM. Their study also suggested that excessive weight and the presence of retinopathy were the predictors of desire and lubrication disorders, respectively. However, treatment with insulin was a protective factor for lack of satisfaction in women with DM [49]. Although there are conflicts in the literature, the duration of diabetes and the presence of neuropathy and nephropathy are believed to impair sexual function in diabetic women [23].

The effects of peripheral neuropathy in women with diabetes include sexual arousal disorders and decreases in lubrication. Neuropathy damages the autonomic nervous system, disrupts the process of orgasm, and causes prolongation of the level of arousal and desire. Painful sexual intercourse occurs due to lack of lubrication [70]. Women with diabetes could be at greater risk for SD due to their higher rates of depression and neuropathy [63]. Neuropathy, vascular impairment and psychological complaints have been implicated in the pathogenesis of decreased libido, low arousability, decreased vaginal lubrication, orgasmic dysfunction, sexual desire, clitoral sensation and intercourse satisfaction among diabetic women [26, 41].

4. Obesity

Obesity has the potential to promote SD through several mechanisms. These include the exacerbation of medical problems which contribute to SD, changes in circulating hormone levels affecting women's sexual interest and response, and changes in body image relating to self-perception of sexual attractiveness. Obese women tend to have greater body image dissatisfaction compared with non-obese women. In addition, when compared with women of normal weight, they may also develop issues related to poorer mental health and impaired sexual functioning [22].

5. Hyperlipidemia

Hyperlipidemia is among the most common risk factors associated with SD [10]. A high percentage of diabetics will have hyperlipidemia, whether it be elevated triglycerides, elevated LDL or low HDL. This carries an additional risk of heart disease but elevated lipids are also related to SD. An important culprit is oxidized LDL which may inactivate nitric oxide or increase its disposal as well as decrease its production. Small particle LDL has been shown to affect NO and decrease blood flow. Diabetics also have elevated free fatty acid levels, especially postprandially [34].

6. Hormonal Status

The other possible cause could be the usage of hormones, either combined oral contraceptive pills or hormonal therapy [49, 61]. Hormone replacement therapy (HRT) has been shown to improve blood flow in post-menopausal women but has been less effective in diabetic women [34]. It is a well-recognized fact, however, that although hormones may have a modulating effect on female sexuality, there are many other powerful influences involved. Relationships, different partners, psychology, sociology, culture, and past experiences all seem at times to override the hormonal milieu [49, 61]. A recent hypothesis proposes that sexual dysfunction in women with diabetes may be related to the imbalance of sex steroid hormones [42].

Menopause was an important risk factor for sexual dysfunctions in DM females in the studies by Enzlin et al. (2009) (only for lubrication disorders) [20], and Olarinoye and Olarinoye (2008) (only for desire disorders) [50]. In a study of 385 healthy women between the ages of 40-65, Yanez et al. determined that SD was 1.8 times more common in women going through the process of menopause [67]. The onset of menopause causes many profound changes in the female body. Women begin to experience a decrease in serum estrogen levels which affects sexual response. Reduction in estrogen levels causes vaginal atrophy, vaginal dryness, and dyspareunia [36].

7. Medication Use

Female stress-related factors and drug use can also induce SD. Indeed, antidepressants, antihypertensives, anticholinergics, diuretics and other commonly prescribed drugs have been associated with female SD [9]. It has been reported that the drugs used in the treatment of diabetes may lead to SD [9, 13, 65]. El-Rufaie et al. also showed that SD was associated with medication use [18].

8. Physical Activity

A higher level of physical activity was protective for female SD. Diabetic women with higher levels of declared physical activity were approximately 10% less likely to have female SD when compared with those with the lowest level [25].

9. Married or Partnered Status

Recent studies show that partner-related status is related to SD in healthy females [49]. Previous studies have found that female SD is associated with married or partnered status [20, 44]. In women with type 2 DM, chronic disease is diagnosed after health professionals first establish whether she is married or partnered. If so, she would be helped to modify her sexual expectations and relationship pattern in order to exert positive change on any problems and/or conflicts [4, 5, 57]. Rosemary Basson (2008) showed that 36% of females with type 2 DM demonstrated fear of becoming dependent on the partner and 29% believed that their body image had suffered due to physical changes from diabetes [4]. Sarkadi and Rosenquist (2003) also presented a focus group interview showing intimacy problems in females with type 2 DM and issues of blame and embarrassment regarding diabetes and sexual functioning [57].

Another factor affecting sexual function is the partner's health status. A study of healthy women by Yanez et al. found SD to be 14.6 times higher in the spouses of patients with ED and more than 9 times higher in the spouses of patients with premature ejaculation [67]. A partner's ideas and preferences are important factors affecting female sexuality [36]. In this context, it seems that the onset of the disease and relationships with the partner and family might explain the relation between the type of DM and the presence of SD [30].

10. Sexual Identity and Body Image

Sexual identity and body image are important components of sexuality that often affect a woman's sexual desire, but are rarely addressed. There are no formal sexology studies pertaining to either delayed psychosexual maturation in women diagnosed with diabetes at an early age, or of the use of insulin manipulation, enemas and laxatives to reduce the weight that is typically gained from insulin. Sexual concerns outside the sphere of hypoactive sexual desire or disordered genital reflexes are commonly ignored [5].

Body image and sexuality are shaped by intrapersonal, interpersonal and social experiences and are defined as a person's internal representation of their own outer appearance. Body image attitudes affect one's appearance as related to cognitions, emotions, and behaviours. Dissatisfaction with one's body or particular aspects of their body is just one facet of body image. Surveys show that many women, regardless of their age or weight, are dissatisfied with their bodies. However, body dissatisfaction may inhibit sexual behavior and interfere with the quality of sexual experiences. Women, who are dissatisfied with their physical appearance, report feeling more self-conscious, and less comfortable and confident about their body during sexual encounters. Body image and feeling attractive are also modified by diseases that affect mobility and physical activity as these inhibit sexual desire, resulting in decreased interest in sexual activity [22].

A woman's negative body image may lead to a decrease in sexual arousal [7]. A study by Stulhofer et al. determined that a negative body image has been associated with arousal and pain disorders in women [62]. Another study by Speer et al. found a relationship between body image and sexual satisfaction as well as a correlation between improved body image and an increase in sexual satisfaction [60].

11. Psychosocial Factors

Female sexuality is a complex phenomenon and may change over time with a woman's life situation. Women are able to respond to social and cultural contexts showing the so-called "erotic plasticity" which enables them to adapt to or to compensate for the biological changes caused by chronic illnesses, such as DM. In that context, the correlation between DM and sexual functions in females may not be direct but more dependent on sociopsychological factors and DM coping skills [20, 49]. Psychological and social factors also have an important impact on therapy adherence and control in chronic diseases [40].

Researchers have categorized psychosocial factors that can contribute to SD into four groups: Intrapersonal conflicts which include social restrictions, sexual identity conflicts, and guilt; interpersonal conflicts such as extra-marital affairs, sexual libido, desire, a partner's different lifestyle habits, and poor sexual communication; historical factors as in past or current abuse, rape, and sexual inexperience; and life stressors with one's family, job problems, and depression ([39]. Indeed, recent studies have highlighted the importance of interpersonal and intrapersonal factors [49].

The effects of DM on female sexual functioning are believed to be multidimensional [49]. Female SD is known to profoundly affect a woman's quality of life [63]. For instance, SD may prompt DM patients to seek nutritional advice from a registered dietician in efforts to change their regular nutrition habits. In addition, the stigma associated with a chronic disease, such as diabetes, may also affect patients' social life and could cause social isolation. This has been identified as an important risk factor for depression [28, 73].

The psychological effects of diabetes may manifest themselves through problems of self-image, loss of self-esteem, feelings of unattractiveness, loneliness, and isolation. Female SD can lead to loss of confidence, deterioration in relationships with others and emotional stress in women [21]. The impact of these symptoms on a woman's life can be significant and may result in psychological distress, altered self-perception, and dysfunctional family dynamics [37]. These consequences may be even more severe in certain cultures which teach women that sex is only for procreation, should not be enjoyed, or that pleasing the male partner at her own expense is most important. These issues are relevant in male-centric cultures [21].

Female sexuality is a complex phenomenon, and sexual disorders in women with diabetes may have more than just a biological etiology [49]. Whereas male SD in most cases is organically related, female SD is most likely due to psychogenic factors including depression/anxiety, stress, and drugs [9]. It has been suggested that female sexual function relies on psychosocial factors, such as mood and family relationships. Women with DM could have difficulties adjusting to their disease, and, therefore, potentially have sexual problems [64]. A significant number of women experience disorders of desire, arousal, lubrication, orgasm and satisfaction, and sexual pain including dyspareunia and vaginismus during intercourse. All categories of female SD correlate with impaired physical and emotional satisfaction [37]. Nobre and Pinto-Gouveia (2006) demonstrated that both men and women with SD had significantly less positive emotional reactions to automatic thoughts during sexual activity. Women with SD also had significantly less pleasure and satisfaction, and more sadness, disillusion, guilt, and anger [47]. Interestingly, the prevalence of anxiety is almost doubled in type 2 diabetic patients compared with healthy individuals [40].

12. Depression

Depression is twice as common in diabetic patients as in nondiabetics. It not only increases the burden of disease and impairs quality of life, but also contributes to increased mortality rates in type 2 diabetes [40]. Studies have determined that depression correlates with diabetes, and it has been shown to be a psychosocial factor involved in SD [39].

Previous studies have also found that female SD is associated with depressive symptoms [19, 44], and depression is a well-known risk factor for female SD. This correlation was aptly described by Enzlin et al., (2009) in the recent analysis of the Diabetes Control and Complications Trial / Epidemiology of Diabetes Interventions and Complications study [20].

Erol et al. also described a correlation between the presence of depression and arousal and orgasmic and satisfaction disorders in females with type 2 DM [23].

Inaccurate or inadequate characterization of diabetes, glycemic control, neurovascular complications, and the coexistence of depression may all be implicated in their connection to SD in women diabetic patients [25]. Salonia et al. (2006) showed that depressive symptoms had a negative impact on all sexual domains in the follicular phase of the cycle, whereas a negative impact was shown only on desire and arousal in the luteal one [56]. At this time the research shows that women with DM are at high risk of developing depression [58]. Although depression is a risk factor for developing SD, it is not clear if psychological disturbances are the cause or the result of sexual dysfunctions [48]. It is worth mentioning that depressive symptoms might be a function of chronically badly controlled DM and thus indirectly influence the sexual dysfunctions.

13. Treatment

SD is very common among patients treated with selective serotonin re-uptake inhibitors. Antidepressant treatment-associated SD occurs in 30%-70% of men and women treated for major depression with first- or second-generation agents. This is a principal reason for a three-fold increased risk of non-adherence that approaches 70% during the first months of treatment and leads to increased relapse, recurrence, disability and resource utilization by affected patients [9]. On the other hand, Kaplan et al. reported that sildenafil is safe, with limited efficacy, in treating postmenopausal women with self-described SD [41].

4. TREATMENT APPROACH IN PATIENTS WITH SEXUAL DYSFUNCTION AND TYPE 2 DIABETES MELLITUS

The general tendency of men with ED to avoid seeking treatment because of ignorance, misinformation, and embarrassment has already been described [11]. Most patients with ED were embarrassed to discuss the topic, thought it was a natural part of aging, or believed the problem would go away. This illustrates the important role of general practitioners and the need for more discussions with patients to determine whether they have ED, and, if so, to inform patients with highly prevalent comorbid conditions of treatment options [31]. Most patients would like their physicians to take the lead in discussing ED, yet only 7.9% of patients with ED had been asked about ED by their doctors [38]. The reality indicates that physicians tend to avoid asking diabetic patients about sexual problems [11]. Although most patients wanted their doctors to initiate discussion of ED, embarrassment related to discussing this topic and misinformation about ED treatment were the main causes for not seeking professional help. Younger men, on the other hand, are likely to believe in the spontaneous recovery from an erectile problem and seek help less often. At this time, doctors caring for diabetic patients recommend a routine screening for erectile problems [38].

The treatment of SD should ensure that health care professionals are thoroughly informed concerning women's perceptions and attitudes about their bodies and physical appearance. They should also become fully knowledgeable about the relationship between body image dissatisfaction and SD [22]. Likewise, women need to become more aware and informed about sexual problems and their solutions. In fact, the incidence of SD is significantly less in women who have information about sexual issues [21].

The ability to access the latest information on diabetes and SD is very important, but even though women patients use more and different strategies for coping with their disease, they claim less satisfaction with social support. Positive social support, particularly by the spouse, was found to improve glycaemic control and better adaptation to the disease [40]. The patient's degree of disease at the time of diagnosis may also be the key to successful psychological and sexual adjustment [4].

Considering the high prevalence of SD among patients with diabetes, it seems the management of these disorders should be more precisely monitored in the health care setting [73]. Possible therapeutic interventions include psychological counseling with cognitive behavioral therapy, individual and couple's therapy, physiotherapy, and the partner's sexual education [48]. Although patient-oriented education geared to self-management improves treatment adherence and glycaemic control in patients with type 2 diabetes, it is still unclear whether sex-specific differences affect compliance with diabetes management and/or strategies for coping with the disease. Strategies include the depressive or active approach, problem-oriented behavior or distraction, and religiosity or wishful thinking [40].

In general, patients with diabetes may benefit from educational interventions to reduce the SD impact on their personal life. In addition, cognitive behaviour therapy, problem solving skills and improvments in family communications might also help to better the outcomes of SD among patients. Indeed, effective interactions with diabetic patients who suffer from sexual problems remain the most important task and challenge of the health care workforce [73]. Depressive symptoms, partner-related factors, reproductive history, and individual perception of sexuality should be evaluated when counseling females with DM as they may be factors mediating their sexual dysfunctions [49].

CONCLUSION

This chapter was written to contribute to the literature on SD in men and women with DM and to alert health professionals to the many issues related to this problem. In conclusion, men and women with type 2 diabetes are at risk for several forms of SD. Understanding sexual functioning in women with diabetes and knowing the possible predictors of female SD are essential in clinical sexual health care, both in prevention and treatment. More research is needed to clarify the mechanisms underlying the evident differences between male and female sexual function. Future studies are also needed to more fully understand the attitudes of men and women on human sexuality, the factors affecting their behavior in getting treatment for SD issues, and the attitudes of health professionals in assessing and treating SD.

REFERENCES

[1] Abu Ali R, Al Hajeri R, Khader Y, Shegem N, Ajlouni K. Sexual dysfunction in Jordanian women. *Diabetes Care* 2008; 31: 1580-1.

[2]   Awad, H, Salem A, Gadalla A, Wafa AE, Mohamed OA. Erectile function in men diabetes type 2: Correlation with glycemic control. *Int J Impot Res* 2010; 22: 36-39.

[3]   Bacon CG, Murray A, Mittlemean A, Kawachi I, Giovannucci E, Glasser DB, Rimm EB. Sexual function in men older than 50 years of age: results from the health professionals follow-up study. *Ann Intern Med* 2003; 139: 161-168.

[4]   Basson R. Women's sexual function and dysfunction: Current uncertainties, future directions. *Int J Impot Res* 2008; 20: 466-78.

[5]   Basson RJ, Rucker BM, Laird PG, Conry R. Sexuality of women with diabetes. *J Sex Reprod Med* 2001; 1: 11-2.

[6]   Caruso S, Rugolo S, Mirabella D, Intelisano G, Di Mari L, Cianci A. Changes in clitoral blood flow in premenopausal women affected by type 1 diabetes after single 100-mg administration of sildenafil. *Urology* 2006; 68: 161-5.

[7]   Cellek S. Kadınlarda cinsel fonksiyon bozuklugunun patofizyolojisi. *Androloji Bulteni* 2002; 11: 9-10.

[8]   Centers for Disease Control and Prevention (2007). Incidence of diagnosed diabetes per 1000 population aged 18-79 years, by sex and age, United States, 1997-2005. Available from: January 28, 2013, http://www.cdc.gov/diabetes/statistics/incidence/fig5.htm.

[9]   Chedraui P, Perez-Lopez FR, Miguel GS, Avila C. Assessment of sexuality among middle-aged women using the Female Sexual Function Index. *Climacteric* 2009; 12: 213-221.

[10]   Corona G, Mannucci E, Mansani R, Petrone L, Bartolini M, Giommi R, Forti G, Maggi M. Organic, relational and psychological factors in erectile dysfunction in men with diabetes mellitus. *Eur Urol* 2004; 46: 222-228.

[11]   De Berardis G, Franciosi M, Belfiglio M, Dı Nardo B, Greenfield S, Kaplan SH, Pellegrini F, Sacco M, Tognoni G, Valentini M, Nicolucci A, for the Quality of Care and Outcomes in Type 2 Diabetes (QUED) Study Group. Erectile Dysfunction and Quality of Life in Type 2 Diabetic Patients. *Diabetes Care* 2002; 25: 284-291.

[12]   De Boer BJ, Bots ML, Lycklama A, Nijeholt AAB, Moors JPC, Pieters HM, Verheij ThJM. Erectile dysfunction in primary care: prevalence and patient characteristics. The ENIGMA study. *Int J Impot Res* 2004; 16: 358-364.

[13]   Delgado PL, Brannan SK, Mallinckrodt CH, Tran PV, McNamara RK, Wang F, Watkin JG, Detke MJ. Sexual functioning assessed in 4 double-blind placebo-and paroxetine-controlled trials of duloexetine for major depressive disorder. *J Clin Psychiatry* 2005; 66: 686-92.

[14]   Dey J, Shepherd MD. Evaluation and treatment of erectile dysfunction in men with diabetes mellitus. *Mayo Clin Proc* 2002; 77: 276-282.

[15]   Doruk H, Akbay E, Cayan S, Akbay E, Bozlu M, Acar D. Effects of diabetes mellitus on female sexual function and risk factors. *Arch Andrology* 2005; 51: 1-6.

[16]   Eardley I, Fisher W, Rosen RC, Niederberger C, Nadel A, Sand M. The multinational Men's Attitudes to Life Events and Sexuality study: the influence of diabetes on self-reported erectile function, attitudes and treatment-seeking patterns in men with erectile dysfunction. *Int J Clin Pract* 2007; 61-9: 1446-1453.

[17]   Ege E, Akın B, Yaralı Arslan S, Bilgili N. Prevalence and risk factors of female sexual dysfunction among healthy women. *TUBAV Bilim Dergisi* 2010; 3: 137-144.

[18]   El-Rufaıe OEF, Bener A, Abuzeid MSO, Ali TA. Sexual dysfunction among type II diabetic men: A controlled study. *J Psychosom Res* 1997; 4: 605-612.

[19] Enzlin P, Mathieu C, Van Den Bruel A, Bosteels J, Vanderschueren D, Demyttenaere K. Sexual dysfunction in women with type 1 diabetes. *Diabetes Care* 2002; 25: 672-677.

[20] Enzlin P, Rosen R, Wiegel M, Brown J, Wessells H, Gatcomb P, Rutledge B, Chan Ka-Ling, Cleary PA, The DCCT/EDIC Research Group. Sexual dysfuntion in women with type 1 diabetes: Long-term findings from the DCCT/EDIC study cohort. *Diabetes Care* 2009; 32: 780-5.

[21] Erbil N. Prevalence and risk factors for female sexual dysfunction among Turkish women attending a maternity and gynecology outpatient clinic. *Sex Disabil* 2011; 29: 377-386.

[22] Erbil N. The relationship between sexual function, body image, and body mass index among women. *Sex Disabil*, 2012 (DOI:10.1007/s11195-012-9258-4).

[23] Erol B, Tefekli A, Ozbey I, Salman F, Dincag N, Kadioglu A, Tellaloglu S. Sexual dysfunction in type II diabetic females: A comparative study. *J Sex Marital Ther* 2002; 28 (suppl.1): 55-62.

[24] Erol B, Tefekli A, Sanli O, Ziylan O, Armagan A, Kendirci M, Eryasar D, Kadioglu A. Does sexual dysfunction correlate with deterioration of somatic sensory system in diabetic women? *Int J Impot Res* 2003; 15: 198-202.

[25] Esposito K, Maiorino MI, Bellastella G, Giugliano F, Romano M, Giugliano D. Determinants of female sexual dysfunction in type 2 diabetes. *Int J Impot Res* 2010; 22:179-184.

[26] Fatemi SS, Taghavi SM. Evaluation of sexual function in women with type 2 diabetes mellitus. *Diabetes Vasc Dis Res* 2009; 6 (1): 38-9.

[27] Feldman HA, Johannes CB, Derby CA, Kleinman KP, Mohr BA, Araujo AB, McKinlay JB. Erectile dysfunction and coronary risk factors: Prospective results from the Massachusetts Male Aging Study. *Prev Med* 2000; 30: 328-38.

[28] Fisher L, Mullan JT, Arean P, Glasgow RE, Hessler D, Masharani U. Diabetes distress and can not clinical depression or depressive symptoms is associated with glycemic control in both cross-sectional and longitudinal analysis. *Diabetes Care* 2010; 33: 23-28.

[29] Gades NM, Nehra A, Jacobson DJ, McGree ME, Girman CJ, Rhodes T, Roberts RO, Lieber MM, Jacobsen SJ. Association between smoking and erectile dysfunction: a population-based study. *Am J Epidemiol*, 2005; 161 (4): 346-51.

[30] Giraldi A, Kristensen E. Sexual dysfunction in women with diabetes mellitus. *J Sex Res* 2010; 47: 199-211.

[31] Giuliano FA, Leriche A, Jaudinot EO, De Gendre AS. Prevalence of erectile dysfunction among 7689 patients with diabetes or hypertension, or both. *Urology* 2004; 64: 1196-1201.

[32] Goldstein I. The mutually reinforcing triad of depressive symptoms, cardiovascular disease and erectile dysfunction. *Am J Cardiol* 2000; 86 (suppl): 41-45.

[33] Gregersen N, Jensen PT, Giraldi EGE. Sexual dysfunction in the peri and postmenopause. *Dan Med Bull* 2006; 53: 349-53.

[34] Guay AT. Sexual dysfunction in the diabetic patient. *Int J Impot Res* 2001; 13 (Suppl 5): 47-50.

[35] Hackett G. The burden and extent of comorbid conditions in patients wiith erectile dysfunction. *Int. Clin Pract* 2009; 63: 1205-1213.

[36]   Howard JR, O'Neill S, Travers C. factors affecting sexuality in older Australian women: sexual interest, sexual arousal, relationships and sexual distress in older Australian women. *Climacteric* 2006; 9: 355-67.

[37]   Isidori AM, Pozza C, Esposito K, Giugliano D, Morano S, Vignozzi L, Corona G, Lenzi A, Jannini EA. Development and validation of a 6-item version of the Female Sexual Function Index (FSFI) as a diagnostic tool for female sexual dysfunction. *J Sex Med* 2010; 7 (3): 1139-1146.

[38]   Jiann BP, Lu CC, Lam HC, Chu CH, Sun CC, Lee JK. Patterns and their correlates of seeking treatment for erectile dysfunction in type 2 diabetic patients. *J Sex Med* 2009; 6: 2008-2016.

[39]   Juarez B, Gonzales C. Sexual dysfunction in women with type 2 diabetes. *Ethnicity & Disease* 2007; 17: 5-11.

[40]   Kacerovsky-Bielesz G, Lienhardt S, Hagenhofer M, Kacerovsky M, Forster E, Roth R, Roden M. Sex-related psychological effects on metabolic control in type 2 diabetes mellitus. *Diabetologia* 2009; 52: 781-788.

[41]   Kaplan SA, Reis RB, Kohn IJ, Ikeguchi EF, Laor E, Te AE, Martins ACP. Safety and efficacy of sildenafil in postmenopauzal women with sexual dysfunction. *J Urol* 1999; 53 (3): 481-486.

[42]   Kim N. Sex steroid hormones in diabetes-induced sexual dysfunction: Focus on the female gender. *J Sex Med* 2009; 6: 239-46.

[43]   Lue TF, Brant W, Shindel AW, Bella AJ. Sexual dysfunction in diabetes. Available from: February 15, 2013, http:www.endotext.org/diabetes/diabetes32/diabetes32htm.

[44]   Lutfey K, Link C, Rosen R, Wiegel M, McKinlay J. Prevalence and correlates of sexual activity and function in women: Results from the Boston Area Community Health (BACH) survey. *Arch Sex Behav* 2008; 38: 514-27.

[45]   Malavige LS, Levy JC. Erectile dysfunction in diabetes mellitus. *J Sex Med* 2009; 6: 1232-1247.

[46]   Moreira ED, Hartmann U, Glasser DB, Gingell C. A population survey of sexual activity, sexual dysfunction and associated help-seeking behavior in middle-aged and older adults in Germany. *Eur J Med Res* 2005; 10: 434-443.

[47]   Nobre PJ, Pinto-Gouveia J. Emotions during sexual activity: Differences between sexually functional and dysfunctional men and women. *Arch Sex Behav* 2006; 35: 491-499.

[48]   Nowosielski K, Drosdzol A, Sipinski A, Kowalczyk R, Skrzy-Pulec V. Diabetes mellitus and sexuality-does it really matter? *J Sex Med* 2010; 7: 723-35.

[49]   Nowosielski K, Skrzypulec-Plinta V. Mediators of sexual functions in women with diabetes. *J Sex Med* 2011; 8: 2532-2545.

[50]   Olarinoye J, Olarinoye A. Determinants of sexual function among women with type 2 diabetes in a Nigerian population. *J Sex Med* 2008; 5: 878-86.

[51]   Owiredu WKBA, Amidu N, Alidu H, Sarpong C, Gyasi-Sarbong CK. Determinants of sexual dysfunction among clinically diagnosed diabetic patients. *Reprod Biol Endocrin* 2011; 9: 70.

[52]   Ozerdogan N, Sayıner FD, Kosgeroglu N, Unsal A. The prevalence of sexual dysfunction and depression and other factors associated in women 40 to 65 years old. Maltepe Universitesi Hemsirelik Bilim ve Sanatı Dergisi 2009; 2: 46-59.

[53]   Polsky JY, Aronson KJ, Heaton JPW, Adams MA. Smoking and other lifestyle factors in relation to erectile dysfunction. *BJU International* 2005; 96: 1355-9.

[54]   Rao K, Du GH, Yang WM. Erectile dysfunction and hyperlipidemia. *NJA* 2006 Jul; 12: 643-6.

[55]   Rosen RC, Riley A, Wagner G, Osterloh IH, Kirkpatrick I, Mishra A. The International Index of Erectile Function (IIEF). A multidimensional scala for assessment of erectile dysfunction. *J Urol* 1997; 49: 822-830.

[56]   Salonia A, Lanzi R, Scavini M, Pontillo M, Gatti E, Petrella G, Licata G, Nappi RE, Bosi E, Briganti A, Rigatti P, Montorsi F. Sexual function and endocrine profile in fertile women with Type 1 diabetes. *Diabetes Care* 2006; 29: 312-6.

[57]   Sarkadi A, Rosenqvist U. Intimacy and women with type 2 diabetes: An exploratory study using focus group interviews. *Diabetes Educ* 2003; 29: 641-52.

[58]   Schram MT, Baan CA, Pouwer F. Depression and quality of life in patients with diabetes: A systematic review from the European depression in Diabetes (EDID) research consortium. *Curr Diabetes Rev* 2009; 5: 12-9.

[59]   Sidi H, Puteh SE, Abdullah N, Midin M. The prevalence of sexual dysfunction and potential risk factors that may impair sexual function in Malaysian women. *J Sex Med* 2007; 4: 311-321.

[60]   Speer JJ, Hillenberg B, Sugrue DP, Blacker C, Kresge CL, Decker VB, Zakalik D, Decker DA. Study of sexual functioning determinants in breast cancer survivors. *Breast J* 2005; 11 (6): 440-447.

[61]   Stuckey BG. Female sexual function and dysfunction in the reproductive years: The influence of endogenous and exogenous sex hormones. *J Sex Med* 2008; 5: 2282-90.

[62]   Stulhofer A, Gregurovic M, Pikic A, Galic I. Sexual problems of urban women in Croatia: prevalence and correlates in a community sample. *Croat Med J* 2005; 46: 45-51.

[63]   Wallner LP, Sarma AV, Kim C. Sexual functioning among Women with and without Diabetes in the Boston Area Community Health Study. *J Sex Med* 2010; 7: 881-887.

[64]   Whitehouse CR. Sexuality in the older female with diabetes mellitus - A review of the literature. *Urol Nurs* 2009; 29: 11-19.

[65]   Williams VS, Baldwin DS, Hogue SL, Fehnel SE, Hollis KA, Edin HM. Estimating the prevalence and impact of antidepressant-induced sexual dysfunction in 2 European countries: a cross-sectional patient survey. *J Clin Psychiatry* 2006; 67: 204-10.

[66]   Yalcın Y, Yalcın F, Ericin O, Safak A, Oguz A. Diabetes mellitus ve erektil disfonksiyon. *Diabet Bilimi* 2003; 1: 127-129.

[67]   Yanez D, Castelo-Branco C, Hidalgo LA, Chedraui PA. Sexual dysfunction and related risk factors in a cohort of middle-aged Ecuadorian women. *J Obstet Gynaecol* 2006; 26: 682-6.

[68]   Yenmez M, Mert M, Karadeniz T, Acar M. Kadınlarda cinsel fonksiyon bozuklugunun patofizyolojisi ve diyabet. *Diabet Bilimi* 2004; 2: 6-8.

[69]   Yenmez M, Mert M, Kepekci P, Karadeniz T, Acar M. Diyabetli kadınlarda cinsel fonksiyon bozuklugunun tanı ve tedavisi. *Diabet Bilimi* 2005; 3: 96-98.

[70]   Yıldız H, Pınar R. Diyabetli kadınlarda ihmal edilen bir konu: Cinsel yasam. *Hemsirelik Forumu* 2004; 7: 11-13.

[71] Zdravko A, Kamenov V, Tsanka G, Yankova M. Erectile dysfunction in diabetic men is libked more to microangiopathic complications and neuropathy than to acroangiopathic disturbances. *J Mens Health* 2007; 4: 64-73.

[72] Zedan H, Hareadei AA, Abd-Elsayed AA, Abdel-Maguid EM. Cigarette smoking, hypertension and diabetes mellitus as a risk factors for erectile dysfunction in upper Egypt. *East Mediterr Health J (EMHJ)* 2010; 16: 281-285.

[73] Ziaei-Rad M, Vahdaninia M, Montazeri A. Sexual dysfunction in patients with diabetes: A study from Iran. *Reprod Biol Endocrin* 2010; 8: 50.

In: Sexual Dysfunctions
Editor: Frédérique Courtois

Chapter 8

ERECTILE DYSFUNCTION IN DIABETIC MEN

*Zdravko Kamenov**

Clinic of Endocrinology, Alexandrovska University Hospital,
Medical University-Sofia, Sofia, Bulgaria

ABSTRACT

The aim of this chapter is to summarize the current state of knowledge about diabetic erectile dysfunction (DED) – epidemiology, pathogenesis, diagnostic and treatment options. Diabetes type 2 (DM2) has become an epidemic affecting one in 10-15 people worldwide. This spread is caused by genetic (population accumulation of predisposing genes), longer life span and environmental (lifestyle – nutrition and hypokinesia, and stress) factors. The prognosis of the International Diabetes Federation is alarming: In 2030 there will be nearly half billion people with diabetes worldwide. ED is more common in men with diabetes. Several large studies were conducted in different countries presenting variable prevalence of DED – from 32 to 90%, dependent on the population age and diabetes type and duration. In 12 to 30% of men, ED is the first sign of diabetes, diagnosed later. All these data suggest an increasing number of men with DED in the future. The main factors playing in the complex pathogenesis of DED are diabetic neuropathy (advanced glucation end-products, oxidative stress, polyol pathway, nerve growth factor deficiency, dysfunction of protein kinase C, tissue remodeling, etc.), macrovascular arterial disease (endothelial dysfunction, abnormal collagen deposition and smooth muscle degeneration, dyslipidemia, arterial hypertension, veno-occlusive dysfunction, etc.), hypogonadism, structural remodeling of the corporeal tissue, psychogenic components and adverse drug reactions. In most studies no evaluation of macro- and microvascular (including neuropathy) complications is presented. The diagnostic process is based on the results of questionnaires, neurological, vascular (Doppler) and other more rarely used investigations. Because of the complex pathogenesis of DED, diabetic men represent "difficult" treatment group. In many studies DM is an exclusion criterion. Elimination of lifestyle unfavorable factors, improvement in glycemic, lipids, and arterial pressure control, and careful re-evaluation of the

*Corresponding author: Prof. Zdravko Kamenov, MD, PhD, DMSc, Head of the Department of Internal diseases Medical Faculty, Medical University – Sofia, Head of the Clinic of Endocrinology, Alexandrovska University Hospital, President of the Bulgarian Association for Sexual Medicine. Adress: 1Georgi Sofiiski Str., 1431 Sofia, Bulgaria, Tel/fax. +35929230275, Mob. +359887726683, Email : zkamenov@hotmail.com.

concomitant medications are necessary general measures. PDE-5 inhibitors are the first line therapy but their effect in men with DED is lower, compared to non-DM men. There are few studies with diabetic populations and even less with head-to-head comparisons. Our results support a similar effect between PDE-5 inhibitors. Men with DM have a higher prevalence of hypogonadism. Testosterone replacement therapy should be started in symptomatic men with demonstrated hypogonadism and no contraindications. Vacuum constrictor devices and intraurethral or intracavernous applications of vasoactive drugs are the second line therapy. Vascular surgery rarely comes into consideration. Penile implants are the last and effective option for men with severe DED.

INTRODUCTION

Over the past two decades, diabetes mellitus (DM) became an epidemic, mostly because of type 2 (DM2), which represents 90-95% of the cases with DM, although the incidence of type 1 (DM1) has also doubled [Ryan, 2009]. Nowadays, there are 366 million people with DM in the world (8.3% of the adult population), and in 2030, their number is expected to be 552 millions and 8.9% respectively [IDF, 2011].

The therapeutic progress in diabetology has led to:

1. Practical elimination of ketoacidosis and other severe diabetic complications as a cause of death.
2. Improvement of the glycemic control to the highest level so far. These favourable factors made it possible today for the people with diabetes to live longer than ever, which increases the chance of developing the late complications of the disease.

Thus, demographic tendencies and epidemiological prognoses highlight the increasing importance of chronic diabetic complications in the future including diabetic erectile dysfunction (DED).

During the last fifteen years the scientific interest towards erectile dysfunction grew significantly (Fig. 1). The most important reasons for this are:

1. Aging of the population and in particular the increasing life expectancy of men. Men live around 5 years less compared to women in developed countries. The prevalence of erectile dysfunction increases with age. According to a WHO report (2008) it is expected 35% of the population to be over 60 years in industrial countries in the year 2025 [NIC, 2008].
2. The global aspects of the problem erectile dysfunction were demonstrated in several large epidemiological studies. ED is common in men of all nations.
3. There is a growing body of evidence about direct links between ED and cardio-vascular diseases. ED is a marker of the vascular and in particular endothelial health of men and it can be considered not only a part of the quality of life but also as a predictor of its length as well.
4. The release of the first PDE-5-inhibitor – sildenafil – on the market about 15 years ago, followed by vardenafil, tadalafil and others, revolutionized the treatment of ED making it more effective, accessible, safe and cheap.

Diabetic erectile dysfunction represents an even more serious problem. To the above-mentioned reasons should be added:

5. Prevalence of diabetes increases dramatically and it has been recognized as a pandemic disease.
6. The prevalence of ED in men with DM is higher compared to healthy men.
7. Pathogenesis of DED is more complex compared to non-diabetic one.
8. ED is more severe and impacts more profoundly the quality of life of diabetic men.
9. The effectiveness of the treatment for DED is lower compared to men without DM.

EPIDEMIOLOGY OF DED

The review of scientific publications indexed in PubMed focused on DED showed an increasing interest during the last years (figure 1).

Epidemiological data about DED vary significantly between different studies depending on the age, duration and type of DM and diagnostic and inclusion criteria. Reviewing the literature Malavige and Levy (2009) estimated a range of 35% to 90% reported in different studies from different countries [Malavige, 2009]. ED is 3-4 times more common in diabetics compared to the general population [Martin-Morales, 2001; Feldman, 1994]. The prevalence of ED in type 1 diabetes (DM1) is 32% and in type 2 (DM2) – 46% [Vickers, 2004]. During the first 10 years after the diagnosis of DM ED is established in more than half of the men [Vinik, 1998]. According to two studies from different countries the prevalence of DED increases from 9% in the age interval 20-29 years and 15% between 30-34 to 95% in 60-70 years old men and this increase correlates with the duration of diabetes, poor metabolic control and diabetic complications [Fedele, 1998; Smith, 1981]. Multivariateanalyses of several population based cohorts show that of all risk factors diabetes imparts thehighest risk for ED with an age adjusted relative risk of 1.3 to 3 depending on diabetes type [Chitaley, 2009a; Chitaley, 2009b.; Bacon, 2002; Johannes, 2000].

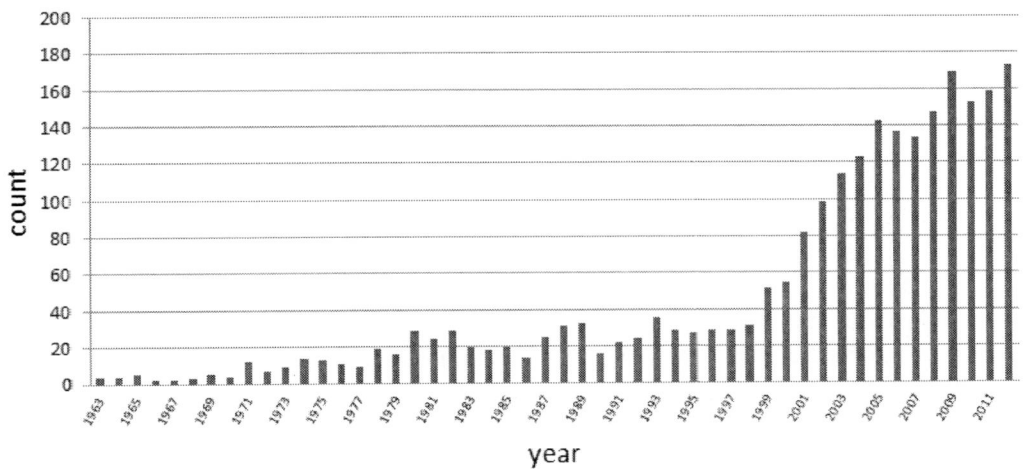

Figure 1. Publications on Diabetes and Erectile Dysfunction indexed in PubMed – 1963-2012.

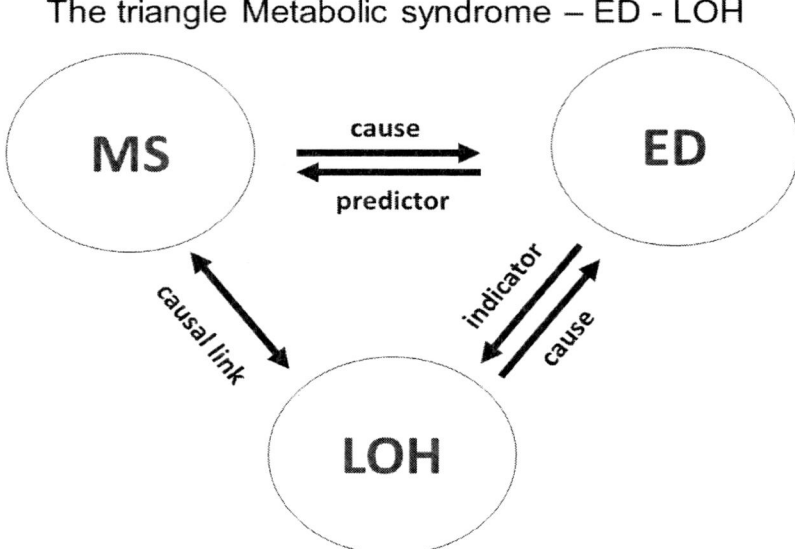

Figure 2.Links between the metabolic syndrome, erectile dysfunction and late onset hypogonadism.

Similar to the prediction of coronary artery disease, ED has been proven to be the first sign of diabetes, diagnosed later in 12 to 30% of men [Lewis, 2001; Adegite, 2009] (figure 2).

Besides ED, other sexual problems are more common in diabetic men. A study from Minnesota demonstrated DM to be associated with a decreased sexual desire, ejaculatory function and sexual satisfaction [Burke, 2006]. Another study reported 80% of the interviewees to have sexual problems, including decreased libido (50.3%), premature ejaculation (19.7%), retrograde ejaculation (19.2%). According to the answer to the question for having problems with the erection it appeared 51.5% to have ED and according to IIEF – 87.9% [Adegite, 2009]. The sexual problem has preceded the diagnosis of diabetes in 30.2%. In 45.3% of the cases no medical consultation has been sought.

PATHOGENESIS OF DED

Detailed description of the process of *erection* is not an object of this chapter. Shortly, erection is a complex physiological process in which psychological, social, endocrine, paracrine, neural, vascular and other factors take part. The penis is a hydraulic organ which state – from relaxation to different phases of erection is determined by the grade of fullness with blood of corpora cavernosa. Their volume is defined by two variables – arterial inflow and venous outflow. The capacity of the filling terminal helical arteries is determined by the NO-dependent smooth muscles relaxation. Different stimuli – psychogenic (visual, auditory, olfactory, memory, fantasy) or reflexogenic (tactile) activate the central and/or peripheral neuronal chains leading to synthesis and secretion of NO from the non-adrenergic–non-cholinergic (NANC) neuronal terminals in the cavernosal bodies through activation of neuronal nitric oxide synthase (nNOS). This small amount of NO triggers initial smooth muscle relaxation starting the hemodynamic process of erection. Further, receptor mechanisms and the shear stress in the vascular wall activate phosphatidylinositol-3-

kinase/protein kinase B (Akt) pathway leading to activation of endothelial nitric oxide synthase (eNOS) and further NO release from the penile endothelial cells. Binding of the released neural and endothelial NO to soluble guanylate cyclase in the smooth muscle cells (SMC) increases cyclicguanosine monophosphate (cGMP) levels andcGMP-dependent protein kinase G (PKG) activity.As a consequence cell membrane Ca-channels are closed decreasing the Ca++ influx in the cell and from the other side cytosolic Ca++ is retained in the endoplasmic reticulum. The opening of the Ca-dependent potassium channels on the membrane leads to potassium outflux and hyperpolarization. Finally, the cytosolic Ca++ depletion causes cavernosal SMC relaxation leading to increased blood inflow through the helical arteries, sinusoidal filling and cavernosaldilation. The volume of corpora cavernosa increases and a compression of the draining venous vessels - emissary veins in subtunical venular plexus against the rigid tunica albuginea occurs with a consequence – venous occlusion,decrease of outflow and further increase of intracavernosal pressure. The process of erection needs an intact cavernosal structure, characterized by abundant elastic fibers and less collagen.

Detumescence is initiated with activation of the sympathetic neurons and liberation of norepinephrine from the adrenergic terminals of the cavernosal nerve, as well as endotelins and $PgF_{2\alpha}$ from the endothelial cells covering the cavernosal sinusoids. An increase in intracellularcalcium activates myosin light chain (MLC) kinaseand phosphorylation of MLC to generate SMCcontraction. Additional pathways such as RhoA/Rho-kinase lead to the sensitization of the SMCcontractile apparatus to calcium, promotingcontraction. Activation of Rho-kinase results ininhibition of MLC phosphatase and continuedexpression of phosphorylated MLC. RhoA/Rho-kinase pathway isa predominant calcium-sensitizing pathway tomediate continuous smooth muscle tone in thepenis. Protein kinase C (PKC) is also calcium sensitizingand acts to inhibit MLC phosphatase, alsopromoting the contractile response [Hidalgo-Tamola, 2009].

Disturbances of each of the described consecutive stages from the erotic stimulus to the venous drainage may compromise the process causing ED. The pathogenic concept about ED evolved from the dominating psychogenic, in the past, to the leading organic currently. It should be mentioned that psychogenic and organic disturbances interplay in every case of ED and cannot be separated definitely even for didactic reasons. The similarities between dilatation mechanisms in the corpora cavernosa and the remaining arterial vessels in the body, based on the key role of NO, explain the common mechanism involved in their deterioration and in endothelial dysfunction. The presence of cardio-vascular disease increases significantly the likelihood for ED [Martin-Morales, 2001] (Fig. 2). On the other hand, ED may be the first sign of existing but undiagnosed CVD [Montorsi, 2003]. During the last years special attention has been paid to the importance of DM as a vascular risk factor. It accelerates the development of endothelial dysfunction – an earlier event of the vascular disease, induces oxidative stress and dyslipidemia, potentiates atherosclerotic process, aggravates arterial hypertension, etc. A vicious pathogenic circle between DM and hypogonadism is perpetuated (Fig. 2): men with DM have lower testosterone levels and men with hypogonadism have increased risk of developing obesity, metabolic syndrome and DM, with the full spectrum of their unfavorable cardiovascular consequences [Mulligan, 2006]. This global vascular disorder takes place in the cavernosal bodies as well, where other more DM-specific pathogenic biochemical mechanisms develop:

- Neuronal impairment

The initial stage of the erection process at penile level – NANC nerve endings nNOS activation and NO release has been shown to be impaired in animal models of DM1 and (although less convincingly) in DM2 [Hidalgo-Tamola, 2009]. Otsuka Long-Evans Tokushima fatty (OLETF) rats represent an appropriate model for spontaneously developing DM2 with its late complications [Kawano, 1992], including DN [Kamenov, 2006]. OLETF rats showdecreased immunofluorescent staining for nNOSin dorsal nerves and40% decrease in nNOS 160 kDa protein expression relative to that ofnon-diabetic controls ($P<0.01$), thus supporting an impaired nNOS effectiveness in DM2 [Jesmin, 2003].

- Endothelial dysfunction

This is probably the most discussed aspect of DED in the literature. Recently, Angulo et al (2010), attempting to shed more light on the reasons for the smaller response to PDE5-inhibitorstherapy in DED patients, investigated the function of NO/cGMP signalling in human erectile tissues[Angulo, 2010]. They usedcorpus cavernosum strips (human corpus cavernosum [HCC]) and penile resistance arteries (HPRA) collected from penile specimens from organ donors (OD) and from diabetic and non-diabetic men with ED undergoing penile prosthesis implantation. The relaxation to acetylcholine, electrical field stimulation, sodium nitroprusside, and sildenafil were evaluated in phenylephrine-contracted HCC and norepinephrine-contracted HPRA, and cGMP content in HCC was also determined.The impairment of endothelium-dependent relaxation in HCC and HPRA from ED patients was exacerbated by diabetes - E(max) 76.1, 62.9, and 49.3% in HCC and 73.1, 59.8, and 46.0% in HPRA from OD, non-diabetic and diabetic ED, respectively. Hypertension, hypercholesterolemia, or aging did not exert further impairment in endothelial relaxation among ED patients. Diabetes also caused further impairment in neurogenic relaxation in HCC and HPRA. The basal and stimulated content of cGMP in HCC was significantly decreased in patients with ED, but specifically reduced in diabetic patients. Diabetes clearly impaired PDE5 inhibitor-induced vasodilation of HPRA from ED patients. The authors concluded that ED is related to impaired vasodilation, reduced relaxant capacity, and diminished cGMP content in penile tissue. These alterations are more severe in diabetes and accompany the reduced relaxant efficacy of PDE5 inhibition. Thus, an exacerbated reduction of nitric oxide/cGMP signaling could be responsible for ED in diabetic men and would explain their reduced response to treatment.

NO bioavailability may be decreased by supresed eNOS expression and/or activity or by increased NO scavenging. Jesmin et al. (2004) reported reduction of eNOS mRNA expression suggesting an eNOS deficient expression at transcriptional level in OLETF rats [Jesmin, 2003]. In the same study a decreased VEGF expression and mRNA transcription in penile tissues were also found. It should be mentioned that the Akt-dependentpathway mediates both shear stress and vascularendothelial growth factor (VEGF) phosphorylationof eNOS [Musicki, 2004]. The effects of VEGF include endothelialcell proliferation, migration, angiogenesis, and anti-apoptosis. VEGF increases eNOS phosphorylation and expression of anti-apoptotic proteins.There is strong evidence that VEGF is a survivalfactor for endothelial cells [Dimmeler, 2000]. At the molecular level, VEGF can upregulateeNOS expression in endothelial cells[Papapetropoulos, 1997]. Furthermore,increased expression of eNOS has been reported inthe rat penis after intracavernosal injection withVEGF [Lin, 2002]. These findings support theimportance of VEGF as an eNOS inducer. Itwould be logical to assume that the reducedexpression of eNOS shown by Jesmin S,et al. (2004) in the OLETF rat penismay be causally related to the decrease in VEGFexpression in the tissue.Unlike eNOS, nNOS does not appear to beinducible by VEGF [Sheehy, 1997]. The penileexpression level of nNOS has been documented toremain unchanged in VEGF-treated rats [Lin, 2002]. Thus, the VEGF-triggered biochemicalevents probably have no targets in the nNOS gene,which continues to produce nNOS transcripts at asteady level.

- Oxidative stress

Oxidative stress is a key pathogenic factor in the development of diabetic complications. Chronic hyperglycemia induces free radical (reactive oxygen species – ROS) production through formation of advance glycation end-products (AGE), lipid peroxidation, polyol pathway activation, superoxide production, and activation of protein kinase C [32]. ROS participates in most studied mechanisms for initiation and maintenance of the functional and structural deterioration. Increased oxidative activity and expression of inflammatory markers are seen in patients with DED. Circulating monocyte activity and expressions of inflammatory markers such as endothelin-1 (ET-1) and intracellular adhesion molecule-1 (ICAM-1) are used as markers for ROS and inflammation [Hidalgo-Tamola, 2009].

- Advanced Glycation End-products (AGEs)

Normally with aging every tissue in the body is glycated to some extent. In hyperglycemic conditions the glycation process is more active and leads to micro-structural changes on molecular level, which can further compromise the function of the tissue and finally lead to macro-structural deterioration. AGEs bond covalently with the vascular collagen leading to thickening of the vascular wall, deceased elasticity, endothelial dysfunction and atherosclerosis [Bucala, 1991; Singh, 2001a]. Interaction between AGEs and endothelial cells up-regulates adhesion molecules that mediate vascular damage. AGE also stimulates cytokine expression on monocytes and macrophages [Yan, 2008]. AGEs are increased in corpora cavernosa of rats and men with DM and cause impaired cavernosal smooth muscle relaxation and ED in diabetic rats [Seftel, 1997; Cartledge, 2001b; Usta, 2003]. One important mechanism for decreasing cavernosal compliance and smooth muscle relaxation is through generation of free radicals which react with NO and decrease its availability. Increased penile levels of ROS were found in diabetic rats. The resultant most reactive peroxinitrite is involved in cell damage and death. Summarizing, AGEs contribute to the development of DED by generating free radicals leading to oxidative cell damage and by quenching NO [Cartledge, 2001b; Bivalacqua, 2005; Khan, 2001].

- Endotelins

Endotelin has three isopeptides (1, 2 and 3) and two receptors bound to G-protein (ETA and ETB). ET-1 is a powerful vasoconstrictor released from the vascular endothelium in the penis [Moore, 2006]. There is evidence that DED is related to a disturbed balance towards increased vasoconstriction, caused by endotelin and its receptors [Bivalacqua, 2003;Christ, 1995]. The plasma levels of ET-1 are increased in diabetic men [Clozel, 1992]. ETA-receptors are located on the smooth muscle cells and induce vasoconstriction and cell proliferation. ETB-receptors are presented mostly on the vascular endothelium and induce vasodilatation through NO- and prostacyclin release [Bivalacqua, 2003; Sima, 1996]. On the contrary, these receptors mediate vasoconstriction in some arteries like coronary in dogs and mammary in men [Clozel, 1992; Teerlink, 1994]. It was found that ETB-receptors are upregulated in the cavernosal bodies of diabetic rabbits where it is supposed to have constrictive role. In this way an increase in ETB receptors and their ligands may cause disbalance and vasoconstriction [Sima, 1996]. It is considered that the mitogenic effect of ETB causes early ultrastructural atherosclerotic changes in diabetics [Lu, 2004].

- RhoA-Rho kinase

RhoA is a GTB-binding protein affected by Rho-kinase. The ET1 induced vasoconstriction is related to RhoA-Rho kinase pathway [Park, 2002; Wang, 2002; Buyukafsar, 2003] the activation of which suppresses eNOS [Ming, 2002]. Rho-kinase is found in cavernosal tissue of rats, rabbits and men and is activated in diabetic rats. It is considered that RhoA-Rho kinase pathway potentiates ED by a decreased production of NO in the penis [Rees, 2002; Bivalacqua, 2004; Chua, 2006].

Several other mechanisms have been described in which hyperglycemia leads to functional and structural changes in cavernosal bodies and arteries. The described complex pathogenetic attack decreases the capacity of smooth muscle relaxation and functional dilatation of cavernosal structures, but also limits the penile arterial inflow through atherosclerotic changes.

- Diabetic neuropathy (DN)

Diabetic neuropathy (DN) is the most common diabetic complication, affecting 10 – 90% of people with diabetes, depending of the diagnostic criteria and the age and duration of DM [Vinik, 1992; Young, 1993; Dyck, 1993; Tesfaye, 1996]. The distal symmetric sensorimotor diabetic polyneuropathy (the most frequent form of somatic DN), combined with the diabetic autonomic neuropathy, are the most important pathogenic factors for the development of diabetic foot with following diabetic ulceration and amputation. Neuropathy is a very important pathogenic factor in the development of DED. Because DN affects all levels of the neural system, disturbances could also happen at all levels in the complex process of erection – from the central initiation to the penis. In the literature much more attention is paid to the vascular aspects of DED compared to the neural ones.

The central aspects of erection have been investigated in some studies, from fundamental investigations of sexual behavior to functional MRI and PET in the phase of REM sleep, associated with nocturnal penile tumescences, as well as the whole sexual cycle in men [Nofzinger, 1997]. It should be mentioned that central aspects of DN and DED have been much less investigated probably because of the insufficient options for selective therapeutic influence.

In the clinical classification of DN DED traditionally is positioned in the genito-urinary autonomic neuropathy [Kamenov, 2012]. By applying different neurological tests it has been shown that diabetics with ED present more common with abnormal NCV, sphincter electromyography and vibration sensitivity compared to those without ED [Hakim, 1996; Hecht, 2001]. The combination of sensory and autonomic disturbances leads to decreased sensory afferentation that is necessary for the initiation and maintenance of erection, but also limits the effect of NO from the intracavernosal nerve terminals and that is critically necessary for erection. In most studies no separate evaluation of the macro- and microvascular (including DN) complications is presented. We investigated 150 diabetic men (74% with type 2) aged 53.0 ±12,5 (18-86) years with diabetes duration of 8.6±6.7 years and mean BMI 29.0±4.3 kg/m2, and found that 44.7% of them had DED [Kamenov, 2007]. In this study microangiopathy and in particular DN appeared to be more important risk factor for DED than macroangiopathy.Presence of ED increased the likelihood of having macrovascular, but to a higher degree, microvascular diabetic complications. These data support the crucial negative role of DN in the complex pathogenesis of DED, and may explain why men with diabetes are more prone to ED compared to men with the same degree of macrovascular disease but without DN.

- Hypogonadism

Testosterone deficiency is very common in diabetic men. Choosing a cut-off of total testosterone (TT) < 10.4 nmol/l for evaluation of 2165 men men aged ≥ 45 years visiting primary care practices in the United States, the investigators of HIM study reported that half of diabetic men with DM were hypogonadal (table 1) [Mulligan, 2006]. Hypogonadism was also very common in other co-morbidities included in the metabolic syndrome, namely obesity, arterial hypertension, hyperlipidemia.

Many studies support the weight-increasing effect of hypogonadism and the testosterone lowering effect of obesity. It is difficult to answer which one is the initial event – hypogonadism or the metabolic syndrome. Even if the cause-consequence dilemma is still not definitely solved, the treatment should be directed to both problems (figure 3).

Table 1. Prevalence of hypogonadism (TT < 10.4) nmol/l in different co-morbidities [Mulligan, 2006]

Risk factor/comdition	Prevalence of hypogonadism (95% CI)	Odds ratio (95% CI)
Obesity	52.4 (47.9-56.9)	2.38 (1.93-2.93)
DM	50.0 (45.5-54.4)	2.09 (1.70-2.58)
Arterial hypertension	42.4 (39.6-45.2)	1.84 (1.53-2.22)
Hyperlipidemia	40.4 (37.6-43.3)	1.47 (1.23-1.76)
Osteoporosis	44.4 (25.5-64.7)	1.41 (0.64-3.01)
Asthma/COPD	43.5 (36.8-50.3)	1.40 (1.04-1.86)
Prostatae diseases	41.3 (36.4-46.2)	1.29 (1.03-1.62)
Chronic pain	38.8 (33.7-44.0)	1.13 (0.89-1.44)
Headache during the last 2 weeks	32.1 (25.3-38.8)	0.81 (0.58-1.11)

The link between the metabolic syndrome and hypogonadism

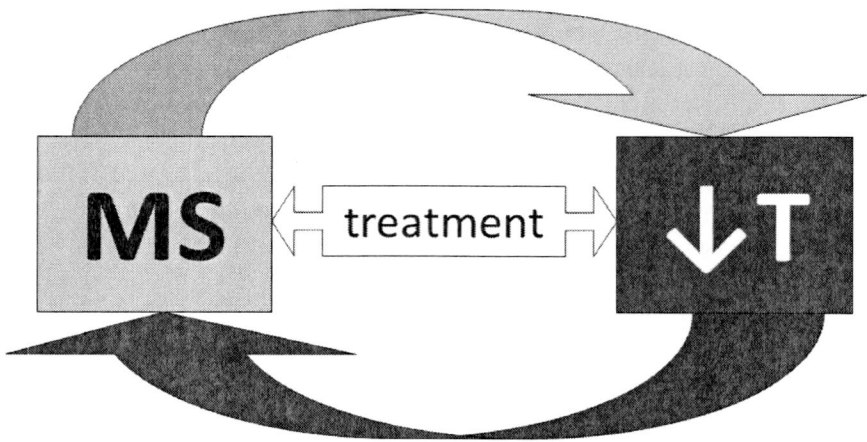

Figure 3.The link between the metabolic syndrome and hypogonadism.

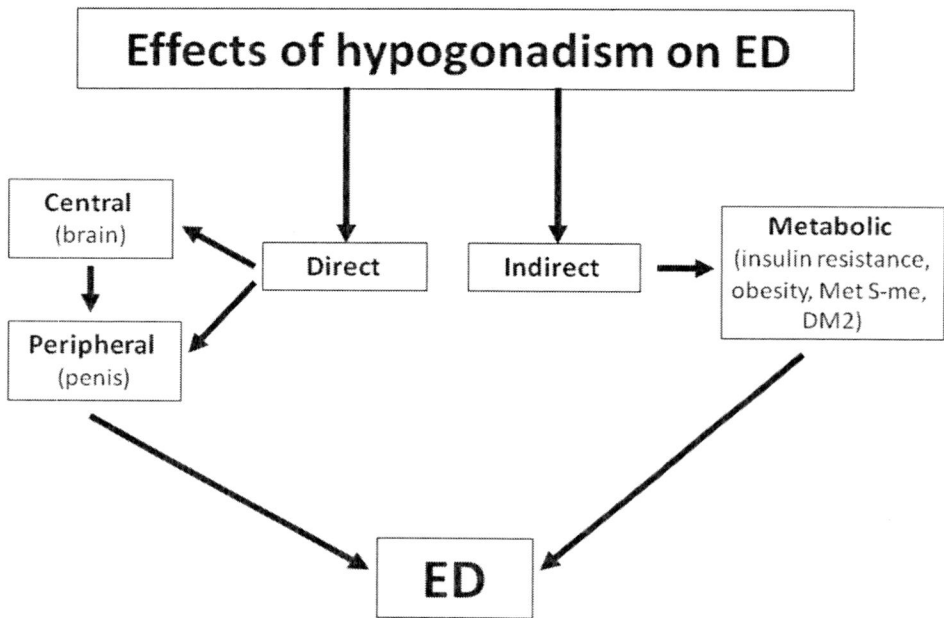

Figure 4. Effects of hypogonadism on erectile dysfunction.

Against the older opinion that testosterone is mostly a trigger of desire with limited importance for the lower levels of erection, a growing body of evidence supports its active participation and importance at all levels of the above described hierarchic structure of the erectile process (figure 4).

At the cerebral level, testosterone acts by itself, but also through its metabolites after appropriate enzymatic transformations to estradiol (aromatase) and dihydrotestosterone (5-alpha reductase). It stimulates the synthesis storage and release of pro-erectogenic neurotransmitters and modulates the neuronal activity, receptor sensitivity, neurotransmitter liberation, socio-sexual behavior (increasing libido) and positively influencing dopamine, NO, oxytocine, etc. At the spinal level, testosterone activates the androgen-sensitive motoneurons innervating the bulbospongiosus and ischiocavernosa muscles, and the androgen receptors in the parasympathetic erectile area S_{2-4}.

It is generally accepted that androgens are critical for the development, growth, and maintenance of penile erectile tissue. Animal studies showed testosterone dependency of the nNOS-containing cavernous parasympathetic fibers [Baba, 2000]. In animal models, androgen deprivation produces penile tissue atrophy concomitant with alterations in dorsal nerve structure, endothelial morphology, reduction in trabecular smooth muscle content, and increased deposition of extracellular matrix. Furthermore, androgen deprivation results in accumulation of fat-containing cells (adipocytes) in the subtunical region of the corpus cavernosum [Traish, 2005]. Testosterone deprivation is followed by programed cell death in the cavernosal smooth muscles [Porst, 2007]. Interestingly, testosterone stimulates both the initiator of the erection (NOS) and its terminator (PDE-5), thus balancing the whole process. Androgen deficiency diminishes protein expression and enzymatic activity of nitric oxide synthases (eNOS and nNOS) and phosphodiesterase type 5 (PDE5) [Vignozzi et al. 2007]. The androgen-dependent loss of erectile response is restored by androgen administration but not by administration of PDE5 inhibitors alone. These data suggest that androgens regulate trabecular smooth muscle growth and connective tissue protein synthesis in the corpus cavernosum. Furthermore, androgens may stimulate the differentiation of progenitor cells into the smooth muscle cells and inhibit their differentiation into adipocytes. Clinical and preclinical studies have suggested that veno-occlusion is modulated by the tone of the vascular smooth muscle in the resistance arteries and cavernosal tissue, and by the balance between trabecular smooth muscle content and connective tissue matrix. In men with erectile dysfunction, venous leakage is thought to be a common condition among nonresponders to medical management and is attributed to penile smooth muscle atrophy. Traish and Kim (2005) concluded that androgens exert a direct effect on penile tissue to maintain erectile function and that androgen-deficiency produces a metabolic and structural imbalance in the corpus cavernosum, resulting in venous leakage and erectile dysfunction [Traish, 2005].

The testosterone level necessary for normal erectile function still needs exact determination. Interventional studies in men have demonstrated favorable effect of testosterone replacement therapy (TRT) on erectile function in men with organic hypogonadism, mostly in the cases where it is the only reason for ED [Shabsigh, 2006]. Hypogonadism is frequently associated with DM2 [Yagihashi, 2007; Bartolini, 2004; Corrales, 2004; Corona, 2007].

Other structural changes related to diabetes include loss of normal cavernosal endothelium and smooth muscle cells [Burchardt, 2000] and increased deposition of collagen and thickening of the basal lamina leading to fibrosis [Jevtich, 1990].

- Other sexual dysfunctions

DM is associated not only with erectile dysfunction but with all aspects of sexual function, including sexual drive, ejaculatory function, sexual problems and sexual satisfaction, etc. [Burke, 2007]. In patients with DM there is a strong association between ED and reduced libido (OR = 4.38, CI = 1.39-13.82) and between ED and premature ejaculation (odds ratio [OR] = 4.41, 95% confidence interval [CI] = 2.08-9.39). The presence of one of these three conditions (ED, PE and reduced libido) requires screening for the other two [Malavige, 2008].

Balanitis is more common in diabetes (16%) compared to the general population (5,8%) [Fakjian, 1990]. It has been shown that 12% of men have had balanitis during the last two years before the diagnosis of DM [Drivsholm, 2005]. Inflammation, pain and discharge, related to mycotic balanitis may have somatic and psychological unfavorable effects on erection and sexual intercourse.

Phimosis is common in diabetes – 32% of men admitted to an urological clinic with phymosis have had DM [Drivsholm, 2005]. Phimosis may cause pain and difficulties with the physical and psychological aspects of coitus.

Peyronie disease (induratio penis plastica) is associated with the presence [El-Sakka, 2005] and duration with DM [Arafa, 2007]. The prevalence in diabetic men varies from 8.1 to 18.3% [El-Sakka, 2005; Schwarzer, 2001; Tefekli, 2006]. In patients with DED prevalence of 20.3% [Arafa, 2007] has been reported and 16 [Kadioglu, 2004] compared to 3.2% [Schwarzer, 2001] and 3.64% [Rhoden, 2001] in non-selected populations.

In most cases patients with DM have several co-morbid conditions. The results of the last clinical mega-studies recommended an early and aggressive therapeutic intervention aiming primary prevention of micro- and macro-vascular diabetic complications. This multimorbidity and the necessity for multifactorial therapy determine a poly-pragmatic medication approach in patients with DM (figure 5).

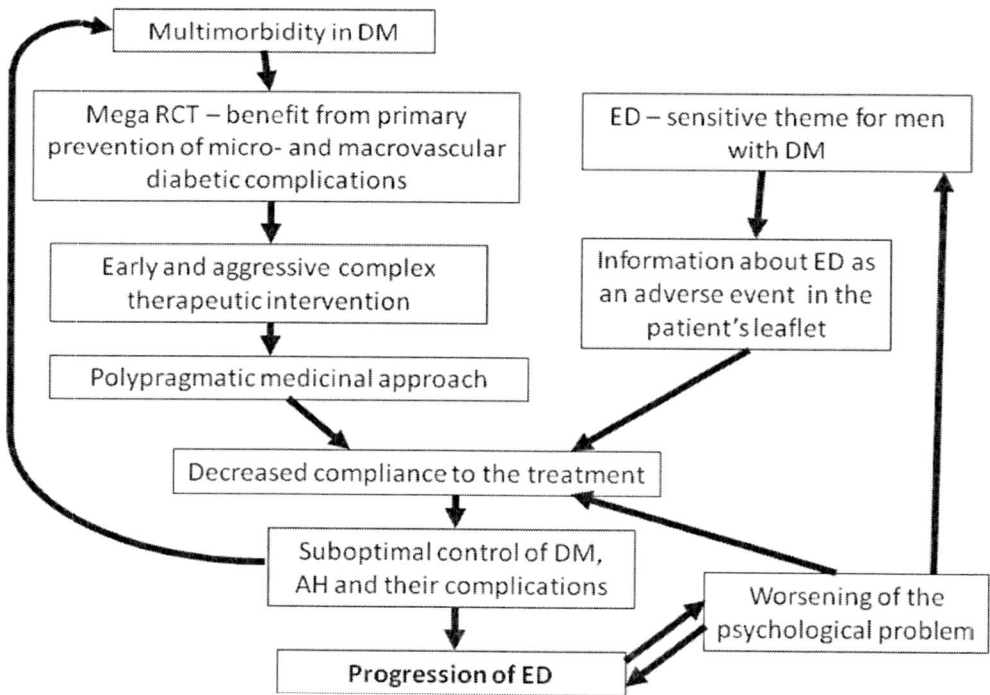

Figure 5. Drugs-associated subjective factors for ED.

A large proportion of the drugs that are used (antihypertensive, neuropathic pain control, etc.) possess unfavorable effects on erectile function. On the other hand, men with DM are psychologically more sensitive to ED. In many cases, the information provided on the patient information leaflet about the possible development of ED as an adverse event of a particular medication, can compromise the understanding of the necessity to keep blood sugar, lipids and blood pressure levels normal, thereby compromising the compliance to treatment with this particular drug. This imposes a careful selection of the treatment options, choosing harmonized therapeutic scheme aiming no between-drug interference, but also no undesirable effects on the different aspects of the metabolic syndrome and ED in patients with DM.

DIAGNOSTIC PROCESS

The diagnostic process in DED does not differ significantly from the usually described diagnostic algorithms for ED. The clinical workout for ED could be divided in two steps: (1) *diagnosis* - confirmation of the presence of ED and (2) *differential diagnosis* – identification of all possible factors and causes for the development of the particular ED. The second step is very important for the decision for treatment of all treatable pathogenetic factors.

1. The *diagnosis of ED* is not a difficult one, but it may be impeded by several mainly subjective obstacles. Men are usually distressed by the disease and ED and shame to speak voluntary about the problem (figure 6).

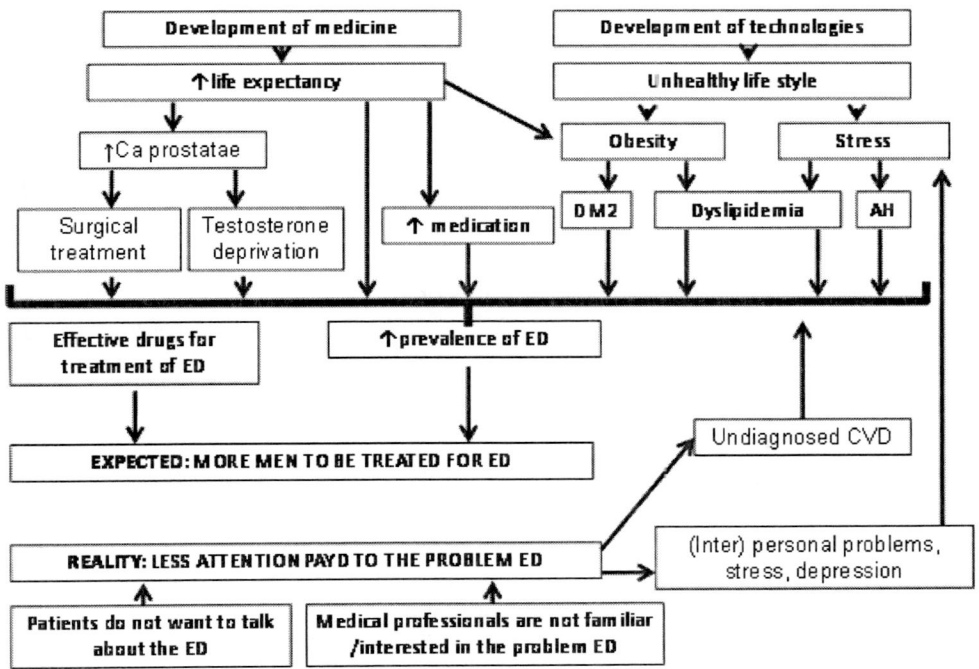

Figure 6. Controversy between expected and real consultations and treatment. Ca prostatae – prostate carcinoma; AH – arterial hypertension; CVD – cardiovascular diseases, DM2 – diabetes type 2; ED – erectile dysfunction.

The medical specialist with a general medical profile does not initiate this conversation as well because of a lack of knowledge, interest, motivation or time. Consultation in this sensitive area needs special skills and practice in the field of sexual medicine – an interdisciplinary specialty with growing number of experts. Several validated questionnaires, described in details elsewhere, may be used for the diagnosis of ED.

- The International Index of Erectile Function (IIEF) [Rosen, 1997] is the currently most widely used questionnaire [Basu, 2004]. Commonly, the domain for erectile function is preferred, including questions 1-5 and 15, aiming the last 4 weeks period. The presence of ED is assumed if the score is less than 26. ED is stratified into severe < 11, moderate < 16, moderate to mild < 21 and mild ≤ 25.
- The sexual Encounter Profile Question-2 (SEP2) – have you been able to insert your penis into partner's vagina?
- Sexual Encounter Profile Question-3 (SEP3) – Was your erection long enough to allow successful sexual encounter?
- Global Assessment Question (GAQ) – Do you think that the treatment improved your erection? (answer yes/no). This question isasked after the use of the drug.

2. The differential diagnosis is based on carefully collecting the patient's history, which may help significantly in the orientation of the main causes for ED in this particular case.

- In DM the origin of ED is organic in most cases, but it should not be forgotten that in young men with diabetes of shorter duration, a psychogenic component may prevail. It should be remembered that psychogenic aspects are necessarily present in different degrees in all patients independent of the stage of the disease (figure 7). When further psychological support and therapy is planned, the patient should be referred to the appropriate specialist.
- Patients with DED need more common vascular investigations with Doppler for diagnostic reasons and therapeutic evaluation.
- More sophisticated investigations like the RigiScan for characterization of nocturnal tumescence might be helpful on some occasions. The simple stamp-test could also be used if doubt exists about the nocturnal tumescences.
- Neurologically focused history and tests are of special interest in DED. It should be mentioned that absence of neurological symptoms and signs does not necessary mean absence of DN. On the other hand, some symptoms and signs caused by other neurological diseases are commonly attributed to DN because medical specialists are expecting the patient to have this diabetic complication. DN is a diagnosis per exclusionem. The most common initial nerve damage usually affects different sensory modalities and autonomic functions. Simple sensory diagnostic devices may be applied for the evaluation of sensory function, like the 128-Hz Rydel-Seiffer tuning fork (vibration perception), the Semmes-Weinstein 5.07 (10 g) monofilament (pressure perception), a thermal discriminator (thermal perception), etc., as well as autonomic tests (Neuropad for sudomotor function). These can be used easily in daily clinical practice in the community to improve diagnostic sensitivity [Kamenov,

2012b; Kamenov, 2010]. Special neurological tests may also be necessary for patients with ED [Diemont, 1997].

- The reported very high prevalence of low testosterone levels in diabetic men makes the exclusion of hypogonadism a more important initial diagnostic step compared to non-diabetic men. Omitting testosterone determination at this point of the evaluation of DED may cause further ineffectiveness of pro-erectogenic medications, loss of confidence and disappointment and worsening of the treatment prognosis and increasing frustration. Early morning testosterone levels below 8 nmol/L, confirmed on a consecutive visit, associated with corresponding symptoms (table 2) usually require testosterone supplementation after exclusion of the respective contraindications. Levels above 12 nmol/L usually are not considered as an indication for TRT. If the patient has testosterone levels in the grey zone (8-12 nmol/L) the case needs further evaluation and determination of free testosterone. In details the diagnostic approach for hypogonadism is described elsewhere [Wang, 2009]. It should not be forgotten that the decrease in testosterone levels may be caused by different endocrine (hypothalamic, pituitary, testicular, etc.) and other diseases or drugs, which makes the full set of differential diagnosis for hypogonadism necessary.

Psycho-organic link in DED

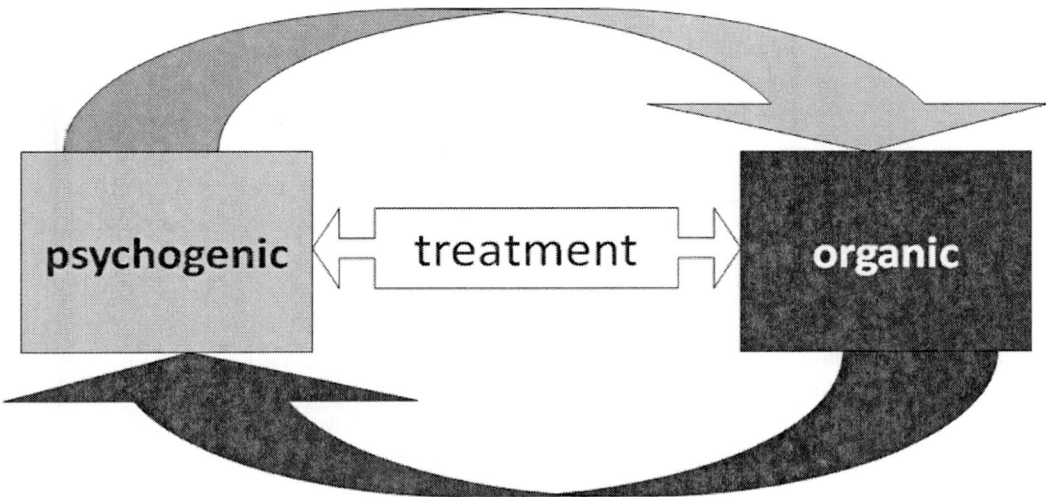

Figure 7. The psycho-organic link in DED (diabetic erectile dysfunction).

TREATMENT OPTIONS FOR DED

The already described mixed pathogenesis of DED requires a complex treatment which can be divided in general and specific measures.

The *general measures* include improvement and control of the main pathogenetic factors leading to DED.

Table 2. Main symptoms and signs of Late onset hypogonadism (LOH) in men

Somatic	Psychologic
↑ fat mass (especially visceral)	↑ irritability and depressiveness
↓ free fat mass	↓ energy
↓ muscle mass, strength and endurance	↓ libido and erections (ED)
↓ bone mineral density	↓ cognitive functions
↓ hair growth and skin thickness	↓ quality of sleep

The therapeutic approach does not differ from the currently accepted options for reaching the appropriate targets in terms of the patient blood glucose, lipids and blood pressure control, as well as for the cessation or limitation of unhealthy lifestyle habits like smoking, alcohol overconsumption, immobilization, stress, use of recreational drugs, etc. Although data about the beneficial effects of life style modification on ED are limited, changes in diet and physical activity should always be recommended for diabetic men with ED. Adherence to a Mediterranean diet has been shown to lower the prevalence of ED in men with DM2 [Giugliano, 2010]. Obesity is one of the strongest risk factors for DM2. Most patients with DM2 are overweight or obese and weight loss has a powerful beneficial effect ranging from improvement of glycaemia, blood pressure, lipids, etc. to disappearance of diabetes in obese patients with recently diagnosed DM2. Nevertheless, studies investigating the effect of weight loss on DED are scarce.

The Look AHEAD (Action for Health in Diabetes) trial examined 1-year changes in erectile function, measured by the International Index of Erectile Function (IIEF) in 372overweight/obese men aged 45–74 with DM2 randomly assigned to a control condition involving diabetes support and education or to intensive lifestyle intervention involving group and individual sessions to reduce weight and increase physical activity. Uncontrolled hyperglycemia($HbA1c > 11\%$), hypertension (blood pressure >160/100 mm Hg), fasting triglycerides $\geq$ 600 mg/dL, a cardiovascular event within the past 3months were exclusion criteria. At 1 year, the intensive group lost a greater percent of initial body weight (9.9% vs. 0.6 %), had greater improvements in fitness (22.7% vs. 4.6%) and erectile function improved more (17.3 ±7.6 at baseline; 18.6 ± 8.1at 1 year) than the control group (18.3 ±7.6 at baseline; 18.4 ± 8.0 at 1 year); $P = 0.04$ and $P = 0.06$ after adjusting for baseline differences.

According to the results of the 306 men (82%) who completed the study the authors concluded that in this sample of older overweight/obese diabetic men, weight loss intervention was mildly helpful in maintaining erectile function [Wing, 2010].

Keeping in mind that hyperglycemia is the trigger for all consecutive metabolic and hemodynamic disturbances in DM, strict glycemic control is the cornerstone of treatment for the disease and for the prevention of its complications, like DED. Patients with poor control are at 2 to 5-fold increased risk for ED compared to patients with good control [Fedele, 1998; Klein, 2005]. In a study including 792 subjects with 83.6% having ED and 43.2% severe ED Lu, et al. (2009) concluded that better glycemic control probably reduces the prevalence of ED and its severity among younger men with DM2, but for the older group, aging is the major determinant for ED risk [Lu, 2009]. It should be mentioned that the results of large scale studies in diabetic populations (ACCORD, ADVANCE, VADT, etc.) recommend to make changes in the therapeutic paradigm for DM2, which are reflected in the recent consensus statements of the American Diabetes Association, European Association for the Study of Diabetes, American Association of Clinical Endocrinologists and other international and national organizations [Inzucchi, 2012; Garber, 2013].

The *specific measures* include the whole therapeutic spectrum covering psychotherapy, oral treatment, intra-cavernosal injections and intra-urethral application of PgE1, vacuum constrictor devices and penile implants. Summarizing the results of the literature, it should be mentioned that:

1. There are not many studies designed for diabetic patients. Usually diabetics are sub-groups of larger patient populations. In some trials DM is even an exclusion criterion.

2. In most series, diabetes (type, duration, control, etc.) and its complications, macro- and micro-angiopathy including DN (presence, stage and treatment), are not described in details.

3. In most cases oral treatment should be applied with the highest dose: sildenafil 100 mg, vardenafil 20 mg, tadalafil 20 mg, avanafil 200 mg, udenafil 200 mg, and mirodenafil 100 mg.

4. The effectiveness of treatment in diabetic men is lower compared to non-diabetics [Price, 2008]. This difference is even underestimated because commonly poor glycemic control is an exclusion criterion upon enrollment in randomized clinical trials (RCT).

5. Patients with DED require more often switching to a higher line of treatment like intracavernosal injections, vacuum constrictor devices and implants compared to healthy men.

6. Vascular reconstruction operations for ED are very rarely performed in diabetic patients.

PSYCHOLOGICAL ASPECTS OF ED IN DM

Detailed description of the psychological therapeutic approach in men with ED, and particularly DED, is above the scope of this review. Although there is a growing number of studies on the association between DED and psychological factors, the prevailing scientific interest remains focused primarily on the organic pathology of DED. Some authors drew the attention to the individual and marital pathology in male diabetic patients and the significance of psychological dimensions on the sexual impact of the illness [Siddiqui, 2012]. ED is associated with higher levels of diabetes-specific health distress and worse psychological adaptation to diabetes, which in turn worsens the metabolic control [Berardis, 2002]. Diabetic patients are more likely to consider their ED to be severe and permanent, compared with men without diabetes [Eardley, 2007]. ED contributes to poorer overall quality of life in diabetic patients [Avasthi, 2011].

PDE-5 INHIBITORS

A new era in the erectology began about 15 years ago with the introduction of the first inhibitor of PDE-5 – sildenafil. The representatives of this group of drugs inhibit the main phosphodiesterase isoform in the cavernosal smooth muscle – type 5 responsible for the degradation of cGMP [Wallis, 1999], which level increases and leads to improvement of the erection. Later PDE-5 inhibitors – vardenafil and tadalafil - have higher specificity to the target iso-enzyme [de Tejada, 2001a]. Further avanafil and udenafil were also introduced on the market. Currently available PDE-5 inhibitors are very effective and safe and represent the first line therapy for the treatment of ED, including DED, although less effective in diabetic men [Ng, 2002; Padma-Nathan, 2003; Goldstein, 2003]. Only 56% of DM2 patients respond to PDE5,compared to 87% response in normal patients [Rendell, 1999]. Even when a good response to treatment is initially reported in DM2 patients, the effects are not sustainable overtime. After 1 year of treatment of men with DED, IIEF scores reverted to baseline values [Penson, 2003].

- Sildenafil

Sildenafil is the first member of the PDE-5 inhibitors family, released on the market in 1998. It is also the most studied drug with an enormous database. Sildenafil has been successfully used in doses 25, 50 and 100 mg in the general population as well as difficult-to-treat subgroups, particularly diabetic men with ED. In one of the first trials - multicenter, randomized, double-blind, placebo-controlled, flexible dose study268 men with DED were randomized to receive sildenafil in escalating dose or placebo for a period of 12 weeks. In the active arm, 56% of the patients had improvement of the erections compared to 10% in the placebo arm [Rendell, 1999].

Sildenafil has also been shown to be effective vs. placebo in DM1 patients. Significant improvements in the ability to achieve erections evaluated by IIEF (35.7% vs. 19.9%) and to maintain erections (68.4% vs. 26.5%), improved erections with treatment (GAQ 66.6% vs. 28.6%), and successful attempts at intercourse (63% vs. 33%) were reported [Stuckey, 2003].

In a randomized, double-blind, placebo-controlled, and fixed-dose study, a total of 282 men were randomized to sildenafil to placebo. Significant improvements from baseline on the IIEF Q3 (55% vs. 29%) and IIEF Q4 (61% vs. 25%) were observed. The author concluded that oral sildenafil is a moderately effective treatment for ED in men with diabetes. The response rate was lower and cardiovascular events were higher than previously reported in nondiabetic patients [Safarinejad, 2004].

Sildenafil has been investigated for potential benefits in different diabetic areas. Investigating the changes in serum levels of biomarkers of vascular function serum cyclic guanosine monophosphate, 8-isoprostane, interleukin-6 and interleukin-8 in men with type 2 diabetes with ED after the use of sildenafil for 12 weeks. Burnett et al. (2009) concluded that the data suggest that short-term, continuous sildenafil treatment causes systemic endothelial function to be enhanced and remain so for a duration after its discontinuation. However, they do not indicate any influence of this treatment on systemic oxidative stress or inflammation, or an effect on long-term erectile function improvement [Burnett, 2009].

In a double-blind, randomized, controlled trial, 40 male patients aged 35-50 with DM2 received sildenafil citrate 50 mg daily or a placebo for 30 days. Levels of hs-CRP, microalbuminuria, homocysteine, A1c and erectile function were measured at baseline and at the end of the study. Men who received sildenafil citrate displayed a significant decrease in the microalbuminuria concentrations ($p<0.01$) versus baseline, ($p<0.02$) versus placebo, and A1c ($p<0.01$) versus baseline, ($p<0.01$) versus placebo[Grover-Páez, 2007].

To evaluate the endothelial function, a double-blind placebo-controlled prospective trial was conducted with 24 men with type 2 diabetes who were randomized into 2 groups: one receiving daily sildenafil 50 mg and the other placebo for 10 weeks. At the conclusion of the 10-week trial, patients who received daily sildenafil had significantly improved erectile rigidity as captured by IIEF-5 ($p<0.001$) and increased endothelial function via brachial artery flow-mediated dilation ($p<0.01$) [Deyoung, 2012].

- Tadalafil

Tadalafil is an effective drug for treatment of ED of different severity and etiology. The most important difference compared to other currently available PDE-5 inhibitors is its long half-life (17.5 hours) allowing (1) a long-lasting clinical effect of 36 hours by on demand dosing with 5, 10 or 20 mg, and (2) full diurnal therapeutic coverage by daily use in lesser dose – 2.5 and 5 mg. The highest amount of data refers to the general population with mild to moderate ED [Brock, 2002; Carson, 2004], but there is also evidence for successful use in difficult-to-treat patients with severe organic ED [Carson, 2005], DED [de Tejada, 2002; Fonseca, 2004], after radical prostatectomy [Carson, 2005; Montorsi, 2004] or radiation therapy [Incrocci, 2007]. In a study with 191 diabetic men tadalafil 10 and 20 mg on demand resulted in 56% and 64% improvement of their erections compared to 25% in the placebo arm [de Tejada, 2002]. Some studies showed a significant benefit for low dose tadalafil use on a daily basis [McMahon, 2004; Porst, 2008] that was approved by FDA in 2008.

Recently the results from a large trial including 726 patients with ED and DM were reported. It represents the diabetic arm of The Scheduled Use vs. on-demand Regimen Evaluation (SURE) – randomized crossover, open study with 4262 patients from 392 centers in 14 European countries [Buvat, 2006]. Tadalafil was used in 20 mg dose in two dose regimens - regularly three times a week irrespective of the sexual activity or on demand. The patients were divided into two groups according to the used regimen and after a 5-6 weeks period the two arms were crossed using the alternative dose regimen for the same period of time. Regarding DM, patients were considered having type 1 or 2 according to the current insulin use and the age of onset of DM – before or after 40 years of age with no pre-selection for diabetic complications. Minimal duration of ED was 3 months. At the end point of both regimens, the mean IIEF EF domain score was 22, and >40% of the patients had a normal EF domain score (≥ 26). The proportion of "yes" responses was $\geq 73\%$ for SEP2 (penetration), $\geq 58\%$ for SEP3 (successful intercourse), >46% for SEP4 (hardness of erection), and $\geq 45\%$ for SEP5 (overall satisfaction). Efficacy was maintained up to 36 hours post-dosing. More than 70% of sexual attempts while on the three-times-per-week regimen and approximately 50% of the attempts on the on-demand treatment occurred >4 hours post-dosing. Treatment preference was 57.2% for on demand and 42.8% for three times per week. The authors concluded that Tadalafil, when taken on demand or three times per week, is effective and safe for men with DM and ED.

In a similar study with 191 diabetic men tadalafil 10 and 20 mg on demand resulted in 56 and 64% improvement of erection compared to 25% in the placebo arm [de Tejada, 2002]. Schulman et al. (2004) studied the difference in effectiveness of a fixed dose use of tadalafil over time [Schulman, 2004]. They combined the data from 5 placebo-controlled 12-week studies including 3 groups of 308, 321 and 258 men on placebo, 10 and 20 mg tadalafil. The very first dose lead to significant improvement in SEP2: 47%, 74%, 79% respectively in the three patients populations; SEP3: 31%, 56%, 67% and SEP5 (satisfied overall with their sexual experience): 15%, 36%, 47% respectively. Later on, the effect was magnified reaching a plateau at 95% (SEP2), 90% (SEP3), and 81% (SEP5) between the 4th and 8th dose.

Fonseca et al. (2004) conducted a meta-analysis of 12 placebo-controlled studies with tadalafil in patients with diabetes including 637 men with a mean age of 57 years and mean baseline IIEF = 12.6 [Fonseca, 2004]. The use of tadalafil 10 or 20 mg for 12 weeks lead to improvement of 7.4 points vs. 0.9 points in the placebo group. In men with diabetes 53% of the sexual attempts were successful vs. 22% in the placebo group. Baseline IIEF showed negative correlation with HbA1c, but the response to tadalafil treatment was not related to the glycemic control, type of treatment or previous use of sildenafil. No analysis was made on the pathogenic factors of ED. Comparison of this population with 1681 men of mean age 56 years with ED (baseline IIEF=15) without diabetes demonstrated more severe ED in DM but independently equal therapeutic effect to tadalafil.

- Vardenafil

Vardenafil is a powerful PDE5 inhibitor which efficacy and tolerability at doses 5, 10 and 20 mg were shown in randomized double-blind placebo-controlled trials including large populations of men with ED [Porst, 2001; Hellstrom, 2002; Hatzichristou, 2004], and men presenting difficult-to-treat groups like DM, after prostatectomy etc. [Goldstein, 2003; Brock, 2003]. Reliability of vardenafil was determined in retrospective analysis of two clinical studies. The results showed increased probability for penetration, maintenance of erection and general satisfaction compared to placebo. The major part of the patients who responded to the first dose of vardenafil reported success during the whole 12-week treatment period. [Montorsi, 2004].

In one open study on 398 non-selected men aged ≥ 18 years with ED the efficacy and tolerability of vardenafil used at initial dose of 10 mg and titrated to 5 or 20 mg were investigated. [Potempa, 2004]. At the end of the 10-week therapeutic period were reported: improvement in erectile function domain of IIEF ranging from 13.9 to 25.9 points, successful penetration SEP2 in 89%, maintenance of erection SEP3 in 78% and general satisfaction of the treatment GAQ in 92%.

Goldstein et al. (2003) conducted a multicenter randomized double-blind placebo-controlled trial with 452 men with diabetes type 1 and 2 [Goldstein, 2003]. The study took place in 47 centers in USA and Canada. Inclusion criteria were: age > 18 years, stable heterosexual relationship > 6 months, HbA1c < 12%. Patients were randomized in 3 groups: use of 10 or 20 mg of vardenafil or placebo over 12 week period. The drug was taken 1 hour before coitus no more than once a day. After the end of this period the patients received 10 or 20 mg vardenafil for another 12 weeks. Treatment efficacy was assessed on 4-week intervals using IIEF and GAQ. Moreover the patients had to fill in a diary describing their sexual attempts according SEP2 and SEP3. Sub-analyses of received data was also made according to the baseline severity of ED, HbA1c (<6, <8 and>8%) and dose-response effect. Special focus was placed on the recording of possible side effects. At the end of the trial, 57% and 72% of the men reported an improvement in erectile function according to GAQ compared to 13% improvement in the placebo group. On the twelfth treatment week IIEF increased by 19.0 points. Successful penetration (SEP2) was achieved by 64%, and successful coitus (SEP3) by 54% of men. The results of this study are summarized in three major conclusions: (1) Vardenafil has a favorable dose-dependent treatment profile on erectile dysfunction in patients with DM. (2) The efficacy of vardenafil is present irrespective of the baseline severity of ED and glycemia. (3) The drug has no serious side effects and has very good tolerability. No disturbances of color vision were reported.

Patient satisfaction with the treatment for ED is critical for his long term compliance [Dean, 2006]. In one international trial with 3291 men with ED 47% of them pointed the constant efficacy as the most important feature of the treatment [Eardley, 2003; Meuleman, 2003]. This is extremely important in men with DM, who report their ED to be severe and permanent, seek medical help more often and are more prone to discontinuation of treatment because of unsatisfactory results, compared to men with ED but with no diabetes. [Eardley, 2007].

Most of the above mentioned research suggests that responsiveness to PDE5i drugs increases with sequential dosing from initiation; eight doses are generally considered an adequate trial of therapy to establish efficacy. The effect of the first intake of a PDE5 inhibitor is a prognostic factor for its treatment efficacy. It can be stated that the initial success and further reliability of the treatment for ED are crucial for patient satisfaction with the treatment that directly affects his compliance. The aim of the study of Valiquette et al. (2005) was to evaluate the efficacy of the first intake of 10 mg vardenafil vs. placebo in a nonselected population of 600 men with a mean age (adjusted mean data for the two groups of placebo and vardenafil) of 54±11 years (20-79), of whom 30% had hypertension, 15% DM and 16% dyslipidemia [Valiquette, 2005]. Baseline IIEF (erectile function domain) is 14.6 ±5 points, and ED duration – about 5.6±5.2 years. Efficacy regarding SEP2 is 87% = 520 of total 600 men reported successful penetration and 85% of them maintained their erection to the end of intercourse (SEP3), which equals 74% success for the first intake of vardenafil regarding SEP3 in the general population. Although the head-to-head comparisons are scarce the data about effectiveness of the PDE-5 inhibitors in diabetic men suggest similar degree. Recently we compared the effect of the first intake of tadalafil 20 mg and vardenafil 20 mg in men from the difficult-to-treat group with DED and proven DN [Kamenov, 2011]. To synchronize the therapeutic windows, sexual intercourse should have been initiated in the interval of 1 to 6 hours after drug intake. In this time frame the effectiveness (IIEF-EF, SEP2, SEP3, GAQ) of both medications was comparable.

- Avanafil

Avanafil was recently approved by the US Food and Drug Administration for the management of ED. Avanafil was studied in over 1300 patients during clinical trials, including patients with DM and those who had undergone radical prostatectomy, and was found to be more effective than placebo in all men who were randomized to the drug. The medication was studied with on-demand dosing as 50, 100, or 200 mg that may occur after food and/or alcohol intake.

Avanafil may differentiate itself from the other phosphodiesterase type 5 inhibitors with its quicker onset and higher specificity for phosphodiesterase type 5 versus other phosphodiesterase subtypesthus, appearing to be as safe as the other available agents in the class [Burke, 2012].

In a 12-week, multicenter, double-blind, placebo-controlled study 390 men with diabetes and erectile dysfunction were randomized 1:1:1 to receive avanafil 100 or 200 mg, or placebo. Compared with placebo IIEF-EF domain, SEP 2 and SEP 3 improved with both avanafil, 100 mg (P≤.002), and avanafil, 200 mg (P<.001). The authors concluded that avanafil was safe and effective for treating erectile dysfunction in men with diabetes and was effective as early as 15 minutes and more than 6 hours after dosing. The adverse events seen with avanafil were similar to those seen with other phosphodiesterase 5 inhibitors [Goldstein, 2012].

- Udenafil

Udenafilis a potent novel PDE-5 inhibitor approved for use in Korea. Udenafil has a T max of 1.0-1.5 h and a T 1/2 of 11-13 h. Therefore, both on-demand and once-daily use of udenafil have been reported. Udenafil's efficacy and tolerability in doses 100 or 200 mg have been evaluated in several studies, and recent and continuing studies have demonstrated udenafil's promise in both dosing regimens. Presently, tadalafil is the only FDA-approved drug for daily dosing, but udenafil can be used as a once-daily dose for erectile dysfunction patients who cannot tolerate tadalafil due to phosphodiesterase subtype selectivity. Udenafil as an on-demand or once-daily dose is effective and tolerable, but more studies are needed in patients of other ethnicities and with comorbid conditions such as diabetes mellitus, hypertension, and benign prostate hyperplasia [Kang, 2013].

A placebo-controlled, randomized, double-blind, double-dummy, fixed-dose parallel-group design multicenter study, was conducted. The trial involved seven study sites in Korea, with 174 ED patients with DM. The subjects, treated with placebo, 100 or 200 mg of udenafil for 12 weeks, were evaluated by IIEF questions 3 (Q3) and Q4 and the rate of achieving normal erectile function (EFD ≥ 26), SEP Q2 and Q3, and the Global Assessment Question (GAQ).

Compared with the placebo, patients receiving both doses of udenafil showed statistically significant improvements in the IIEF-EFD score. However, significant difference was not observed between the udenafil 100 mg and 200mg groups. Similar results were observed in the comparison of Q3 and Q4 of IIEF, SEP diary, and GAQ. The percentages of subjects experiencing at least one adverse event related to the study drugs were 3.6%, 15.8%, and 22.4% for the placebo, udenafil 100 mg and 200 mg groups, respectively. However, these events were all mild in severity. Major adverse events were flushing, headache, nausea, and conjunctival hyperemia. The study concluded that udenafil was effective for the treatment of ED, demonstrating statistically significant improvement in erectile function in patients with DM. The incidence of adverse events was relatively low and well tolerated in patients with DM [Moon, 2011].

- Mirodenafil

A multicenter, randomized, double-blind, placebo-controlled, parallel-group, fixed-dose study was conducted with 112 subjects who were randomized to either placebo or mirodenafil 100 mg on demand for 12 weeks. Mirodenafil group showed significantly greater change from baseline compared with the placebo group in the following indicators: IIEF-EF domain score (9.3 vs. 1.4, P < 0.0001), IIEF Q3 (1.7 vs. 0.4, P < 0.0001) and Q4 (1.7 vs. 0.3, P < 0.0001), SEP2 (82.0% vs. 55.2%, P = 0.0003), SEP3 (68.9% vs. 22.3%, P < 0.0001) positive answer to GAQ (76.9% vs. 19.1%, P < 0.0001). Normal EF domain scores (≥ 26) at study end were achieved by 32.7% and 9.4% in the mirodeniafl and placebo groups, respectively (P = 0.0031). As for the Life Satisfaction Checklist scores, the mirodenafil group showed significantly greater improvements in sexual life and partner relationship than the placebo group. Most treatment-associated AEs were mild and resolved spontaneously. The conclusion of this study was that mirodenafil is an effective and well-tolerated agent for the treatment of diabetic patients with ED in Korea [Park, 2010].

- Adverse effects of PDE-5 inhibitors

The tolerance and safety of PDS-5 inhibitors is very good. A Cochrane Database Report analyzing the randomized placebo-controlled studies did not find any lethal case of men with DM and ED. In only one study cardiovascular adverse events were reported. The most common side effects (with decreasing rate) are: headache, flush, respiratory tract complains and flu-like symptoms, dyspepsia, myalgia, vision disturbances and back pain [Vardi, 2007]. More concise data about the adverse events are available for the "older" PDE-5 inhibitors. After a systematic review and meta-analysis [Tsertsvadze, 2009] the following conclusions about (1) vs. placebo and (2) head-to-head comparisons were made: (1) A greater proportion of men treated with PDE-5 inhibitors than men who received placebo had at least one adverse event. The most commonly reported adverse events were headache, flushing, rhinitis, and dyspepsia. Other reported events were visual disturbances, myalgia, nausea, diarrhea, vomiting, dizziness, and chest pain. In general, these events were mild to moderate and were transient. Serious adverse events were reported in fewer than 2.0% of participants, and incidence did not differ between PDE-5 inhibitor recipients and placebo recipients. (2) Differences in the incidence of any adverse events among men treated with sildenafil (range, 24.0% to 34.0%), tadalafil (range, 28.0% to 35.0%), and vardenafil (27.0%) were not statistically significant. Discontinuation due to adverse effects ranged from 0.5% to 3.8% during tadalafil treatment, 0.5% to 3.8% during sildenafil treatment, and 1.0% during vardenafil treatment. The frequency of specific adverse events (headache, flushing, dyspepsia, and nasal congestion) seemed similar among treatments.

- Non-responders

In real *non-responders* to a particular PDE-5 inhibitor the following could be attempted: test for low testosterone level (if not already done at the initiation of treatment) and if hypogonadal – TRT should be started (more details in [Nieschlag, 2006]); metabolic optimization (also an earlier target); escalation of the dose of PDE-5 inhibitor ad maximal; change of the PDE-5 inhibitor; daily dosing of tadalafil; second and third line treatment.

- Second and third line therapy

Second line treatment options include intracavernosal injections of individual or combined (bimix, trimix) drugs – papaverine, phentolamine and PGE1 and vacuum constrictor devices. Penile prostheses (implants) are the *third-line therapy* for ED.

Intracavernosal injections of vasoactive drugs - prostaglandin E1, phentolamine, papaverine. PGE1 stimulates adenylate cyclase, thereby increasing levels of cAMP, which results in smooth muscle relaxation and vasodilatation. Erection appears after 5 to 15 minutes and lasts for a period that depends on the dose injected. The patient should be enrolled in an office-based training programme (requiring one or two visits) to learn the correct injection procedure [Phé, 2012].

The efficacy rate is approximately 70%, with reported sexual activity after 94% of injections, and satisfaction rates are high [Moore, 2006]. However, dropout rates of 41–68% have been reported, with most dropouts occurring within the first 2 to 3 months [Verdi, 2000]. Complications with intracavernous alprostadil include penile pain (50% of patients after 11% of injections), prolonged erections (5%), priapism (1%) and fibrosis (2%) [Hatzimouratidis, 2005]. Drug combinations such as alprostadil plus papaverine, a non-specific PDE inhibitor resulting in increased levels of cAMP and/or cGMP, and alprostadil plus phentolamine, a competitive antagonist of alpha-1 and alpha-2 adrenoreceptors, may increase efficacy by up to 90%.

Vacuum constriction devices (VCDs): VCDs apply negative pressure to draw blood into the penis that is then retained by the application of a visible constricting band at the base of the penis. This method appears to be more acceptable to older patients [Levine, 2001]. There are few recognized complications, and there are low-cost treatment options for selected diabetic ED patients.

It was reported that VCDs achieved satisfactory erections in more than 70% of diabetic men [Price, 1991]. Problems with VCDs include pain from the constriction ring, lack of spontaneity, decrease in the quality of orgasm and ejaculatory discomfort. In addition, up to 30% of patients discontinue its use as the result of inadequate rigidity, penile pain, failure to ejaculate and the appearance of the penis while using the device [Price, 1991; Sidi, 1990]. Other disadvantages include lack of spontaneity and, in a minority of cases, the partner deemed it an unacceptable method.

Penile implants: When pharmacotherapy fails, surgical implantation of a penile prosthesis may be considered. Prostheses are either malleable (semi rigid) or inflatable (two- or three-piece). Penile implants provide a predictable and reliable erection, and have the highest satisfaction rate among both patients and their partners of all the available treatments for waning erections [Phé, 2012]. The two main complications associated with penile prosthesis implantation are mechanical failure (< 5% after a 5-year follow-up with the currently available three-piece prostheses) and infection. Since the introduction of a three-piece inflatable penile implant impregnated with the antibiotics minocycline and rifampin, there has been a significant reduction in infection rates among those with an antibiotic-impregnated penile implant; currently, the infection rate is 1% [Carson, 2011]. For nonimpregnated implants, the infection risk rate is 2.5% in this population [Montague, 2001].

Some research has indicated that diabetics have an increased risk of infection *vs* non-diabetics, but other studies have indicated no differences in infection rates [Montague, 2001; Wilson, 1998; Wilson, 1995; Jarow, 1996].

CONCLUSION

Due to its complex pathogenesis DED is more common and difficult for treatment compared to healthy men. Its presentation commonly precedes the clinical manifestation of the vascular diseases in other arterial areas and might be a predictor of more serious micro-vascular problems. Therapeutic schemes for co-morbidities like hypertension, dyslipidemia, pain relief, psychological problems, etc., should be composed carefully and harmonized with the aspect of metabolic syndrome and erectile dysfunction. Treatment of DED includes correction of metabolic disturbances and possible hypogonadism. Although effective and safe medications already exist, very often DED is not adequately diagnosed and treated which leads further to aggravation of the psychological and micro social distress. In most cases the reason for this is the communicative problem – the physician does not ask and the patient does not share spontaneously the presence of DED. PDE-5 inhibitors are the first line therapy in DED. Switching to second and third line therapy – intracavernosal injections, vacuum constrictor devices, implants, is more common in men with DED.

REFERENCES

Adegite A., Aniekwensi E., Ohihoin A., Puepet F. Perception about aettiology of sexual problems, health seeking behavior and treatment for sexual problems among type 2 diabetic men. 20th IDF World Congress, 18-22.10.2009, Montreal, Canada; P-1370, *Book of abstracts* p.462.

Angulo J, González-Corrochano R, Cuevas P, Fernández A, La Fuente JM, Rolo F, Allona A, Sáenz de Tejada I. Diabetes exacerbates the functional deficiency of NO/cGMP pathway associated with erectile dysfunction in human corpus cavernosum and penile arteries.*J. Sex Med.* 2010 Feb;7(2 Pt 1):758-68.

Arafa M, Eid H, El-Badry A et al. The prevalence of Peyronie's disease in diabetic patients with erectile dysfunction.*Int. J. Impot. Res.;*2007;19:213–7.

Avasthi A, Grover S, Bhansali A, Dash RJ, Gupta N, Sharan P, Sharma S. Erectile dysfunction in diabetes mellitus contributes to poor quality of life. *Int. Rev. Psychiatry.* 2011;23(1):93-9.

Baba K, Yajima M, Carrier S et al. Effect of testosterone on the number of NADPH diaphorase-stained nerve fibers in the rat corpus cavernosum and dorsal nerve.*Urology*;2000;56:533–8.

Bacon CG, Hu FB, Giovannucci E, et al. Association of type and duration of diabetes with erectiledysfunction in a large cohort of men. *Diabetes Care* 2002;25:1458.

Bartolini M, Giommi R, Forti G et al. Organic, relational and psychological factors in erectile dysfunction in men with diabetes mellitus. *Eur. Urol.* 2004;46:222–8.

Basu A, Ryder RE.New treatment options for erectile dysfunction in patients with diabetes mellitus. *Drugs.* 2004;64(23):2667-88

Berardis GD, Franciosi M, Belfigli M. et al.. Erectile Dys-function and Quality of Life in Type 2 Diabetic Patients: A serious problem too often overlooked. *Diabetes Care*2002, 25:284–291.

Bivalacqua TJ, Champion HC, Usta MF et al. RhoA/Rhokinase suppresses endothelial nitric oxide synthase in the penis: a mechanism for diabetes-associated erectile dysfunction. *Proc. Natl. Acad. Sci. USA* 2004; 101: 9121–6.

Bivalacqua TJ, Usta MF, Champion HC et al. Endothelial dysfunction in erectile dysfunction: role of the endothelium in erectile physiology and disease. *J. Androl.* 2003; 24 (Suppl 6): S17–37.

Bivalacqua TJ, Usta MF, Kendirci M et al. Superoxide anion production in the rat penis impairs erectile function in diabetes: influence of in vivo extracellular superoxide dismutase gene therapy. *J. Sex Med.* 2005; 2: 187–97.

Brock G, Nehra A, Lipshultz LI, et al. Safety and efficacy of vardenafil for the treatment of men with erectile dysfunction after radical retropubic prostatectomy. *J. Urol.* 2003;170(4, pt 1):1278-1283.

Brock GB, McMahon CG, Chen KK, et al. Efficacy and safety of tadalafi l for the treatment of erectile dysfunction: results of integrated analyses. *J. Urol.* 2002;168:1332–6.

Bucala R, Tracey KJ, Cerami A. Advanced glycosylation products quench nitric oxide and mediate defective endothe-lium-dependent vasodilation in experimental diabetes. *J. Clin.Invest.*1991; 87: 432–8.

Burchardt T, Burchardt M, Karden J et al. Reduction of endothelial and smooth muscle density in the corpora cavernosa of the streptozotocin induced diabetic rat. *J. Urol.* 2000;164:1807–11.

Burke FP, Jacobson DF, McGree ME et al. Diabetes and sexual dysfunction in Olmsted County, Minnesota. *J. Sex Med.* 2006; 3 (Suppl 1): 19.

Burke JP, Jacobson DJ, McGree ME, Nehra A, Roberts RO, Lieber MM, Jacobsen SJ. Diabetes and sexual dysfunction: Result from Olmsted county study of urinary symptoms and health status among men. *The journal of urology* 2007, 177(4):1438-1442.

Burke RM, Evans JD. Avanafil for treatment of erectile dysfunction: review of its potential.*Vasc.Health Risk Manag.* 2012;8:517-23.

Burnett AL, Strong TD, Trock BJ, Jin L, Bivalacqua TJ, Musicki B. Serum biomarker measurements of endothelial function and oxidative stress after daily dosing ofsildenafil in type 2 diabetic men with erectile dysfunction.*J. Urol.* 2009 Jan;181(1):245-51.

Buvat J, H.van Ahlen, H.Schmitt et al. Efficacy and safety of two dosing regimens of tadalafil and patterns of sexual activity in men with diabetes mellitus and erectile dysfunction: Scheduled use vs. on-demand regimen evaluation (SURE) study in 14 European countries. *J. Sex Med.* 2006;May;3(3):512-20.

Buyukafsar K, Un I. Effects of the Rho-kinase inhibitors, Y-27632 and fasudil, on the corpus cavernosum from diabetic mice.*Eur. J. Pharmacol.*2003; 472: 235–8.

Carson 3rd CC, Mulcahy JJ, Harsch MR. Long-term infection outcomes after original antibiotic impregnated inflatable penile prosthesis implants: up to 7.7 years of follow-up. *J. Urol.* 2011;185:614–8.

Carson CC, Rajfer J, Eardley I, et al. The efficacy and safety of tadalafi l: an update. BJU Int. 2004;93:1276–81.

Carson CC, Shabsigh R, Segal S, et al. Efficacy, safety, and treatment satisfaction of tadalafi l versus placebo in patients with erectile dysfunction evaluated at tertiary-care academic centers. *Urology.* 2005;65:353–9.

Cartledge JJ, Eardley I, Morrison JF. Advanced glycation end-products are responsible for the impairment of corpus cavernosal smooth muscle relaxation seen in diabetes. *B. J. U. Int.* 2001b; 87: 402–7.

Chitaley K, Kupelian V, Subak L, Wessells H.Diabetes, obesity and erectiledysfunction: fieldoverview and researchpriorities. *J. Urol.* 2009a Dec;182(6 Suppl):S45-50.

Chitaley K. Type 1 and type 2 diabetic-erectile dysfunction: same diagnosis (ICD-9), different disease?*J. Sex Med.*6(suppl):262. 2009b.

Christ GJ, Lerner SE, Kim DC et al. Endothelin-1 as a putative modulator of erectile dysfunction: I. Characteristics of contraction of isolated corporal tissue strips. *J. Urol.* 1995; 153: 1998–2003.

Chua R, Tar M, Melman A et al. Streptozotocin-induced diabetes results in time-dependent upregulation of the endothelin/rho-kinase pathway in rat corpus cavernosum smooth muscle.*J. Sex Med.* 2006; 3 (Suppl 1): 25.

Clozel M, Gray GA, Breu V et al. The endothelin ETB receptor mediates both vasodilation and vasoconstriction in vivo. *Biochem.Biophys. Res. Commun.*1992; 186: 867–73.

Corona G, Mannucci E, Petrone L et al. NCEP-ATPIII-defined metabolic syndrome, type 2 diabetes mellitus, and prevalence of hypogonadism in male patients with sexual dysfunction. *J. Sex Med* 2007;4:1038–45.

Corrales JJ, Burgo RM, Garca-Berrocal B et al. Partial androgen deficiency in aging type 2 diabetic men and its relationship to glycemic control. *Metabolism* 2004;53:666–72.

Dean J, Hackett GI, Gentile V, Pirozzi-Farina F, Rosen RC, Zhao Y, Warner MR, Beardsworth A. Psychosocial outcomes and drug attributes affecting treatment choice in men receiving sildenafil citrate and tadalafil for the treatment of erectile dysfunction: results of a multicenter, randomized, open-label, crossover study. *J. Sex Med.* 2006 *Jul;3(4):650-61.*

Deyoung L, Chung E, Kovac JR, Romano W, Brock GB. Daily use of sildenafil improves endothelial function in men with type 2 diabetes.*J. Androl.* 2012 Mar-Apr;33(2):176-80.

Diemont W. Meuleman E. Neurological testing in erectile dysfunction.*J. Androl.* 1997;18(4):345-50.

Dimmeler S & Zeiher AM Endothelial cell apoptosis inangiogenesis and vessel regression.*Circulation Research* 2000;87:434–9.

Drivsholm T, de Fine Olivarius N, Nielsen AB et al. Symptoms, signs and complications in newly diagnosed type 2 diabetic patients, and their relationship to glycaemia, blood pressure and weight. *Diabetologia* 2005;48:210–4.

Dyck PJ, Kratz KM, Karnes JL, Litchy WJ, Klein R, Pach JM, Wilson DM, O'Brien PC, Melton LJ 3rd, Service FJ. The prevalence by staged severity of various types of diabetic neuropathy, retinopathy, and nephropathy in a population-based cohort: the Rochester Diabetic Neuropathy Study. *Neurology.* 1993;43:817-24.

Eardley I, Fisher W, Rosen RC, Niederberger C, Nadel A, Sand M. The multinational Men's Attitudes to Life Events and Sexuality study: the influence of diabetes on self-reported erectile function, attitudes and treatment-seeking patterns in men with erectile dysfunction. *Int. J. Clin.Pract.* 2007 Sep;61(9):1446-53.

Eardley I, Rosen R, Fisher WA, Niederberger C, Sand M. Attitudes toward treatment of erectile dysfunction: results from the MALES study. *Eur. Urol. Suppl.* 2003;2:97. Abstract 377.

El-Sakka AI, Tayeb KA.Peyronie's disease in diabetic patients being screened for erectile dysfunction.*J. Urol.* 2005;174:1026–30.

Fakjian N, Hunter S, Cole GW et al. An argument for circumcision.Prevention of balanitis in the adult.*Arch. Dermatol.* 1990;126:1046–7.

Fedele D, Coscelli C, Santeusanio F et al. Erectile dysfunction in diabetic subjects in Italy. Gruppo Italiano Studio Deficit Erettile nei Diabetici.*Diabetes Care* 1998;21(11):1973–7.

Feldman HA, Goldstein I, Hatzichristou DG et al. Impotence and its medical and psychosocial correlates: results of the Massachusetts Male Aging Study. *J. Urol.* 1994; 151: 54–61.

FonsecaV., A.Seftel, J.Denne, Fredlund P.. Impact of diabetes mellitus on the severity of erectile dysfunction and response to treatment: analysis of data from tadalafil clinical trials.*Diabetologia.* 2004 Nov;47(11):1914-23.

Garber AJ, Abrahamson MJ, Barzilay JI, Blonde L, Bloomgarden ZT, Bush MA, Dagogo-Jack S, Davidson MB, Einhorn D, Garvey WT, Grunberger G, Handelsman Y, Hirsch IB, Jellinger PS, McGill JB, Mechanick JI, Rosenblit PD, Umpierrez G, Davidson MH.AACE Comprehensive DiabetesManagement Algorithm 2013.*Endocr.Pract.*2013 Mar-Apr;19(2):327-36.

Giugliano F, Maiorino MI, Bellastella G, Autorino R, De SioM, Giugliano D, Esposito K. Adherence to Mediterranean dietand erectile dysfunction in men with type 2 Diabetes. *J. Sex Med.*2010;7:1911–7.

Goldstein I, Young JM, Fischer J, Bangerter K, Segerson T, Taylor T, Vardenafil Diabetes Study Group. Vardenafil, a new phosphodiesterase type 5 inhibitor, in the treatment of erectile dysfunction in men with diabetes: a multicenter double-blind placebo-controlled fixed-dose study. *Diabetes Care*.2003;26:777-783.

Goldstein I, Jones LA, Belkoff LH, Karlin GS, Bowden CH, Peterson CA, Trask BA, Day WW. Avanafil for the treatment of erectile dysfunction: a multicenter, randomized, double-blind study in men with diabetes mellitus.*Mayo.Clin. Proc.* 2012 Sep;87(9):843-52.

Grover-Páez F, Villegas Rivera G, Guillén Ortíz R. Sildenafil citrate diminishes microalbuminuria and the percentage of A1c in male patients with type 2diabetes.*Diabetes Res. Clin.Pract.* 2007 Oct;78(1):136-40.

Hakim LS, Goldstein I. Diabetic sexual dysfunction.*Endocrinol.Metab.Clin.North Am.* 1996; 25: 379–400.

Hatzichristou D, Montorsi F, Buvat J, Laferriere N, Bandel TJ, Porst H, European Vardenafil Study Group. The efficacy and safety of flexible-dose vardenafil (levitra) in a broad population of European men.*Eur. Urol.*2004;45:634-641.

Hatzimouratidis K, Hatzichristou DG. A comparative review of the options for treatment of erectile dysfunction: which treatment for which patient? *Drugs* 2005;65:1621–50.

Hecht MJ, Neundorfer B, Kiesewetter F et al. Neuropathy is a major contributing factor to diabetic erectile dysfunction. *Neurol. Res.* 2001; 23: 651–4.

Hellstrom WJ, Gittelman M, Karlin G, et al. Vardenafil for treatment of men with erectile dysfunction: efficacy and safety in a randomized, doubleblind, placebo-controlled trial. *J. Androl.* 2002;23:763-771.

Hidalgo-Tamola J, and Chitaley K. Type 2 diabetes mellitus and erectile dysfunction.*J. SexMed.*2009;6:916–926.

Incrocci L, Slob AK, Hop WC. Tadalafi l (Cialis) and erectile dysfunction after radiotherapy for prostate cancer: an open-label extension of a blinded trial. Urology, 2007;70:1190–3.

InternationalDiabetesFederation, IDF Diabetes atlas, 11th edition, 2011.

Inzucchi SE, Bergenstal RM, Buse JB, Diamant M, Ferrannini E, Nauck M, Peters AL, Tsapas A, Wender R, Matthews DR. Management of hyperglycaemia in type 2 diabetes: a patient-centered approach. Positionstatement of the American Diabetes Association (ADA) and the European Association for the Study of Diabetes (EASD).*Diabetologia.* 2012Jun;55(6):1577-96 and *Diabetes Care.* 2012Jun;35(6):1364-79.

Jarow JP. Risk factors for penile prosthetic infection.*J. Urol.* 1996;156(2 Pt 1):402–4.

Jesmin S, Sakuma I, Salah-Eldin A, Nonomura K,Hattori Y, Kitabatake A. Diminished penile expressionof vascular endothelial growth factor and itsreceptors at the insulin-resistant stage of a type IIdiabetic rat model: a possible cause for erectile dysfunctionin diabetes. *J. Mol. Endocrinol.* 2003;31:401–18.

Jevtich MJ, Khawand NY, Vidic B. Clinical significance of ultrastructural findings in the corpora cavernosa of normal and impotent men.*J. Urol.* 1990; 143:289–93.

Johannes CB, Araujo AB, Feldman HA, et al. Incidence of erectile dysfunction in men 40 to 69 yearsold: longitudinal results from the Massachusetts Male Aging Study. *J. Urol.*2000;163:460.

Kadioglu A, Oktar T, Kandirali E et al. Incidentally diagnosed Peyronie's disease in men presenting with erectile dysfunction. *Int. J. Impot. Res.* 2004;16:540–3.

Kamenov Z, Christov V, Yankova T. Erectile dysfunction in diabetic men - linked more to microangiopathic complications and neuropathy than to macroangiopathic disturbances. *Journal of Men's Health and Gender*; 2007; 4(1):64-73.

Kamenov Z, Higashino H, Todorova M, Kajimoto N, Suzuki A. Physiological characteristics of diabetic neuropathy in sucrose-fed Otsuka Long-Evans Tokushima fatty rats.*Methods Find Exp Clin Pharmacol.* 2006 Jan-Feb;28(1):13-8.

Kamenov Z. Comparison of the first intake of vardenafil and tadalafil in patients with diabetic neuropathy and diabetic erectile dysfunction.*JSM,* 2011;8(3):851–864.

Kamenov ZA, Petrova JJ, Christov VG. Diagnosis of diabetic neuropathy using simple somatic and a new autonomic (neuropad) tests in the clinical practice.*Exp. Clin.Endocrinol.Diabetes.* 2010 Apr;118(4):226-33.

Kamenov ZA, Traykov LD. Diabetic autonomic neuropathy. Adv Exp Med Biol. 2012;771:176-93.

Kamenov ZA, Traykov LD. Diabetic somaticneuropathy.*Adv. Exp. Med. Biol.* 2012b;771:155-75.

Kang SG, Kim JJ. Udenafil: efficacy and tolerability in the management of erectile dysfunction.*Ther. Adv. Urol.* 2013 Apr;5(2):101-10.

Kawano K, Hirashima T, Mori S, Saitoh Y, KurosumiM, Natori T. Spontaneous long-term yperglycemicrat with diabetic complications.OtsukaLong-Evans Tokushima Fatty (OLETF) strain.*Diabetes* 1992;41:1422–8.

Khan MA, Thompson CS, Jeremy JY et al.The effect of superoxide dismutase on nitric oxide-mediated and electrical field-stimulated diabetic rabbit cavernosal smooth muscle relaxation.*BJU Int*;2001; 87: 98–103.

Klein R, Klein BE, Moss SE. Ten-year incidence of self-reported erectile dysfunction in people withlong-term type 1 diabetes.*J. Diabetes Compl.* 2005;19:35.

Levine LA, Dimitriou RJ. Vacuum constriction and external erection devices in erectile dysfunction.*Urol. Clin. North Am.* 2001;28:335–41 [ix-x]

Lewis RW. Epidemiology of erectile dysfunction. Urol Clin North Am 2001; 28: 209–16.

Lin C-S, Ho H-C, Chen K-C, Lin G, Nunes L & Lue TF. Intracavernosal injection of vascular endothelial growth factor induces nitric oxide synthase isoforms. *BJU International* 2002;89:955–960.

Lu C-C, Jiann B-P, Sun C-C, Lam H-C, Chu C-H, Lee J-K.Association ofglycemic control with risk of erectile dysfunction in men with type 2 diabetes.*J. Sex Med.* 2009;6:1719–1728.

Lu YL, Shen ZJ, Wang H et al. Ultrastructural changes of penile tunica albuginea in diabetic rats.*Asian J. Androl.*2004; 6: 365–8.

Malavige LS, and Levy JC. Erectile dysfunction in diabetes mellitus.*J. Sex Med.* 2009;6:1232–1247.

Malavige LS, Jayaratne SD, Kathriarachchi ST, Sivayogan S, Fernando DJ, Levy JC. Erectile dysfunction among men with diabetes is strongly associated with premature ejaculation and reduced libido. *J. Sex Med.* 2008 Sep;5(9):2125-34.

Martin-Morales, A., J.J.Sanchez-Cruz, I.Saenz de Tejada et al. Prevalence and independent risk factors for erectile dysfunction in Spain: results of the Epidemiologia de la Disfuncion Erectil Masculina Study. *J. Urol.* 2001 Aug;166(2):569-74.

McMahon C. Efficacy and safety of daily tadalafil in men with erectile dysfunction previously unresponsive to on-demand tadalafil.*J. Sex Med.* 2004;1: 292–300.

Meuleman EJ, Eardley I, Rosen R, Fisher W, Niederberger C, Sand M. Attitudes toward treatment of erectile dysfunction: results from the MALES (Men's Attitudes toward Life Events and Sexuality) study. Presented at: Annual Meeting of the Asian Pacific Society of Sexual and Impotence Research; Cebu, Philippines; October 1-4, 2003.

Ming XF, Viswambharan H, Barandier C et al. Rho GTPase/Rho kinase negatively regu- lates endothelial nitric oxide synthase phosphorylation through the inhibition of protein kinase B/Akt in human endothelial cells.*Mol. Cell Biol.* 2002; 22: 8467–77.

Montague DK, Angermeier KW, Lakin MM. Penile prosthesis infections.*Int. J. Impot. Res.* 2001;13:326–8.

Montorsi F, Hellstrom WJ, Valiquette L, et al, North American and European Vardenafil Groups. Vardenafil provides reliable efficacy over time in men with erectile dysfunction. *Urology.*2004;64:1187-1195.

Montorsi P, Montorsi F, Schulman CC. Is erectile dysfunction the ''tip of the iceberg'' of a systemic vascular disorder? *Eur. Urol.* 2003;44(3):352–4.

Moon du G, Yang DY, Lee CH, Ahn TY, Min KS, Park K, Park JK, Kim JJ.A therapeutic confirmatory study to assess the safety and efficacy of Zydena (udenafil) for the treatment of erectile dysfunction in male patients with diabetes mellitus.*J. Sex Med.* 2011 Jul;8(7):2048-61.

Moore CR, Wang R. Pathophysiology and treatment of diabetic erectile dysfunction. *Asian J. Androl.* 2006;8:675–84.

Mulligan T, Frick MF, Zuraw QC et al. Prevalence of hypogonadism in males aged at least 45 years: the HIM study. *Int. J. Clin.Pract.* 2006 Jul;60(7):762-9.

Musicki B, Palese MA, Crone JK, Burnett AL.Phosphorylated endothelial nitric oxide synthasemediates vascular endothelial growth factor-inducedpenile erection. *Biol. Reprod* 2004;70:282–9.

National Intelligence Council. Global trends 2025: *A Transformed World.* 2008.

Ng KK, Lim HC, Ng FC et al.The use of sildenafil in patients with erectile dysfunction in relation to diabetes mellitus—a study of 1,511 patients.*Singapore Med. J.* 2002;43:387–90.

Nieschlag E, Swerdloff R, Behre HM, Gooren LJ, Kaufman JM, Legros JJ, Lunenfeld B, Morley JE, Schulman C, Wang C, Weidner W, Wu FC. Investigation, treatment, and monitoring of late-onset hypogonadism in males: ISA, ISSAM, and EAU recommendations. *J. Androl.* 2006 Mar-Apr;27(2):135-7.

Nofzinger EA. Sexual Dysfunction in Patients with Diabetes Mellitus: The Role of a "Central" Neuropathy. *Semin.Clin.Neuropsychiatry.* 1997 Jan;2(1):31-39.

Padma-Nathan H. Efficacy and tolerability of tadalafil, a novel phosphodiesterase 5 inhibitor, in treatment of erectile dysfunction.*Am. J. Cardiol.* 2003;92:19M–25M.

Papapetropoulos A, García-Cardeña G, Madri JA & Sessa WC Nitric oxide production contributes to the angiogenic properties ofvascular endothelial growth factor in human endothelial cells.*Journal of Clinical Investigation* 1997;100:3131–39.

Park HJ, Choi HK, Ahn TY, Park JK, Chung WS, Lee SW, Kim SW, Hyun JS, Park NC. Efficacy and safety of oral mirodenafil in the treatment of erectile dysfunction in diabetic men in Korea: a multicenter, randomized, double-blind, placebo-controlled clinical trial. *J. Sex Med.* 2010 Aug;7(8):2842-50.

Park JK, Lee SO, Kim YG et al. Role of rho-kinase activity in angiotensin II-induced contraction of rabbit clitoral cavernosum smooth muscle.*Int. J. Impot.Res.* 2002; 14: 472–7.

Penson DF, Latini DM, Lubeck DP, Wallace KL,Henning JM, Lue TF. Do impotent men with diabeteshave more severe erectile dysfunction andworse quality of life than the general population ofimpotent patients? Results from the ExploratoryComprehensive Evaluation of Erectile Dysfunction(ExCEED) database.*Diabetes Care* 2003;26:1093–9.

Phé V, Rouprêt M. Erectile dysfunction and diabetes: a review of the current evidence-based medicine and a synthesis of the main available therapies. *Diabetes Metab.* 2012 Feb;38(1):1-13.

Porst H, Rajfer J, Casabй A, et al. Long-term safety and effi cacy of tadalafil 5 mg dosed once daily in men with erectile dysfunction. *J. Sex. Med.,* 2008;Sep;5(9):2160-9.

Porst H, Rosen R, Padma-Nathan H, et al. The efficacy and tolerability of vardenafil, a new, oral, selective phosphodiesterase type 5 inhibitor, in patients with erectile dysfunction: the first at-home clinical trial. *Int. J. Impot. Res.*2001;13:192-199.

Porst HJB (ed.) Standard practice in sexual medicine.1st edition. Oxford: Blackwell; 2007

Potempa AJ, Ulbrich E, Bernard I, Beneke M, Vardenafil Study Group. Efficacy of vardenafil in men with erectile dysfunction: a flexible-dose community practice study. *Eur. Urol.*2004;46:73-79.

Price D, Hackett G. Management of erectile dysfunction in diabetes: an update for 2008. *Curr.Diab. Rep.* 2008 Dec;8(6):437-43.

Price DE, Cooksey G, Jehu D, Bentley S, Hearnshaw JR, Osborn DE.The management of impotence in diabetic men by vacuum tumescence therapy.*Diabet Med.* 1991;8:964–7.

Rees RW, Ziessen T, Ralph DJ et al. Human and rabbit cavernosal smooth muscle cells express Rho-kinase. *Int. J. Impot. Res.;*2002; 14: 1–7.

Rendell MS, Rajfer J, Wicker PA, Smith MD. Sildenafil fortreatment of erectile dysfunction in men with diabetes: a randomizedcontrolled trial. Sildenafil Diabetes Study Group.*JAMA* 1999; 281: 421–6.

Rhoden EL, Teloken C, Ting HY et al. Prevalence of Peyronie's disease in men over 50-year-old from Southern Brazil. *Int. J. Impot. Res.* 2001;13:291–3.

Rosen RC, A.Riley, G.Wagner, I.H.Osterloh , J.Kirkpatrick, A.Mishra. The international index of erectile function (IIEF): a multidimensional scale for assessment of erectile function. *Urology.* 1997;49:822-830.

Ryan JG. Cost and policy implications from the increasing prevalence of obesity and diabetes mellitus.*Gender Medicine,* 2009;6(1):86-108.

Saenz de Tejada I, Anglin G, Knight JR, Emmick JT. Effects of tadalafil on erectile dysfunction in men with diabetes. *Diabetes Care* 2002;25:2159–64.

Saenz de Tejada I, Emmick J, Anglin G et al. The effect of IC351 taken as needed for treatment of erectile dysfunction in men with diabetes. Eur Urol 2001a; 39: 16,abstract 55.

Safarinejad MR. Oral sildenafil in the treatment of erectiledysfunctionin diabetic men: a randomized double-blind andplacebo-controlled study. *J. Diabetes Complications* 2004;18: 205–10.

Schulman CC, W.Shen, D.R.Stothard et al. Integrated analysis examining first-dose success, success by dose, and maintenance of success among men taking tadalafil for erectile dysfunction.*Urology.* 2004;Oct;64(4):783-8.

Schwarzer U, Sommer F, Klotz T et al. The prevalence of Peyronie's disease: Results of a large survey. *BJU Int.* 2001;88:727–30.

Seftel AD, Vaziri ND, Ni Z et al. Advanced glycation end products in human penis: elevation in diabetic tissue, site of deposition, and possible effect through iNOS oreNOS. *Urology* 1997; 50: 1016–26.

Sheehy AM, Phung YT, Riemer RK & Black SM Growthfactor induction of nitric oxide synthase in rat pheochromocytomacells. *Molecular Brain Research* 1997;52:71–77.

Siddiqui MA, Ahmed Z, Khan AA. Psychological Impact on Sexual Health among Diabetic Patients: A Review. International Journal of Diabetes Research 2012, 1(2): 28-31.

Sidi AA, Becher EF, Zhang G, Lewis JH. Patient acceptance of and satisfaction with an external negative pressure device for impotence.*J. Urol.* 1990;144:1154–6.

Sima AAF, Ristic H, Merry A et al. The primary preventional and secondary in-terventative effects of acetyl-L-carnitine on diabetic neuropathy in the BB/W-rat. *J. Clin. Invest.* 1996;97:1900-7.

Singh R, Barden A, Mori T et al. Advanced glycation end-products: a review. *Diabetologia* 2001a; 44: 129–46.

Smith AD. Causes and classification of impotence.*Urol. Clin.North.Am.* 1981; 8: 79–89.

Stuckey BG, Jadzinsky MN, Murphy LJ, Montorsi F,Kadioglu A, Fraige F, Manzano P, Deerochanawong C.Sildenafil citrate for treatment oferectile dysfunction in men with type 1 diabetes: results of arandomized controlled trial. *Diabetes Care* 2003; 26: 279–84.

Teerlink JR, Breu V, Sprecher U et al. Potent vasoconstriction mediated by endothelin ETB receptors in canine coronary arteries. *Circ. Res.* 1994; 74: 105–14.

Tefekli A, Kandirali E, Erol B et al. Peyronie's disease: A silent consequence of diabetes mellitus. *Asian J. Androl.* 2006;8:75–9.

Tesfaye S, Stevens LK, Stephenson JM, et al. Prevalence of diabetic peripheral neuropathy and its relation to glycaemic control and potential risk factors: the EURODIAB IDDM Complications Study. *Diabetologia.* 1996;39:1377-84.

Traish A, Kim N. The physiological role of androgens in penile erection: regulation of corpus cavernosum structure and function. *J. Sex Med.* 2005 Nov;2(6):759-70.

Tsertsvadze A, Fink HA, Yazdi F, MacDonald R, Bella AJ, Ansari MT, Garritty C, Soares-Weiser K, Daniel R, Sampson M, Fox S, Moher D, Wilt TJ. Oral phosphodiesterase-5 inhibitors and hormonal treatments for erectile dysfunction: a systematic review and meta-analysis. *Ann. Intern. Med.* 2009 Nov 3;151(9):650-61.

Usta MF, Bivalacqua TJ, Yang DY et al. The protective effect of aminoguanidine on erectile function in streptozotocin diabetic rats.*J. Urol.*2003; 170: 1437–42.

Valiquette L, Young JM, Moncada I et al. Sustained efficacy and safety of vardenafil for treatment of erectile dysfunction: a randomized, double-blind, placebo-controlled study. *Mayo.Clin.Proc.* 2005; 80: 1291–7.

Vardi M, Nini A. Phosphodiesterase inhibitors for erectile dysfunction in patients with diabetes mellitus. *Cochrane Database Syst. Rev.* 2007 Jan 24;(1):CD002187.

Vardi Y, Sprecher E, Gruenwald I. Logistic regression and survival analysis of 450 impotent patients treated with injection therapy: long-term dropout parameters. *J. Urol.* 2000;163:467–70.

Vickers MA, Wright EA. Erectile dysfunction in the patient with diabetes mellitus. *Am. J. Manag. Care* 2004; 10 (1 Suppl): S3–11.

Vignozzi L, Morelli A, Filippi S, Ambrosini S, Mancina R, Luconi M, Mungai S, Vannelli GB, Zhang XH, Forti G, Maggi M. Testosterone regulates RhoA/Rho-kinase signaling in two distinct animal models of chemical diabetes. *J. Sex Med.* 2007;4(3):620-30.

Vinik A, Richardson D. Erectile dysfunction in diabetes. *Diabetes Rev.;*1998;6:16–33.

Vinik AI, Holland MT, Le Beau JM, Liuzzi FJ, Stansberry KB, Colen LB. Diabetic neuropathies. *Diabetes Care.* 1992;15:1926-75;

Wallis RM, Corbin JD, Francis SH et al. Tissue distribution of phosphodiesterase families and the effects of sildenafil on tissue cyclic nucleotides, platelet function, and the contractile responses of trabeculae carneae and aortic rings in vitro. *Am. J. Cardiol.* 1999;83:3C–12C.

Wang C, Nieschlag E, Swerdloff R, Behre HM, Hellstrom WJ, Gooren LJ, Kaufman JM, Legros JJ, Lunenfeld B, Morales A, Morley JE, Schulman C, Thompson IM, Weidner W, Wu FC; International Society of Andrology (ISA); International Society for the Study of Aging Male (ISSAM); European Association of Urology (EAU); European Academy of Andrology (EAA); American Society of Andrology (ASA). Investigation, treatment, and monitoring of late-onset hypogonadism in males: ISA, ISSAM, EAU, EAA, and ASA recommendations. *J. Androl.* 2009 Jan-Feb;30(1):1-9.

Wang H, Eto M, Steers WD et al. RhoA-mediated Ca2+ sensitization in erectile function.*J. Biol. Chem.* 2002; 277: 30614–21.

Wilson SK, Carson CC, Cleves MA, Delk JR2nd. Quantifying risk of penile prosthesis infection with elevated glycosylated haemoglobin.*J. Urol.* 1998;159:1537–9 [discussion 1539–40].

Wilson SK, Delk JR2nd. Inflatable penile implant infection: predisposing factors and treatment suggestions. *J. Urol.*1995;153(3 Pt 1):659–61.

Wing RR, Rosen RC, Fava JL, Bahnson J, Brancati F, Gendrano INC, Kitabchi A, SchneiderSH, and Wadden TA. Effects of weight loss intervention on erectile function in older men with type 2diabetes in the look AHEAD trial.*J. Sex. Med* 2010;7:156–165.

Yagihashi S, Yamagishi S, Wada R. Pathology and pathogenetic mechanisms of diabetic neuropathy: Correlation with clinical signs and symptoms. *Diabetes Res. Clin.Pract.* 2007;77(1 suppl):S184–9.

Yan SF, Ramasamy R, Schmidt AM. Mechanisms of disease: advanced glycation end-products and their receptor in inflammation and diabetes complications. *Nat. Clin.Pract.Endocrinol.Metab.* 2008;4:285–93.

Young MJ, Boulton AJM, McLeod AF, Williams DRR, Sonksen PH: A multicentre study of the prevalence of diabetic peripheral neuropathy in the UK hospital clinic population. *Diabetologia*, 1993, 36:150–156.

In: Sexual Dysfunctions
Editor: Frédérique Courtois

ISBN: 978-1-62808-765-9
© 2013 Nova Science Publishers, Inc.

Chapter 9

EFFECTIVE TREATMENT OF MAJOR DEPRESSION AND ACCOMPANYING SEXUAL DYSFUNCTION

*Louis F. Fabre and Louis C. Smith**

Fabre Kramer Pharmaceuticals, Inc., Houston, TX, US

ABSTRACT

Currently the treatment of Major Depression Disorder is in disarray. Only 30% of treated subjects attain remission, with another 30% receiving some benefit and 40% receiving no benefit at all. Prior to treatment, 70-80% of depressed subjects have significant sexual dysfunction. Although it is known that sexual dysfunction is common in major depression, current treatments of depression do not improve sexual function. In fact, the Serotonin Reuptake Inhibitors (SSRIs) and the Serotonin Norepinephrine Reuptake Inhibitors (SNRIs) further compromise sexual function. Studies claim that, should sexual dysfunction occur with SSRIs, up to 90% of depressed subjects receiving these drugs will discontinue treatment. Further, it is claimed that the sexual dysfunction created by SSRIs and SNRIs continues after the drugs are stopped and may become a permanent dysfunction. We believe it is time to revise the concept of major depression and its treatment. The DSM-IV requires 5 of 9 symptoms to diagnose a major depressive episode. Sexual dysfunction is not among these 9 symptoms. Sexual dysfunction is an integral part of major depression and must be diagnosed and treated to achieve effective treatment of major depression. Historically, physicians have not been concerned with (or aware of) sexual dysfunction. The problem has been that to date there have been no approved pharmacologic treatments or combinations of treatments that will achieve effective relief of sexual dysfunction. Over the past 20 years we have been working on the development of gepirone-ER, a drug that does treat both major depression and the accompanying sexual dysfunction. Gepirone-ER is a 5-HT$_{1A}$ partial agonist not an SSRI. In two registrational studies of gepirone-ER in major depression, statistically significant antidepressant improvement was noted as measured by the Hamilton Rating Scale for Depression. Further, statistically significant improvement was found in sexual function as measured by the Derogatis Inventory of Sexual Function (DISF) for total score as well as the domains for desire and orgasm. Gepirone-ER appears to improve sexual function by

---

* Corresponding author: Louis F Fabre MD PhD, Fabre Kramer Pharmaceuticals, Inc. Houston TX USA, Email: lfabre@fabrekramer.com.

three mechanisms: a prosexual effect, and antidepressant effect, and an anxiolytic effect. Improvement in both depression and sexual dysfunction are not only statistically but also clinically significant. The concept of the treatment of major depression must be changed. The physician must understand, diagnose, and treat all the symptoms of major depression including sexual dysfunction. Gepirone-ER would seem to be the first pharmacologic agent capable of adequate treatment.

INTRODUCTION

Antidepressants were the third-most common drugs used by Americans of all ages between 2005 and 2008 and they were the most common drugs among people aged 18 to 44, according to an analysis by the U.S. Centers for Disease Control and Prevention's National Center for Health Statistics (1). Antidepressant use in the United States jumped nearly 400 percent in the 2005-2008 survey period compared with the 1988-1994 period, with 11 percent of those over age 12 taking the drugs. U.S. women are 2-1/2 times more likely than men to take antidepressants, and whites are more likely than blacks to take the drugs [1].

However, According to STAR*D (Sequenced Treatment Alternatives to Relieve Depression) data, a study designed to measure the effectiveness of antidepressants, only 30% of depressed subjects reach remission after treatment with an antidepressant [2]. Possible reasons for this poor performance are the following. Antidepressants work best in severe depression; most subjects have mild to moderate depression; antidepressants have adverse effects such as sexual dysfunction, weight gain, and interference with sleep. Any of these adverse events may cause the subject to discontinue treatment. Antidepressants can interfere with concomitant medications or vice versa. Antidepressants can cause birth defects causing women to be reluctant to use them. Finally, antidepressants can take up to a month to have an effect.

It is common knowledge that loss of interest in sex or some other sexual dysfunction occurs in patients with depression [3-23]. However, this knowledge seems to be lost in the evaluation, diagnosis, and treatment of depressive illnesses. Physicians rarely ask patients complaining of depression about sexual function [24, 25] and patients are reluctant to provide such information.

Depressive illnesses are syndromes diagnosed by DSM-IV (Diagnostic and Statistical Manual Forth ed.) by the presence of symptoms. For major depressive disorder [26], the presence of 5 of 9 identified symptoms is necessary for diagnosis according to DSM-IV. The 9 symptoms in brief are: depressed mood, loss of interest in activities, weight loss, insomnia or hypersomnia, agitation or retardation, loss of energy, worthlessness, or guilt, diminished ability to concentrate, and recurrent thoughts of death. Sexual dysfunction is not represented in this group of symptoms, unless it is subsumed in loss of interest (which would be one form of sexual dysfunction).

Rarely has sexual dysfunction been measured by appropriate rating scales prior to treatment and improvement or lack of improvement after treatment has not been routinely measured by appropriate rating scales [27].

However, recent studies have shown that sexual dysfunction is present in 70-80% of depressed subjects [13, 27-29]. Failure of physicians to recognize this prior to treatment may be due to the fact that up until now physicians had no way to improve sexual dysfunction. In fact, most common treatments of depression make sexual dysfunction worse. SSRIs cause further sexual dysfunction in 40-70% of subjects [30-33]. Ninety per cent of subjects experiencing this sexual dysfunction will prematurely discontinue the drug [34]. But the sexual dysfunction may continue long after the discontinuation and may even be permanent [35].

When the SSRIs were introduced with Prozac (fluoxetine), it was known that efficacy treating depression was not better than the tricyclics [36, 37]. However, the SSRIs were judged to be safer although, at the time, the profound negative effect on sexual function was not appreciated. Considering the effect on sexual function, perhaps the SSRIs are not really safer.

If the sexual dysfunction present with depression prior to treatment is appreciated and antidepressants do not treat this symptom, what current treatment could improve sexual dysfunction? Historically, sexual steroid hormones have been the treatment of sexual dysfunction, with testosterone used successfully in both men and women [38]. However the possibility of increase risk of cancer with steroid hormones concerns both physicians and patients [39]. There are no FDA approved testosterone preparations for women.

While the PDE5 inhibitors have been successful in men to aid erections, they do nothing for desire and orgasm and have not been found useful in women [40].

There is a great medical need for a drug that improves sexual dysfunction in both men and women. Flibanserin showed promise as a drug to improve sexual performance [41]. However, it was not approved by the FDA although it may be under reconsideration [42].

Gepirone-ER was originally designed as an antidepressant [43, 44]. While gepirone-ER is not currently approved in any country for any indication, not only does it have antidepressant activity, it improves sexual activity.

Progress in finding treatments for sexual dysfunctions rely heavily on the methods by which sexual dysfunction is measured. Several rating scales have been devised. A critical issue is the measurement of sexual dysfunction in a normal population. The only rating scale which has proven adequate in this area is the Derogatis Inventory of Sexual Function (DISF) [45, 46]. The DISF has advantages to other scales in that it has norms for a normal non-patient population. Figure 1 depicts the contrast between the normal population and the depressed population. As may be seen the depressed population has much poorer sexual function with little overlap with the non-patient population.

METHODS

Five short term (8 week) studies (134001, 134002, 134004, 134006, FKGBE007) were conducted from 2000 - 2006 in 32 US research sites, funded by Organon. Prior to any study related activity, each subject signed an informed consent that had been approved by an Institutional Review Board. The trials were conducted in compliance with the current revision of the Declaration of Helsinki, International Committee on Harmonization (ICH) guidelines; Good Clinical Practice (GCP), and current regulatory requirements. The data analyses and report writing were done by Fabre-Kramer Pharmaceuticals.

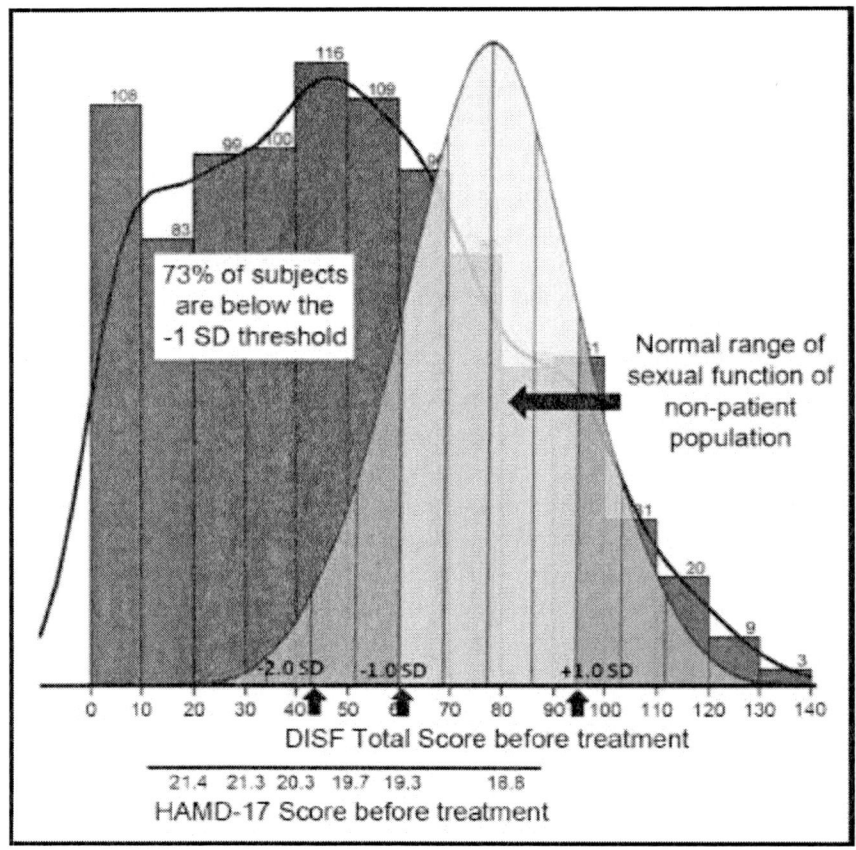

Figure 1. Close Relationship between Severity of Depression and Severity of Sexual Dysfunction.

Each of the 32 sites had one primary psychiatrist rater and one psychiatrist back up. Prior to initiation of the trial an investigator's meeting was held during which the psychiatrists were trained to evaluate sexual function (except 2 studies where only a self rating was used, and one study in which no sexual function data was collected).

Inclusion criteria for all 5 studies included a primary diagnosis of recurrent major depressive disorder (DSM-IV 296.3) [47]. Subjects were at least 18 years and not older than 70 years of age. Three studies involved subjects with classic major depressive disorder (weight loss, poor appetite, insomnia, etc) and two studies were in subjects with atypical depression (ADD) (increased weight, increased appetite, and hypersomnia). The severity of depression was measured by the Hamilton Rating Scale for Depression (HAMD-17). Screening and baseline HAMD-17 score were to be greater than or equal to 18, except for the 2 studies in ADD, for which there were no HAMD-17 entry criteria.

In the 2 studies for those with Atypical Features, the presence of Atypical Features Specifier according to the DSM-IV criteria was assessed using the Atypical Depression Diagnostic Scale (ADDS) [48] administered at baseline. To fulfill atypical depression criteria, subjects must maintain mood reactivity while depressed and have at least 2 of the following features: long standing interpersonal rejection sensitivity, weight gain/increased appetite, hypersomnia, and leaden paralysis.

Exclusion criteria consisted of a history of treatment refractory depression, a history of seizure disorder or bipolar disorder, use of illicit drugs or alcohol abuse, significant suicidal risk (according to the investigator), renal, hepatic, cardiovascular, respiratory, cerebrovascular, or other serious, progressive physical disease and/or clinically meaningful abnormal laboratory findings identified at screening. The exclusion criteria required that subjects be off all psychotropic medications from 2 to 4 weeks prior to the baseline evaluation.

In these 5 short-term (8 week) studies, baseline evaluations included psychiatric evaluation including Hamilton Depression Rating Scale [49], physical examination, clinical laboratory, and electrocardiogram evaluations [50]. Patients taking concomitant medications were excluded, as were those with positive medical, laboratory, or electrocardiogram findings. Although sexual dysfunction was not an entry criterion, sexual function was measured using the DISF or DISF-SR (self report) [46] at baseline and each subsequent clinic visit.

The studies were double blind randomized, placebo controlled studies of gepirone-ER (40 - 80 mg/day) in patients with depressive illnesses. Two of the studies also had selective serotonin reuptake inhibitor (SSRI) controls, either fluoxetine 20 – 40 mg/day or paroxetine 10-40 mg/day. Subjects meeting entry criteria were randomized in a double-blind fashion to treatment with placebo, gepirone-ER, or an SSRI. For all three drugs medication was initiated at the lowest dose given once daily in the morning and escalated over a two-week period.

At each clinic visit after randomization (weeks 2, 4, 8, or end of treatment EOT), depressive symptoms were measured by the HAMD-31 allowing calculation of the HAMD-17 and HAMD-25. The HAMD-25 includes items regarding atypical depression. Secondary efficacy measures included the MADRS (Montgomery-Åsberg Depression Rating Scale (a more modern depression rating scale) [51], the Bech 6 (a measure of core antidepressant symptoms) [52], and the HAMD item 1 (a measure of depressed mood).

The DISF has been normed to the general non-patient population [46, 47] and the number of subjects below one standard deviation has been used as an indication of sexual dysfunction.

The primary efficacy parameter was change from baseline in the HAMD-17 or HAMD-25 total score at endpoint. A HAMD-17 or HAMD-25 responder is defined as a subject who has a score of 50% or more decrease from baseline level. A non-responder did not decrease at least 50%.

HAMD item 12 psychic anxiety was used to determine anxiety responders and non-responders. This item is scored: 0, no difficulty; 1, subjective tension and irritability; 2, worrying about minor matters; 3, apprehensive attitude apparent in face or speech; and 4, fears expressed without questioning. An anxiolytic responder is defined as a subject who scores 0 or 1 after treatment at endpoint and an anxiolytic non-responder as a subject who has a 2, 3, or 4 at endpoint.

The analyses of continuous variables were done by a one way analysis of variance (ANOVA) of the SAS database by a JMP-7.02 program, with means compared by t-test. Categorical data were analyzed with an odds ratio program.

In the studies with sexual function questionnaires, the protocol specified that the results would be analyzed but failed to indicate what kind of analyses would be performed. For this reason, many of the results of these analyses can be considered post-hoc. Eight individual analyses are presented.

A. The Distribution of Sexual Function in Normal and Major Depression Subjects

In a population of 1085 depressed subjects, the presence of sexual dysfunction was defined as those subjects 1 standard deviation or more below the mean of the DISF total score of the normal non-patient population.

B. Percent of Subjects with DSM-IV Specified Symptoms Indicating Depression and Sexual Dysfunction

In a population of 1791 subjects, major depression was diagnosed by DSM-IV criteria. The presence or absence of each of the 9 symptoms was indicated. The DISF total score, one standard deviation or more below normal, identified subjects with sexual dysfunction.

C. The Effect of Fluoxetine on Sexual Function: When to Use SSRIs

The effect of fluoxetine on sexual function as measured by the DISF was determined in a double blind placebo controlled trial in which fluoxetine was the comparator. The DISF at baseline was stratified by ½ standard deviation (SD) increments and the negative effect of fluoxetine was quantified.

D. The Effect of Gepirone-ER on Antidepressant Efficacy Measures

The effect of gepirone-ER treatment of depressive symptoms was measured in the 5 studies. The primary efficacy parameter was the HAMD17 or HAMD-25. Secondary efficacy parameters included MADRS, Bech 6 core depression items, and HAMD item 1 – depressed mood.

E. The Effect of Gepirone-ER on Sexual Function Symptoms in Major Depression Compared to Fluoxetine and Placebo

Of the 5 studies, 4 had sexual function measures and only two had comparator SSRI treatment groups. The DISF total score is made up of 5 domain scores: arousal, behavior, desire, drive, and orgasm.

F. The Effect of Gepirone-ER on Depression in Groups of Depressed Subjects with Differing Levels of Sexual Dysfunction at Baseline

Sexual dysfunction at baseline was defined as 1 or more standard deviations below normal. In study 134001, a study that had positive antidepressant activity, the effect gepirone-

ER on sexual dysfunction at baseline was studied by stratifying the DISF into ½ (SD) increments.

G. The Effect of Gepirone-ER on Sexual Function in Subjects with and without Sexual Dysfunction at Baseline

The effect of gepirone-ER was measured in subjects with sexual dysfunction at baseline and in those without. The effect of gepirone-ER on sexual function was measured in patient groups stratified by baseline sexual dysfunction by ½ SD increments.

H. Gepirone-ER Antidepressant and Anxiolytic Effects on Sexual Function

In one study 134006, the effect of gepirone-ER on the DISF domain for desire was measured. This group was then subdivided into those who were and were not HAMD-25 responders and those who were or were not HAMD item 12 (psychic anxiety) responders or non responders.

I. Clinical Significance of Treatment with Gepirone-ER

In two studies, 134001 and 134004, the results for gepirone-ER and fluoxetine (134004) for antidepressant and sexual function activity are superimposed on the normal distribution chart for depressive symptoms and the DISF.

RESULTS

A. The Distribution of Sexual Function in Normal and Major Depression Subjects

In the Figure 1 below the Gaussian curve (light gray) indicates the distribution of DISF total score results for a normal population [46, 47]. The lighter areas represent the DISF scores for the subjects with major depression. As may be seen, 73% of depressed subjects have DISF scores one standard deviation or more below normal. For HAMD-17 scores of these subjects, the difference between normal sexual function (18.8) and sexual dysfunction (-2 standard deviations below normal) (20.3) is less than 2 points at baseline.

B. Percent of subjects with DSM-IV specified symptoms indicating depression or sexual dysfunction

The results presented in Table 1 indicate that almost all depressed subjects have symptoms of depressed mood, loss of interest in activities, insomnia or hypersomnia, fatigue, worthlessness, and diminished ability to think. Three symptoms, however, did not occur for all depressed patients. The percentage of patients with weight loss or gain was 58%, psychomotor agitation 69.8%, and recurrent thoughts of death 39.5%.

Sexual dysfunction, diagnosed as at least one standard deviation below normal, is present in 73% of subjects with major depression. While not universally ascribed to, sexual dysfunction is present more often than weight issues, agitation, or thoughts of death.

It must be concluded that sexual dysfunction is an integral part of major depression and that it should be evaluated and treated in the course of adequate treatment of depression.

Table 1. Percent Positive Symptoms for Diagnosis of Major Depression

Study	Percent of all depressed subjects (n = 1791)								
	Depressed mood	Loss of Interest	Weight change	Sleep change	Agitation	Fatigue	Worthlessness	Diminished ability to think	Suicidal thoughts
134001	99.5	99	60	95	55	97	93	91	40
134002	100	99	51	96	70	99	90	99	37
FK007	100	100	56	97	79	98	93	96	45
FK008	99	100	65	98	75	99	91	94	36
average	*99.6%*	*99.5%*	*58.0%*	*96.8%*	*69.8%*	*98.3%*	*91.8%*	*95%*	*39.5%*

C. Effect of Fluoxetine on Sexual Function - When to use SSRIs

Figure 2 shows the magnitude of the negative effect of fluoxetine depends on the baseline value of sexual function. In the group of subjects selected with DISF scores ± 0.5 SD of the mean of the non-patient population, the baseline score is almost 80, about the middle of the normal range of sexual function. The upper solid line (▲—▲) displays the baseline DISF total score values (left hand y axis) for each group of the 1 SD windows (x axis). The dotted line (•••••) is the linear regression fit of decreasing sexual function as a function of the standard deviation windows, $R^2 = 0.964$. The end-of-treatment negative effect of fluoxetine on each group is shown at the bottom of *Figure 2*. The lower solid line (◆—◆) indicates the DISF total point decrease caused by fluoxetine after 8 weeks of treatment (right hand y axis). Those depressed subjects with normal sexual function or little sexual dysfunction at baseline show a greater negative effect caused by fluoxetine. At the best level of baseline sexual function (least severe sexual dysfunction), fluoxetine negatively affects DISF total scores by 10 points. Those with a higher level of sexual dysfunction at baseline have a lesser or no negative effect of fluoxetine.

Of course, if sexual function is 3 or more standard deviations below normal, it is not likely that the subjects can become more dysfunction.

SSRIs such as fluoxetine have a greater antidepressant effect in patients with high levels of depression. High levels of depression correlate with high levels of sexual dysfunction. In subjects with high levels of depression and sexual dysfunction fluoxetine causes little negative effect on sexual function. The subject may not notice the negative effect on sexual function. Therefore this situation may be where SSRIs should be used appropriately.

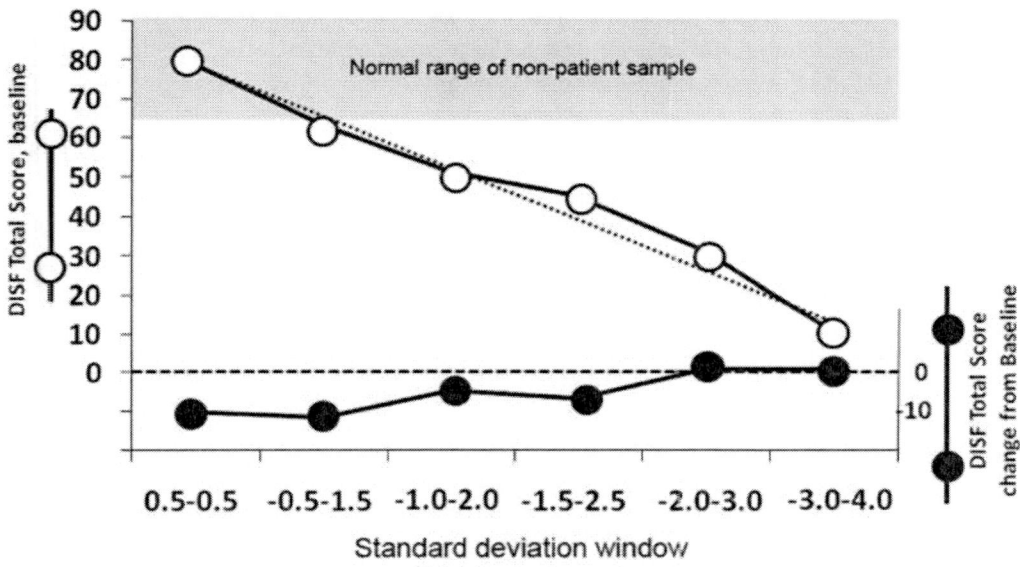

Figure 2. Negative Effect of Fluoxetine on Sexual Function Decreases with Increasing Severity of Baseline Sexual Dysfunction.

D. The Effect of Gepirone-ER on Depressive Symptoms in Major Depression

Of 5 studies of gepirone-ER in major depression (Table 2), two studies showed statistically significant antidepressant activity as measured by the HAMD-17 (134001 and FKGBE007). Study 134001 had a HAMD-17 effect size of -2.47, p = 0.013, and FKGBE007 an effect size of -2.45, p = 0.018. These two studies did not have SSRI comparators and only 1 (134001) had sexual function measurement.

Table 2. Antidepressant Efficacy Studies of Gepirone-ER in Major Depression
Primary Efficacy Parameter: HAMD-17 Change from Baseline

Studies in Classic Major Depression						
			HAMD-17 Change from Baseline			
Study	n, gepirone-ER	n, placebo	gepirone-ER	placebo	effect size	p-value*
134001	101	101	-9.04	-6.57	-2.47	0.013
FKGBE007	116	122	-10.24	-7.79	-2.45	0.018
134002	102	103	-9.95	-9.24	-0.71	0.417
Studies in Atypical Depression						
134004	124	130	-5.63	-6.66	1.03	0.199
134006	140	143	-6.89	-7.13	0.24	0.742
*vs. placebo						

One other study, 134002, did not have positive results on the primary efficacy endpoint but did have positive results on the secondary endpoints.

The gepirone-ER treated group did not have significant antidepressant results in the atypical depression studies for any of the primary or secondary efficacy measures. The comparator SSRI did not have significant results in any of the primary or secondary efficacy parameters as well.

The effect sizes for gepirone-ER in studies 134001 and FKGBE007 are comparable to FDA approved SSRI antidepressant [53].

The antidepressant effect of gepirone-ER in patients with classic major depression is confirmed by the statistically significant effects on the secondary end points (Table 3). Gepirone-ER was not effective in atypical depression.

Table 3. Antidepressant Efficacy Studies of Gepirone-ER in Major Depression Secondary Efficacy Parameters

MADRS						
Studies in Classic Major Depression						
			MADRS change from baseline			
Study	n, Gepirone-ER	n, Placebo	gepirone-ER	placebo	Effect size	p-value
134001	101	101	-11.34	-8.08	-3.26	0.018
FKGBE007	116	121	-13.90	-9.73	-4.17	0.003
134002	102	103	-11.68	-9.42	-2.27	0.083
Studies in Atypical Depression						
134004	124	130	Not done			
134006	140	143	Not done			
Bech-6						
Studies in Classic Major Depression						
			Bech-6 change from baseline			
134001	101	101	-5.09	-3.61	-1.48	0.010
FKGBE007	116	122	-5.75	-4.12	-1.63	0.004
134002	102	103	-5.93	-4.95	-0.98	0.064
Studies in Atypical Depression						
134004	124	130	-4.19	-4.36	0.17	0.727
134006	140	143	-4.61	-4.58	-0.03	0.953
HAMD item 1						
Studies in Classic Major Depression						
			HAMD item 1			
134001	101	101	-1.15	-0.74	-0.41	0.003
FKGBE007	116	122	-1.24	-0.95	-0.29	0.047
134002	102	103	-1.30	-1.01	-0.29	0.032
Studies in Atypical Depression						
134004	124	130	-0.98	-1.11	0.13	0.322
134006	140	143	-1.11	-1.07	-0.04	0.739

E. The Effect of Gepirone-ER on Sexual Function Symptoms in Major Depression Compared to Fluoxetine and Placebo

The results (Table 4) indicate for total DISF score gepirone-ER treated patients have a statistically significant (p = 0.04) positive effect, while fluoxetine treated patients show a statistically significant negative effect (placebo better than fluoxetine p = 0.01). For the individual domains of the DISF, gepirone-ER treated patients have a significantly positive effect on desire (p = 0.003) whereas fluoxetine has statistically significant negative effects on all domains except desire (arousal p = 0.01, behavior p = 0.09, drive p = 0.02, and orgasm p<0.0001.

Table 4. The Effect of Gepirone-ER and SSRIs on DISF Total Score and Domains in All Subjects (Male and Female) Studies 134001 134002 134004 134006 Pooled

| DISF domain | Change from baseline | | | | |
	gepirone-ER Δ mean	p value*	fluoxetine Δ mean	p value*	placebo Δ mean
n	352		128		379
All	5.33	0.04	-4.25	0.01**	1.73
Arousal	1.19	0.27	-0.85	0.01**	0.70
Behavior	0.72	0.17	-0.76	0.10	0.17
Desire	1.32	0.003	-0.78	0.95	-0.73
Drive	1.20	0.13	-0.10	0.02**	0.79
Orgasm	0.90	0.85	-1.76	<0.0001**	0.81

*vs. placebo.
**worse than placebo.

F. The Effect of Gepirone-ER on Depression in groups of Depressed Subjects with Differing Levels of Sexual Dysfunction at Baseline

In study 134001, a study that had positive antidepressant activity, sexual dysfunction at baseline was defined as 1 or more standard deviations below normal. Gepirone-ER treated subjects showed statistically significant antidepressant activity in the group with sexual dysfunction at baseline and did not in the group without sexual dysfunction at baseline, although the results for this group trended in a positive direction. In the group with no sexual dysfunction, the effect size (the HAMD point difference between the effect of gepirone-ER and placebo) was -1.65 points compared to -3.41 points in the group with sexual dysfunction (Table 5).

If all subjects are stratified by their level of sexual dysfunction at baseline, the results (Figure 3) shows that, the more sexual dysfunction present at baseline, the better gepirone-ER worked as an antidepressant. As the level of sexual dysfunction at baseline increases, the antidepressant effect size of gepirone increases. At a sexual dysfunction level at baseline of -2.5 SD below normal, the gepirone-ER effect size is -5.7 points. This difference is three times what is usually seen in antidepressant trials.

Table 5.The Effect of Sexual Dysfunction on HAMD-17 Antidepressant Efficacy Study 134001

DISF Domain	MDD with normal sexual function*			MDD with sexual dysfunction**		
	n Above -1SD G/P	Gepirone-ER HAMD-17 CFB Δ means†	p value†	n Below -1SD G/P	Gepirone-ER HAMD-17 CFB Δ means†	p value†
Total	18/17	-1.65	0.383	49/62	-3.41	0.017

*above the minus 1 SD from mean threshold of normal non-patient population.
**below the minus 1 SD from mean of normal threshold of non-patient population.
†gepirone-ER vs. placebo.

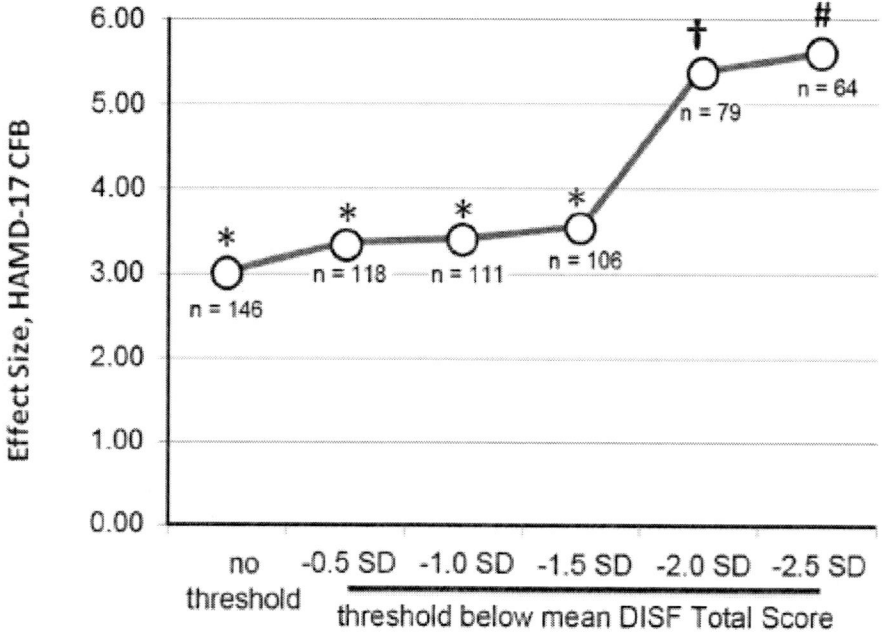

p-values gepirone-ER vs. placebo *
p <0.050
# p<0.010
† p<0.005

Figure 3. Effect of Sexual Dysfunction Threshold on HAMD-17 Effect Size for Gepirone-ER vs. Placebo.

G. The Effect of Gepirone-ER on Sexual Function in Subjects with and without Sexual Dysfunction at Baseline

Table 6 shows that subjects with sexual dysfunction responded better to gepirone-ER, i.e., greater improvement in sexual function, than those without sexual dysfunction at baseline. Fluoxetine has more negative effects on the group with no sexual dysfunction at baseline.

Table 6.Effect of Gepirone-ER and Fluoxetine on Sexual Function in All Subjects (Male and Female) With and Without Sexual Dysfunction at Baseline

Group: Sexual Dysfunction at Baseline			
	DISF Total Score		
Treatment	Mean CFB	SD	p-value
gepirone-ER	9.80*	23.4	<0.0001
fluoxetine	3.65	18.2	0.279
Group: No Sexual Dysfunction at Baseline			
gepirone-ER	-3.10	23.8	0.250
fluoxetine	-16.98**	30.3	<0.0001

*better sexual function.
**worse sexual function.

If all subjects are stratified by their level of sexual dysfunction at baseline (Table 7), the results shows that, the more sexual dysfunction present at baseline, the better gepirone-ER worked to improve sexual function. Ata baseline DISF total score of -3 SD, the effect size of gepirone-ER treatment is 6.7.

Table 7. The Effect of Stratifying DISF Baseline Scores on Sexual Dysfunction after Treatment

	Gepirone-ER		Placebo			with "normal" sexual function		with sexual dysfunction	
DISF total score	n		n		percent above				
threshold	above/below	threshold	above/below	threshold	threshold	above threshold		below threshold	
none	67		79			effect size	p-value	effect size	p-value
-0.5 SD*	15/52	21%	13/66	16%		1.32	0.538	3.37	0.014
-1.0 SD*	18/49	27%	17/62	22%		1.65	0.383	3.41	0.017
-1.5 SD*	20/47	30%	20/59	25%		1.40	0.424	3.56	0.016
-2.0 SD*	30/37	45%	37/42	47%		0.29	0.843	5.38	0.002
-2.5 SD*	36/31	54%	46/33	58%		1.02	0.447	5.61	0.007
-3.0 SD*	48/19	72%	60/19	76%		1.84	0.127	6.68	0.022

H. Gepirone-ER Antidepressant and Anxiolytic Effects on Sexual Function

There are large placebo effects in studies of depression and anxiety. With placebo treatment, the HAMD-17 scores in depression studies and the HAMA scores in anxiety studies decrease. That is the patients have a placebo effect and the depression or anxiety improves. Our studies [55, 56] have shown that this is true for sexual dysfunction as well. That is, with placebo treatment sexual dysfunction improves.

In spite of the placebo improvement the drug placebo difference at endpoint of treatment indicates that gepirone-ER has anxiolytic, antidepressant, and pro-sexual effects. The question then becomes: are the improvements in sexual function due to the anxiolytic and/or antidepressant effects.

Figure 4 shows the effect of gepirone-ER on the entire population of female subjects in studies 134006 and 134503. Gepirone-ER has a statistically positive effect on desire at each time point.

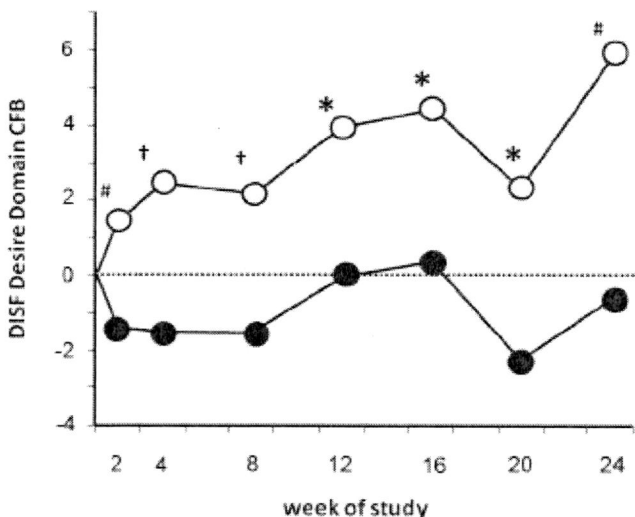

All Females, Studies 134006 and 134503, OC
Gepirone-ER open circles
Placebo filled circles
p-values gepirone-ER vs. placebo
* p <0.050
# p<0.010
† p<0.005

Figure 4. The Effect of Gepirone-ER on DISF Desire Domain in study 134006 and its Extension 134503.

To assess the reason for improvement in depression on the DISF desire domain, at each time point, the subjects were divided into antidepressant responders (HAMD-17 50% of baseline or more) and antidepressant non-responders (HAMD-17 less than 50%). The results are shown in Figures 5 and 6.

Gepirone increases sexual desire in both responders and non-responders indicating that the effect on sexual function is independent of an anti-depressant effect.

To determine whether gepirone-ER's effect on anxiety was not wholly responsible for the positive effect on desire, subjects were divided into anxiolytic responders (score 0 or 1 for HAMD item 12) and anxiolytic non-responders (score 2 or more HAMD item 12). The results are shown in Figures 7 and 8.

Once again, gepirone-ER has a positive effect on subjects who were HAMD item 12 responders and those who were non-responders. Therefore, the effect of gepirone-ER on desire is independent of the anxiolytic effect.

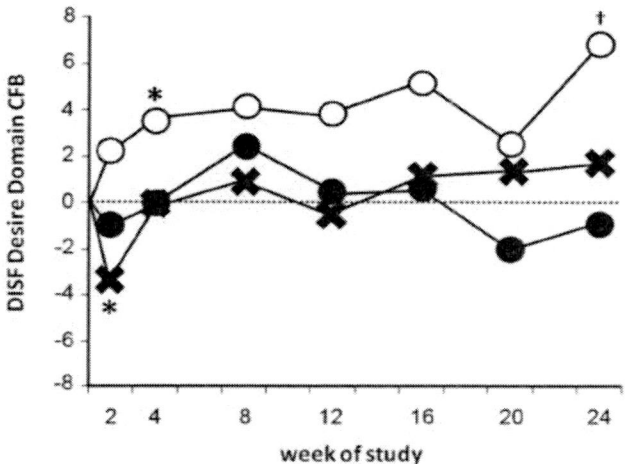

All Females, Studies 134006 and 134503, OC
Gepirone-ER open circles
Placebo filled circles
p-values gepirone-ER vs. placebo
* p <0.050
† p<0.005

Figure 5. DISF Desire Domain Change from Baseline of HAMD-17 Responders.

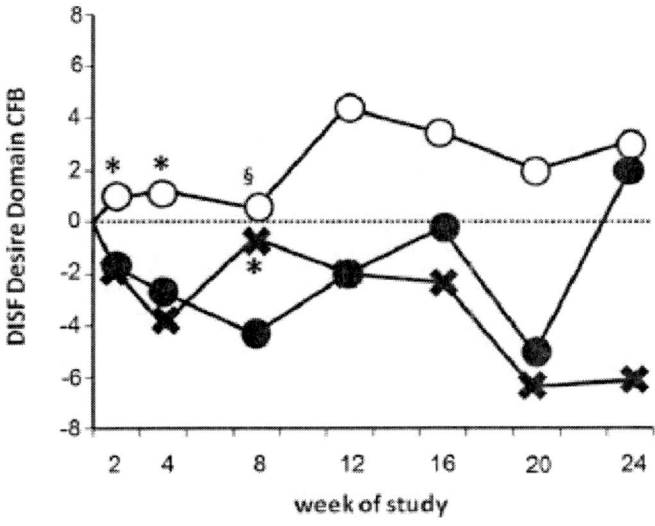

All Females, Studies 134006 and 134503, OC.
Gepirone-ER open circles.
Placebo filled circles.
p-values gepirone-ER vs. placebo.
* p <0.050.
§ p<0.001.

Figure 6. DISF Desire Domain Change from Baseline of HAMD-17 Non-Responders.

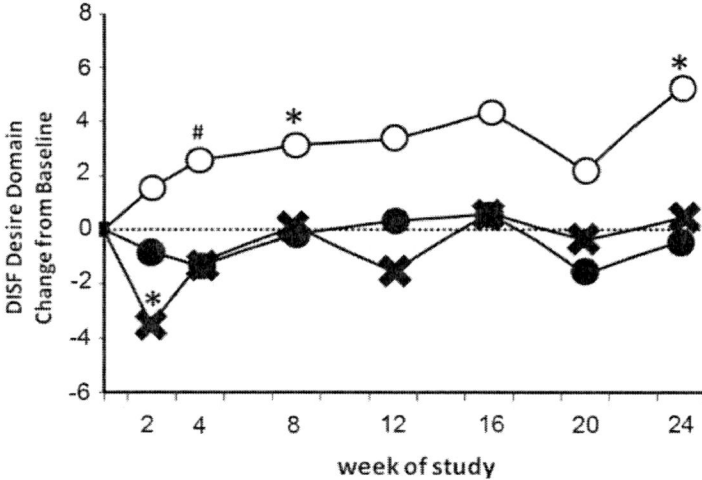

All Females, Studies 134006 and 134503, OC
Gepirone-ER open circles
Placebo filled circles
p-values gepirone-ER vs. placebo
* p <0.050
# p<0.010

Figure 7. DISF Desire Domain Change from Baseline of HAMD item 12 Responders.

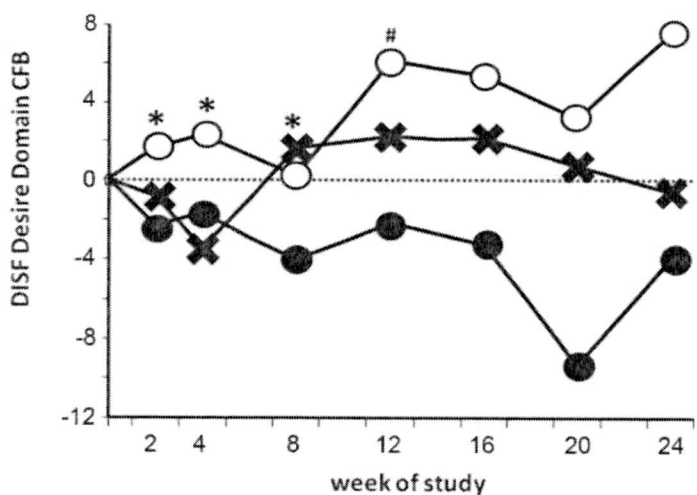

All Females, Studies 134006 and 134503, OC
Gepirone-ER open circles
Placebo filled circles
p-values gepirone-ER vs. placebo
* p <0.050
# p<0.010

Figure 8. DISF Desire Domain Change from Baseline of HAMD item 12 Non-Responders

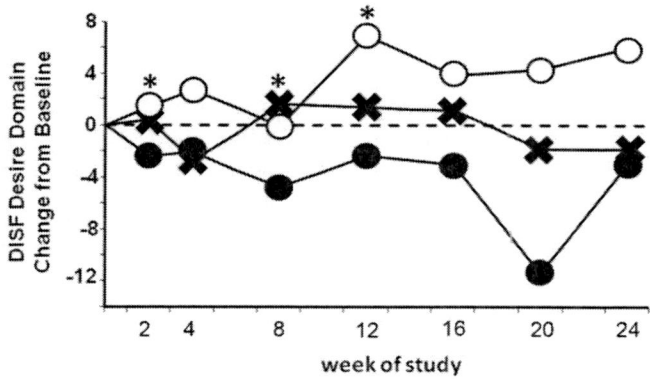

All Females, Studies 134006 and 134503, OC
p-values gepirone-ER vs. placebo
Gepirone-ER open circles
Placebo filled circles
*p <0.050

Figure 9. DISF Desire Domain Change from Baseline of Depressed Subjects who are both
Antidepressant and Anxiolytic Non-Responders.

For completeness, a group of gepirone-ER treated depressed subjects who are both
antidepressant and anxiolytic non-responders was identified. The results in Figure 9 show that
those who experienced neither an antidepressant nor anxiolytic response nevertheless showed
a prosexual effect as the result of gepirone-ER treatment.

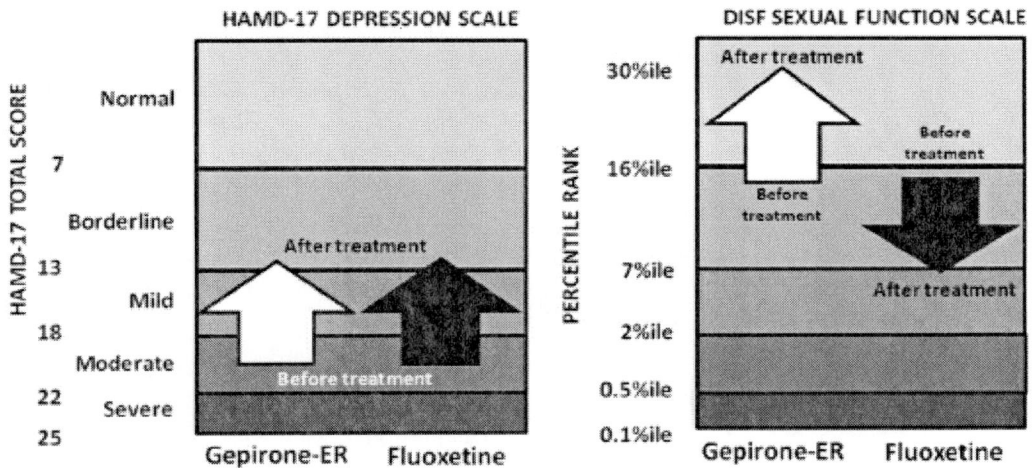

Gepirone-ER n = 116.
Fluoxetine n = 128.
Placebo n = 127.
Left scale HAMD-17 CFB, p-value gepirone-ER vs. placebo not significant.
HAMD-17 CFB, p-value fluoxetine vs. placebo not significant.
Right scale DISF Total Score CFB, p-value gepirone-ER vs. fluoxetine 0.022.

Figure 10. Comparison of Treatment of Major Depression and Sexual Dysfunction with Gepirone-ER
and Fluoxetine.

I. Clinical Significance of Treatment with Gepirone-ER

Figure 10 shows the results of study 134004. As may be seen, both fluoxetine and gepirone-ER improve depression, going from the severely depressed up to the bottom of the normal range. By contrast, gepirone-ER improves sexual function into the normal range while fluoxetine has an opposite effect and causes an even further decline in sexual function.

In study 134001 (Figure 11), gepirone-ER improves depression from the severe range up into the normal range and also improves sexual function into the normal range. In this study, the gepirone-ER effects on depression and sexual function are both statistically significantly positive.

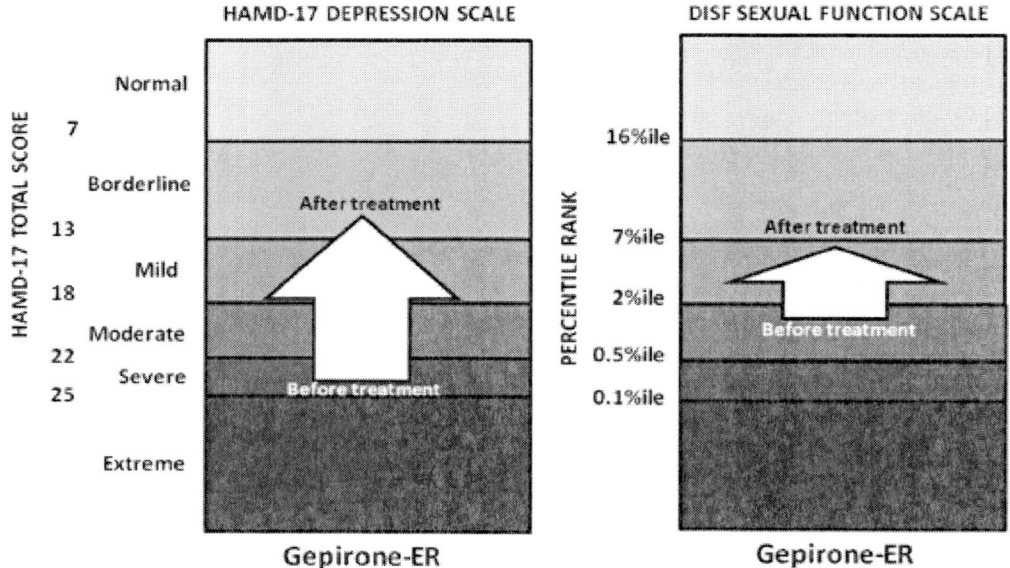

Gepirone-ER n = 67.
Placebo n = 79.
Left scale HAMD-17 CFB, p-value gepirone-ER vs. placebo 0.010.
Right scale DISF Total Score CFB, p-value gepirone-ER vs. placebo 0.025.

Figure 11. Gepirone-ER Treatment Improves both Depression and Sexual Function..

CONCLUSION

In this group of depressed subjects, sexual dysfunction was common. About 80% of subjects with classic major depression had DISF scores below 1 standard deviation from normal. The population distribution for the depressed subjects is different from that of the normal non-patient population, with little over-lap.

The percent of depressed subjects with sexual dysfunction is greater than 3 of the 9 possible DSM-IV symptoms for the diagnosis of major depression. Only 5 are needed for diagnosis of depression. This evidence does not necessarily mean that sexual dysfunction should be used as a criterion for the diagnosis of major depression. However, it does suggest that sexual dysfunction is at least as important as other criteria used to diagnose depression.

Antidepressant medications are not very effective at relieving depression. Recent data like STAR*D have taught us that with antidepressant medications only 30% of patients achieve remission. Another 30% have some relief of symptoms and 40% receive no benefit at all. Antidepressants work best in severe depression [56]. Most patients have mild-moderate depression. Adverse events: sexual side effects, weight gain, somnolence, etc., cause patients to discontinue. Concomitant medications interfere. SSRIs cause birth defects: women of child-bearing potential are afraid to take them. The drugs take as long as a month to have an antidepressant effect.

Currently there is not much data that will allow prediction of whether a patient will respond to an antidepressant or not. At present, indications of a positive response to antidepressants are greater severity of depression, and baseline cholesterol level over 200 mg/dl [57]. Some also believe that if a blood family member responded to a particular drug the patient is likely to also be a responder. The data here suggest that presence of sexual dysfunction at baseline may be a useful indicator of potential antidepressant efficacy.

The serotonin reuptake inhibitors (fluoxetine et al) do not have better efficacy than the tricyclics (imipramine et al). They were approved because they have a better side effect profile. A month's tablets of imipramine taken all at once might be fatal whereas a month of fluoxetine tablets is not. But the SSRIs cause sexual dysfunction in up to 80% of depressed patients, both men and women. Ninety per cent of those with sexual side effects discontinue the SSRI or SNRI. This fact probably contributes to the lack of efficacy.

However, stopping the drug does not stop the sexual dysfunction. Sexual dysfunction can persist after discontinuation. In one study, 79% still had sexual dysfunction 6 months later [30]. Other studies suggest that the dysfunction may last for years or even be permanent.

However, these data are in question because it is rare that sexual function is measured at baseline. If a patient who has sexual dysfunction at baseline, which has not been discovered, develops sexual dysfunction after starting on fluoxetine, fluoxetine may not be the entire cause of the sexual dysfunction. If then fluoxetine is discontinued and the patient continues to have sexual dysfunction as they did prior to drug treatment, it is unlikely that fluoxetine is the cause of the long-term problem.

Therefore, current antidepressant treatments not only do not improve sexual dysfunction, they make sexual dysfunction worse. This fact may explain why subjects with lower levels of depression (and lower levels of sexual dysfunction at baseline) have a lesser antidepressant effect to SSRIs.

Gepirone-ER improves sexual function in both men and women. Gepirone-ER improves DISF total score and the DISF domain score measuring desire. On the other hand fluoxetine causes sexual function to be worse in both men and women affecting total score and most domains of the DISF.

Gepirone-ER has greater antidepressant activity in subjects with sexual dysfunction at baseline, than subjects without sexual dysfunction at baseline. In fact, analyses reveal that the greater the sexual dysfunction at baseline the greater the antidepressant effect size.

Similarly gepirone-ER has a greater positive effect on sexual function in subjects with greater sexual dysfunction at baseline. Fluoxetine and SSRIs or SNRIs have a greater negative effect on sexual function in those subjects with little or no sexual dysfunction at baseline.

In one study, 134006, gepirone-ER was effective in improving the DISF domain of desire at almost every time point out to week 24. In a subgroup of subjects who were not HAMD responders gepirone-ER continued to have a positive effect on sexual function. Similarly, in a subgroup of subjects that were anxiolytic non-responders, gepirone-ER still had positive effects on sexual function. Both groups of responders also showed improvement in sexual function. These results indicate that gepirone-ER may have 3 mechanisms of action a prosexual effect, an antidepressant effect, and an anxiolytic effect.

In one study 134001, gepirone-ER statistically significantly improved both HAMD-17 score measuring depression and DISF score measuring desire. The result was more pronounced in the group of depressed subjects that had sexual dysfunction at baseline than in the group that did not have sexual dysfunction at baseline. Gepirone-ER treatment improved both depression and sexual dysfunction into or almost into the normal range. The results are both statistically and clinically significant.

Sexual dysfunction should be measured in depressed subjects prior to treatment. The treatment of depression should include the treatment of sexual dysfunction. Gepirone-ER shows promise as a new treatment for both depression and sexual dysfunction.

REFERENCES

[1]   Pratt LA, Brody DJ, Gu Q. Antidepressant use in persons aged 12 and over: United States, 2005–2008. NCHS data brief, no 76. Hyattsville, MD: National Center for Health Statistics. 2011.

[2]   Fava M, Rush AJ, Trivedi MH, Nierenberg AA, Thase ME, Sackeim HA, Quitkin FM, Wisniewski S, Lavori PW, Rosenbaum JF, Kupfer DJ. Background and rationale for the sequenced treatment alternatives to relieve depression (STAR*D) study. *Psychiatr. Clin. North Am.* 2003; 26:457-94.

[3]   Derogatis LR, Meyer JK, King KM. Psychopathology in individuals with sexual dysfunction. *Am. J. Psychiatry.* 1981; 138(6):757-63.

[4]   RJ, Weinman ML. Sexual dysfunctions in depression. Arch Sex Behav 1982; 11:323-8.

[5]   Howell JR, Reynolds CF 3rd, Thase ME, Frank E, Jennings JR, Houck PR, Berman S, Jacobs E, Kupfer DJ. Assessment of sexual function, interest and activity in depressed men. *J. Affect. Disord.* 1987; 13:61-6.

[6]   Reynolds CF 3rd, Frank E, Thase ME, Houck PR, Jennings JR, Howell JR, Lilienfeld SO, Kupfer DJ. Assessment of sexual function in depressed, impotent, and healthy men: factor analysis of a Brief Sexual Function Questionnaire for men. *Psychiatry Res.* 1988; 24:231-50.

[7]   Angst J. Sexual problems in healthy and depressed persons. *Int. Clin. Psychopharmacol.* 1998; 13(Suppl 6):S1-4.

[8]   Halvorsen JG, Metz ME. Sexual dysfunction, Part I: Classification, etiology, and pathogenesis. *J. Am. Board Fam. Pract.* 1992; 5:51-61.

[9]   Kennedy SH, Dickens SE, Eisfeld BS, Bagby RM. Sexual dysfunction before antidepressant therapy in major depression. *J. Affect. Disord.* 1999; 56:201-8.

[10]   Bartlik B, Kocsis JH, Legere R, Villaluz J, Kossoy A, Gelenberg AJ. Sexual dysfunction secondary to depressive disorders. J Gend Specif Med. 1999; 2:52-60.

[11] Seidman SN, Roose SP. Sexual dysfunction and depression. *Curr. Psychiatry Rep.* 2001; 3:202-8.

[12] Baldwin DS. Depression and sexual dysfunction. Br Med Bull. 2001; 57:81-99.

[13] Bonierbale M, Lançon C, Tignol J. The ELIXIR study: evaluation of sexual dysfunction in 4557 depressed patients in France. *Curr. Med. Res. Opin.* 2003; 19:114-24.

[14] Cyranowski JM, Frank E, Cherry C, Houck P, Kupfer DJ. Prospective assessment of sexual function in women treated for recurrent major depression. *J. Psychiatr. Res.* 2004; 38:267-73.

[15] Williams K, Reynolds MF. Sexual dysfunction in major depression. *CNS Spectr.* 2006; 11(Suppl 9):19-23.

[16] Clayton AH, Montejo AL. Major depressive disorder, antidepressants, and sexual dysfunction. J Clin Psychiatry. 2006; 67 Suppl 6:33-7.

[17] Kennedy SH, Rizvi S. Sexual dysfunction, depression, and the impact of antidepressants. *J. Clin. Psychopharmacol.* 2009; 29:157-64.

[18] Johannes CB, Clayton AH, Odom DM, Rosen RC, Russo PA, Shifren JL, Monz BU. Distressing sexual problems in United States women revisited: prevalence after accounting for depression. *J. Clin. Psychiatry.* 2009;70:1698-706.

[19] Laurent SM, Simons AD. Sexual dysfunction in depression and anxiety: conceptualizing sexual dysfunction as part of an internalizing dimension. *Clin. Psychol. Rev.* 2009; 29:573-85.

[20] Smith JF, Breyer BN, Eisenberg ML, Sharlip ID, Shindel AW. Sexual function and depressive symptoms among male North American medical students. *J. Sex Med* 2010; 7(12):3909-17.

[21] Atlantis E, Sullivan T. Bidirectional association between depression and sexual dysfunction: a systematic review and meta-analysis. *J. Sex Med.* 2012; 9:1497-507.

[22] Fabre LF, Smith LC. The effect of major depression on sexual function in women. *J. Sex Med.* 2012; 9:231-9.

[23] Clayton AH, Maserejian NN, Connor MK, Huang L, Heiman JR, Rosen RC. Depression in premenopausal women with HSDD: baseline findings from the HSDD Registry for Women. *Psychosom. Med.* 2012; 74:305-11.

[24] Kingsberg SA. *Just ask!* Talking to patients about sexual function. Sexuality, Reproduction & Menopause 2004; 2:199-203.

[25] Kingsberg SA. Identifying HSDD in the family medicine setting. *J. Fam. Pract.* 2009; 58(7 Suppl Hypoactive):S22-5.

[26] American Psychiatry Association: Diagnostic and Statistical Manual of Mental Disorders, Fourth Edition, American Psychiatry Association: Washington, D.C. 1994 pp 496 - 498.

[27] Clayton AH, Pradko JF, Croft HA, Montano CB, Leadbetter RA, Bolden-Watson C, Bass KI, Donahue RM, Jamerson BD, Metz A. Prevalence of sexual dysfunction among newer antidepressants. *J. Clin. Psychiatry.* 2002; 63:357-66.

[28] Casper RC, Redmond DE Jr, Katz MM, Schaffer CB, Davis JM, Koslow SH. Somatic symptoms in primary affective disorder. Presence and relationship to the classification of depression. *Arch. Gen. Psychiatry.* 1985; 42:1098-104.

[29] Clayton AH. Female sexual dysfunction related to depression and antidepressant medications. *Curr. Womens Health Rep.* 2002; 2:182-7.

[30] Montejo AL, Llorca G, Izquierdo JA, Rico-Villademoros F. Incidence of sexual dysfunction associated with antidepressant agents: a prospective multicenter study of 1022 outpatients. Spanish Working Group for the Study of Psychotropic-Related Sexual Dysfunction. *J. Clin. Psychiatry.* 2001; 62 Suppl 3:10-21.

[31] Clayton AH, Pradko JF, Croft HA, Montano CB, Leadbetter RA, Bolden-Watson C, Bass KI, Donahue RM, Jamerson BD, Metz A. Prevalence of sexual dysfunction among newer antidepressants. *J. Clin. Psychiatry.* 2002; 63:357-66.

[32] Gregorian RS, Golden KA, Bahce A, Goodman C, Kwong WJ, Khan ZM. Antidepressant-induced sexual dysfunction. *Ann. Pharmacother.* 2002; 36:1577-89.

[33] Delgado PL, Brannan SK, Mallinckrodt CH, Tran PV, McNamara RK, Wang F, Watkin JG, Detke MJ. Sexual functioning assessed in 4 double-blind placebo- and paroxetine-controlled trials of duloxetine for major depressive disorder. *J. Clin. Psychiatry.* 2005; 66:686-92.

[34] Nurnberg HG, Hensley PL. Selective phosphodiesterase type-5 inhibitor treatment of serotonergic reuptake inhibitor antidepressant-associated sexual dysfunction: a review of diagnosis, treatment, and relevance. *CNS Spectr.* 2003; 8:194-202.

[35] Csoka AB, Bahrick A, Mehtonen OP. Persistent sexual dysfunction after discontinuation of selective serotonin reuptake inhibitors. *J. Sex Med.* 2008; 5:227-33.

[36] Mandrioli R, Mercolini L, Saracino MA, Raggi MA. Selective serotonin reuptake inhibitors (SSRIs): therapeutic drug monitoring and pharmacological interactions. *Curr. Med. Chem.* 2012; 19:1846-63.

[37] Laux G. Cost-benefit analysis of newer versus older antidepressants--pharmacoeconomic studies comparing SSRIs/SNRIs with tricyclic antidepressants. *Pharmacopsychiatry.* 2001; 34:1-5.

[38] Andersen ML, Alvarenga TF, Mazaro-Costa R, Hachul HC, Tufik S. The association of testosterone, sleep, and sexual function in men and women. *Brain Res.* 2011; 1416:80-104.

[39] Fooladi E, Davis SR. An update on the pharmacological management of female sexual dysfunction. *Expert. Opin. Pharmacother.* 2012; 13:2131-42.

[40] Chivers ML, Rosen RC. Phosphodiesterase type 5 inhibitors and female sexual response: faulty protocols or paradigms? *J. Sex Med.* 2010; 7:858-72.

[41] Kennedy S. Flibanserin: initial evidence of efficacy on sexual dysfunction, in patients with major depressive disorder. *J. Sex Med.* 2010; 7:3449-59.

[42] Sand M. Errata by Fabre et al. in gepirone-ER treatment of hypoactive sexual desire disorder associated with depression in women. *J. Sex Med.* 2011; 8:2954.

[43] Feiger AD, Heister JF, Shrivastava RK, Weiss KJ, Smith WT, Sitsen JMA, Gilbertini M. Gepirone extended release: new evidence for efficacy in the treatment of major depressive disorder. *J. Clin. Psychiatr.* 2003; 64:243-249.

[44] Alpert JE, Franznick DA, Hollander SB, Fava M. Gepirone extended-release treatment of anxious depression: evidence from a retrospective subgroup analysis in patients with major depressive disorder. *J. Clin. Psychiatr.* 2004; 65:1069-1075.

[45] Derogatis LR. The Derogatis Interview for Sexual Functioning (DISF/DISF-SR): an introductory report. *J. Sex Marital Ther.* 1997; 23:291-304.

[46] DeRogatis LR. Administration, Procedures, and Scoring Manual (Preliminary) for the DeRogatis Interview for Sexual Functioning (DISF). Baltimore, MD. Clinical Psychometric Research, Inc. 1992.

[47] American Psychiatry Association: Diagnostic and Statistical Manual of Mental Disorders, Fourth Edition, American Psychiatry Association: Washington, D.C. 1994 pp 496 - 498.

[48] American Psychiatry Association: Diagnostic and Statistical Manual of Mental Disorders, Fourth Edition, American Psychiatry Association: Washington, D.C. 1994 pp. 384 - 386.

[49] Hamilton M. A rating scale for depression. *J. Neurol. Neurosurg. Psychiatr.* 1960; 23:56-62

[50] Camm AJ. The design and conduct of human studies to detect and quantify QT interval prolongation induced by new chemical entities. *Fundam. Clin. Pharmacol.* 2002; 16:141-5.

[51] Montgomery SA, Asberg M. A new depression scale designed to be sensitive to change. Br J Psychiatry. 1979; 134:382-9.

[52] Bech P, Gram LF, Dein E, Jacobsen O, Vitger J, Bolwig TG. Quantitative rating of depressive states. *Acta Psychiatr. Scand.* 1975; 51:161-70.

[53] Khin NA, Chen YF, Yang Y, Yang P, Laughren TP. Exploratory analyses of efficacy data from major depressive disorder trials submitted to the US Food and Drug Administration in support of new drug applications. *J. Clin. Psychiatry.* 2011; 72:464-72. Erratum in: J Clin Psychiatry. 2011; 72:874.

[54] Fabre LF, Smith LC, DeRogatis LR. Gepirone-ER treatment of low sexual desire associated with depression in women as measured by the DeRogatis Inventory of Sexual Function (DISF) fantasy/cognition (desire) domain--a post hoc analysis. *J. Sex Med.* 2011; 8:2569-81.

[55] Fabre LF, Clayton AH, Smith LC, Goldstein I, Derogatis LR. The effect of gepirone-ER in the treatment of sexual dysfunction in depressed men. *J. Sex Med.* 2012; 9:821-9.

[56] Fournier JC, DeRubeis RJ, Hollon SD, Dimidjian S, Amsterdam JD, Shelton RC, Fawcett J. Antidepressant drug effects and depression severity: a patient-level meta-analysis. *JAMA.* 2010; 303:47-53.

[57] Fabre LF, Smith LC. Data on file.

CONFLICT OF INTEREST

Data were generated from protocols sponsored by Organon, Inc. Dr. Fabre is a full time employee of and a stockholder in Fabre Kramer Pharmaceuticals, Inc. Dr. Smith is a paid consultant to Fabre Kramer Pharmaceuticals, Inc.

In: Sexual Dysfunctions
Editor: Frédérique Courtois

ISBN: 978-1-62808-765-9
© 2013 Nova Science Publishers, Inc.

Chapter 10

NORMAL SEXUAL FUNCTION IN WOMEN

Frédérique Courtois[1], and Kathleen Charvier[2]*
[1]Université du Québec à Montréal, Sexology Department, Montreal, Canada
[2]Hospices civils de Lyon, Saint-Genis Laval, France

ABSTRACT

This chapter describes the bases of normal sexual functioning in women. It begins with a review of the anatomy of the female genitals, starting with the structure of the clitoris, consisting of its glans and body, but also its vestibular bulbs and crura as recently revealed by ultrasonic and MRI studies. Also revealed by ultrasonic and MRI studies is the clitoro-uretho-vaginal complex which supports the existence of the G spot as an anatomo-physiological region more than a strict anatomo-neural structure. Follows a description of the female reproductive organs, along with the vascular supply and neural innervation of the female genitals. The female sexual response as originally described by Masters and Johnson (1966), followed by Kaplan (1974), and adding the more recent model from Basson (2000), follows including a description of the bodily responses and genital changes associated with the phase of arousal and that of orgasm. The neurophysiology and neuropharmacology of the female sexual responses, including the process of clitoral erection and vaginal lubrication, are then explained and shown to result from the same nitric oxide process than erection in men and involving the same neurotransmitters. The neurophysiology of climax is then described along with the supraspinal modulation of the female sexual responses. These descriptions generally help understanding normal functioning in women, but also help understanding the aetiology of various sexual dysfunctions, as they can develop in women with aging and pathological conditions that are covered throughout the chapters of this book.

---

* Corresponding author: Frédérique Courtois PhD., Université du Québec à Montréal, Department of Sexology Department, CP 8888, succ centre ville, Montreal Canada. H3C 3P8. Phone: 1 514 835-6784, Fax: 1 514 987-6787. Email: courtois.frederique@uqam.ca.

Sexual function in women has been described according to various phases starting with desire (Kaplan, 1974), followed by arousal (Kaplan, 1974; Masters & Johnson 1965), culminating into a plateau phase (Masters & Johnson 1966) immediately precedes orgasm (Kaplan, 1974; Masters & Johnson 1966) and terminating with a resolution phase (Masters & Johnson 1966). Each phase is characterized by specific bodily changes. Sexual dysfunctions can develop on any stage of the female sexual response and affect the neurophysiological events characterizing any of these phases. This chapter describes the basics of normal sexual function in women.

ANATOMY OF THE FEMALE GENITALS

The female genital anatomy is composed of the vulva, globally including the clitoris, the labia majora, the labia minora, the urethra and the vaginal opening (figure 1). The vulva begins below the pubic bone and extends from the anterior commissure to the posterior commissure. The later is followed by the perineal area and the anal region, and is composed of many muscles including the transverse perineal muscle, the anal elevator muscle, and the anal sphincter (Netter 1984), which are involved in the climactic response.

Recent studies on ultrasound (Buisson et al 2008; Caruso et al 2011; Deng et al 2006; Foldes & Buisson, 2009; Khalifé et al 2000; Kukkonen et al 2006) and on magnetic resonance imagery (Deliganis et al 2002; O'Connell et al 2005; 2008; Suh et al 2003) show that the clitoris is a more complex structure that its glans, the latter being only the "tip of the iceberg" from a much large structure running along the labia majora and surrounding the anterolateral aspect of the vagina (figure 2). Most anteriorly, the clitoris is characterized by its glans covered with the clitoral hood or prepuce and prolonged with a body attached to the symphysis pubis by the suspensory ligament.

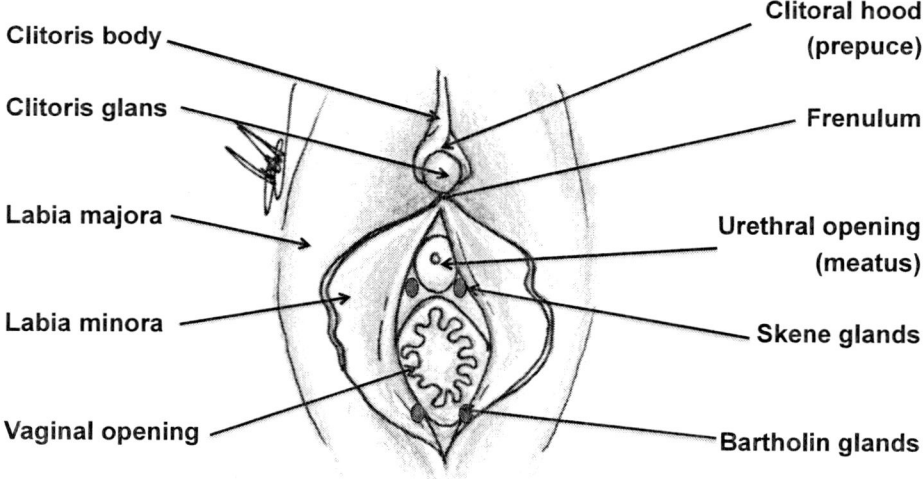

Figure 1. Female genitalia.

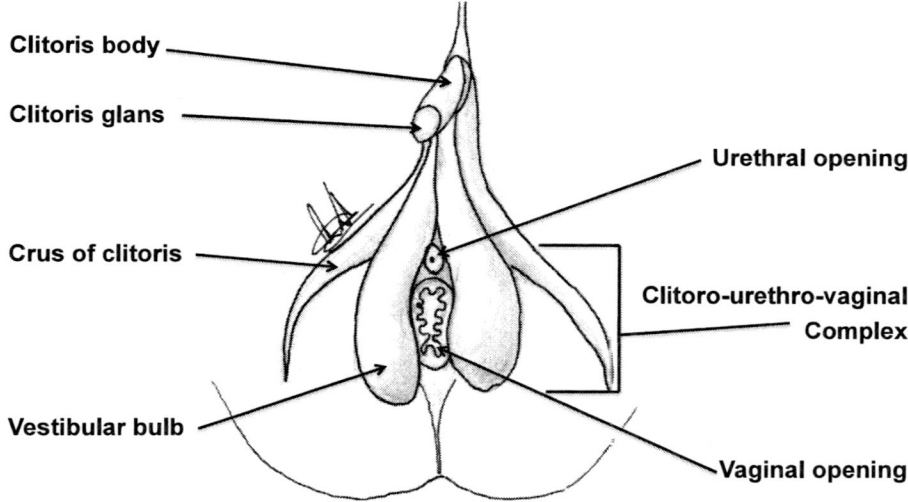

Figure 2. Structure of the clitoris.

On its ventral aspect, the labia minora join the clitoris at the level of the frenulum. Beyond its body, the clitoris shows two internal cavities, equivalent to men's ischiocavernosa and bulbospongiosum cavities, and including the crura (left and right) running laterally, and the vestibular bulbs (equivalent to the bulbospongiosum cavity of the penis) running medially along each side of the vulva. As for men, the clitoral cavities are surrounded by muscles, the ischiocavernosus muscle surrounding the base of each crura, and the bulbospongiosum muscle covering and surrounding the vestibular bulbs.

Given the internal structure of the clitoris, which runs along the vulva, the external third of the vagina is surrounded by erectile tissue arising from the vestibular bulbs (and which become congested during sexual arousal – see below). The urethral opening is also surrounded by some erectile tissue. The vaginal opening is covered by the hymen, a membrane that partially blocks its entry, especially before the first penetration. On each side of the vaginal opening lie Bartholin glands, which contribute to (but do not explain) vaginal lubrication (see below). On each side of the urethral opening also lie two small glands, called the para-urethral or Skene glands. The internal urethral canal is surrounded by peri-urethral glands which, along with Skene glands, represent embryological remnants of the male prostate gland.

Recent studies show that the structures of the clitoris surrounding the anterolateral wall of the vagina support the existence of the G spot as an anatomophysiological location responding to sexual stimulation (Battaglia et al 2010; Deliganis et al 2002; Gravina et al 2008; O'Connell et al 2005; 2008; Suh et al 2003). The erectile tissue composing the clitoral structures and surrounding the urethra compose a more general complex, called the clitoro-urethro-vaginal complex (figure 2), globally responding to sexual stimulation.

The vaginal canal is composed of convoluted layers of smooth muscle fibres allowing stretching of the canal, essential for child delivery. Given the position of the uterus, between the bladder and the rectum, organ descent can occur and exert pressure against the vaginal wall, giving rise to cystocele with bladder descent, rectocele with rectum descent, and prolapsus with uterus descent following childbirth.

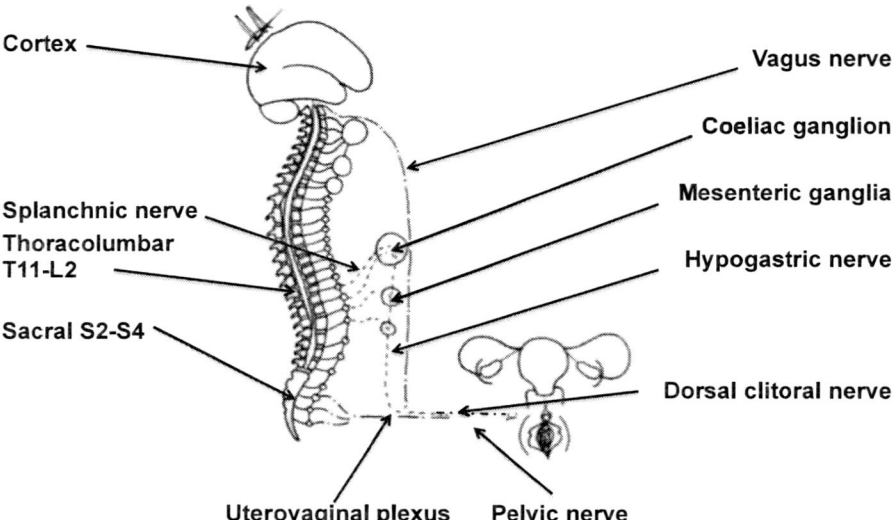

Figure 3. Female genital innervation.

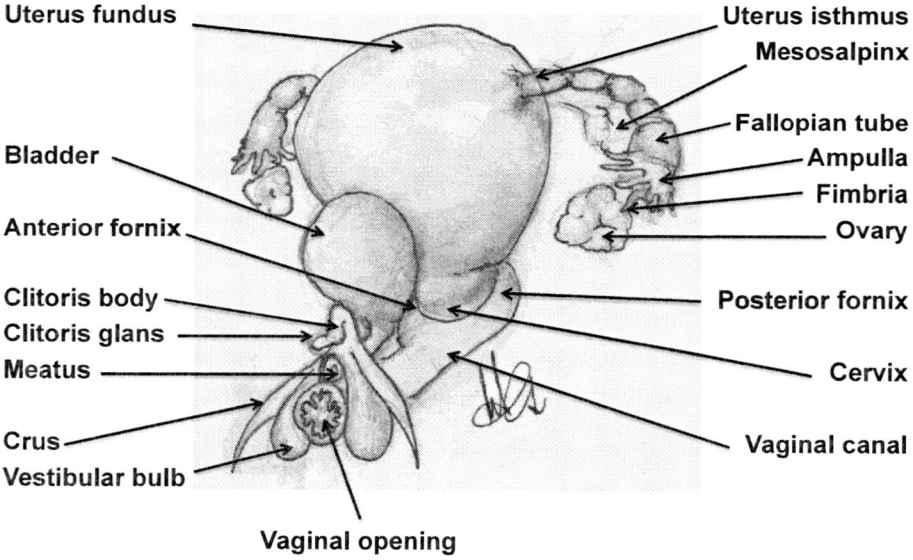

Figure 4. Internal Reproductive Organs in women.

The vaginal canal gives access to the internal reproductive organs, delineated by the cervix or neck of the uterus at the end of the vagina and which slightly penetrates the vagina to create a cul-de-sac, called the anterior and the posterior fornix of the vagina. The uterus itself is composed of a fundus and a body, and is surrounded by several layers of muscles that are essential for child delivery. The internal layer of the uterus is covered with the endometrium, a tissue responding to hormonal stimulation, and showing physiological changes characterizing the various phases of the menstrual cycle (and pregnancy). Within the abdominal cavity, the uterus is sustained by several ligaments, the round ligament anteriorly, the sacro-uterine ligament posteriorly, and the large ligament, which offers a kind of web maintaining the internal reproductive organs together from the ovaries to the cervix. Within the abdominal cavity the uterus normally presents an anterior angulation, facilitating the expansion of the uterus and abdominal skin during pregnancy (figure 4). Other uterine positions are possible including various degrees of anteflexion, retroflexion and retrocession (Netter, 1984).

On each side of the uterus fundus, the isthmus give access to the Fallopian tubes, which run from the uterus to each ovary. At the level of the ovaries, each Fallopian tube enlarges to form an ampulla covered with fimbria that are involved in the process of ovulation. Between the Fallopian tubes and the ovaries, a membrane called the mesosalpinx can be observed, where epoophoron, which are embryological remnants of the male vas deferens, can be found.

The vascular supply of the female genitals arises from three major arteries showing some overlap in their distribution. The internal pudendal artery supplies the external genitalia, the vaginal artery the vaginal canal, and the uterine artery the uterus and cervix. The internal pudendal artery running through Alcock's canal, subdivides into the clitoral and the perineal artery (Graziottin 2006). The clitoral artery gives off many subdivisions, starting with an early branch to the bulbar artery, followed by the a branch to the posterior labial artery and continuing toward the clitoris to give two final subdivision, the dorsal artery of the clitoris and the deep artery of the clitoris (Netter, 1984).

The nerve fibres mediating genital responses are composed of three types of nerves, as in men: the somatic pudendal nerve, the parasympathetic pelvic nerve and the sympathetic hypogastric nerve (Rees et al 2007). The somatic pudendal nerve is composed of a sensory fibre called the dorsal nerve of the clitoris and a motor component called the perineal nerve. The perineal nerve also has sensory fibres, innervating the labia majora and the labia minora, giving rise to the labial nerve in the latter case. The parasympathetic pelvic nerve arises from the sacral segment S2, S3, S4 of the spinal cord and runs up to and through the uterovaginal plexus (equivalent to the male pelvic plexus) to synapse with the cavernous nerve (Kato et al 2008) and innervate the vaginal wall and clitoral cavities. The sympathetic hypogastric nerve originates from the thoracolumbar segments T11,T12, L1,L2, where pre-ganglionic splanchnic nerves synapse in the celiac and mesenteric ganglia with the hypogastric nerve innervating the uterus, cervix and vagina (Netter, 1984).

THE FEMALE SEXUAL RESPONSE

Since the work of Masters and Johnson (1966), the female sexual response has been subdivided into phases, still considered today as the normal female sexual function. According to the authors, the female responses begin with arousal, followed by a phase of maximal excitability called the plateau phase and characterized by an orgasmic plateform, followed by orgasm and by a resolution phase. Kaplan later (1974) revised Master and Johnson's model to include an early stage of desire, essential for sexual responsiveness, and followed by arousal, and climax. Each phase is characterized by specific bodily and genital responses. These responses are, as in men, governed by primary reflexes, but modulated by brain influences. Basson's model (2000) emphasizes these supraspinal influences, both cognitive and emotional, and suggests a circular process where the subjective evaluation of a positive sexual experience reinforces the physiological process of desire and arousal, while negative sexual experiences can inhibit the process of desire and arousal.

The arousal phase of the female sexual response is characterized by vasodilation of the internal pudendal artery and vaginal artery, which result in the erection of the clitoris - glans and body -, and in the vasocongestion of the vestibular bulbs and crura (Cuzin, 2012). Immediately accompanying this vasodilation and vasocongestion, is vaginal lubrication, a transudation process, which begins with arousal and continues throughout this phase of female sexual response. As a result of vasodilation of the vaginal arterioles, an osmotic gradient liberates sodium ions from the vaginal wall into the vaginal lumen in an amount exceeding the reabsorption capacity of the vaginal wall, and resulting in the release of plasma throughout the vaginal canal, explaining the transudation process (Cuzin, 2012).

Contrary to previous beliefs, Bartholin glands' secretions participate to sexual arousal, but are not responsible for vaginal lubrication per se. Bartholin glands secretions only begin upon the final stage of sexual arousal (immediately preceding the plateau phase), and involve only transient secretions of a mucus substance that facilitates vaginal penetration.

Sexual arousal is also characterized by congestion of the labia minora and labia majora. In the former case, the congested labia minora separate from each other and give better access to the vaginal opening (Masters & Johnson 1966). In the latter case, vasocongestion of the labia majora along with the contraction of the bulbocavernosus muscles covering the vestibular bulbs give an impression of flattening of the labia which, along with the congested labia minora, facilitates vaginal penetration. Within the vagina, congestion of the vaginal epithelium smoothens the rugosity of the vaginal wall and offers a smoother surface during penile thrusting of intercourse.

According to Masters and Johnson (1966), sexual arousal is further accompanied by uterine movements, which are responsible for the elevation of the cervix and its retraction from the vagina canal. As tension from the uterine ligaments pulls the uterus upward, it clears the cul-de-sac and elongates the vaginal which offers a receptacle where the partner's semen. This elevation and wearing off of the cervix during sexual arousal also allows deeper thrusting during intercourse without pain.

The plateau phase of the female sexual response described by Masters and Johnson's (1966) is characterized by an orgasmic platform defined as a maximal congestion of the genitals, which turn to a dark purple colour, and maximal congestion of the external third of the vagina, which practically closes the vaginal entry. This maximal congestion of the outer third of the vagina can be attributed to the congestion of the clitoral vestibular bulbs surrounding the anterolateral aspect of the vagina. This congested anterolateral aspect of the vagina which contributes to sexual stimulation explains the origin and location of the G spot (Grafenberg 1950; Jannini et al. 2010).

The orgasmic plateform described by Masters and Johnson's (1966) announces the imminence of climax, the latter being characterized by rhythmic involuntary contractions of the perineal muscles, including the bulbospongiosum and ischiocavernosa muscles surrounding the vagina. The recorded muscular responses in electromyographic studies (Gerstenberg et al 1990; Gillan & Brindley 1979; Littler et al 1974; Masters & Johnson 1966;) result in the perceptual experience of pulsations in the clitoris and in the vagina, and in the contractions of the anal and the urethral sphincters. Some women during this phase of the female sexual cycle experience what has been referred to female ejaculation, arising from the secretion of the peri-urethral glands surrounding the female urethra. These glands attributed to vestigial remains of the male prostate glands in women are not consistently present in every women (Battaglia et al, 2010; Gravina et al 2008; Jannini et al 2010).

To these genital responses are added extragenital events which Masters and Johnson (1966) and others (Bohlen et al. 1982; 1984; Carmichael et al. 1994; Hite, 1976; Kinsey et al 1953; Levin 2004; 2006; Meston et al. 2004a; 2004b) recorded during climax and which includes hypertension, tachycardia, hyperventilation, red skin spots, goose bumps and other signs of autonomic activity (Courtois et al 2011; 2013).

According to Masters and Johnson's (1966), orgasm is followed by a resolution phase, which is not characterized in women by a refractory period as described in men. The resolution phase is usually associated with a decrease of all bodily responses, which return back to their normal baseline level. Detumescence of the clitoris occurs, along with decongestion of the vulva and of the vaginal canal. The uterus returns to its normal position, with the cervix diving into the vaginal canal, and the anterior and posterior fornix of the vagina reappear. All signs of autonomic activity slowly disappear and cardiovascular parameters return back to normal. Following the massive muscular contractions of climax, the resolution phase is accompanied with a sense of muscular relaxation.

THE NEUROPHYSIOLOGY OF THE FEMALE SEXUAL RESPONSES

The innervation of the female genitals explains how various sources of stimulation can produce sexual arousal and climax. Similar to men, the women sexual responses are reflexes, which are modulated by the brain. These reflexes mediate erection of the clitoris, vaginal lubrication, vulvar congestion and arise from stimulation of the clitoris, vagina, G spot, cervix, or the overall clitoro-urethro-vaginal complex (Rees et al 2007). Recent studies on fMRI show that women, during sexual arousal, clitoral, vaginal, and also cervix stimulation can lead to orgasm (Komisaruk et al 2004; Whipple et al 2002) (figure 3).

Upon genital stimulation, the dorsal nerve of the clitoris transmits the sensory information to the spinal segments S2, S3, S4 (Giuliano et al 2002). In the cord, sensory inputs 1) send the information to the brain to allow perception of genital arousal and 2) establish synapses with the efferent fibres initiating spinal reflexes responsible for the erection of the clitoris, vulvar congestion and vaginal lubrication. In the first case, sensory information from the genitals to the brain travels up the dorsal column system and the anterolateral spinal thalamic tracts to convey the sensory experience of genital stimulation and the perceptual experience of sexual (genital) arousal. In the second case, incoming sensory information from the dorsal nerve of the clitoris synapse with the intermediolateral pre-ganglionic parasympathetic fibers of the pelvic nerve, which run back to the genitals to produce the simultaneous relaxation of the clitoral smooth muscles and the vasodilation of the pudendal artery and vaginal arteries, resulting in the erection of the clitoris (glans and body), and vasocongestion of the overall clitoro-urethra-vaginal complex, and vaginal lubrication.

The precise mechanism involves both nitric oxide synthase (NOS) described in the previous chapter on erection in men (chapter 1), and vasointestinal peptide (VIP) that is released from the nerve endings and that activates a similar process than the cyclic guanosine monophophase (cGMP) in men (Burnett et al 1997; Gragasin et al 2004; Kim et al 2003; Musicki et al 2009). VIP released from the nerve endings activates the soluble adenylyl cyclase, which transforms adenosine triphosphate (ATP) into cyclic adenosine monophophase (cAMP), which raises the intracellular concentration of cAMP. This increased intracellular content triggers the hyperpolarization of the smooth muscle cells, which then relax and produces vasodilation of the pudendal artery and the relaxation of clitoral trabeculae, resulting in the erection of the clitoris and genital congestion (Cuzin, 2012).

At the same time as parasympathetic activity triggers vulvar vasocongestion, parasympathetic secretion of Bartholin's glands stimulates the release of its mucus substance along the vulva and upon the entry of the vaginal canal to facilitate penetration.

Also accompanying genital vasocongestion, contractions of the bulbospongiosum and ischiocavernosa muscles, which are mediated by the perineal nerve (motor branch of the pudendal nerve), maximize the congestion of arousal and maintains its throughout the arousal and plateau phases.

THE NEUROPHYSIOLOGY OF CLIMAX

The neural mediation of orgasm and its accompanying genital and extragenital responses is still not clearly understood despite decades of research (Mah & Binik 2001; 2002). The nature of orgasm itself is still open to debate (Courtois et al 2011; 2013). A recent consensus on men suggests that the perceptual experience of orgasm results from the contractions of the internal reproductive organs upon emission, the distension of the urethra upon semen accumulation, and the contractions of perineal muscles upon ejaculation (McMahon et al 2004) The corresponding consensus on women suggests that the perceptual experience of orgasm result from an intense peak of pleasure, contractions of the perineal muscles and myotonia, and feelings of well-being and contentment, accompanied with an altered state of consciousness (Meston et al 2004a; 2004b). While the descriptions slightly differ, the underlying physiological changes recorded in both sexes at orgasm are very similar if not identical (Alzate et al 1989; Bohlen et al. 1980; 1982; 1984; Carmichael et al. 1994; Gerstenberg et al, 1990; Hite, 1976; Levin 2004; 2006; Littler et al, 1974; Masters & Johnson, 1966; Meston et al. 2004a; 2004b; Nemec, et al, 1976; Pollock & Schmidt 1995). Furthermore, while the above definition of orgasm in men emphasizes its link with ejaculation, prostatectomized patients report orgasm despite the absence of ejaculation (and hence lack of perceived congestion of the internal reproductive organs and lack of perceived distension of the urethra upon semen accumulation) (Barnas et al 2004; Dubbelman et al 2009; Newman et al 1982; Perelman 2008), and prepubertal boys can report experiencing orgasm before having reached the physiological maturity for ejaculation. The very nature of orgasm is therefore unclear. Its underlying characteristics, along with their neural transmission, have to await a clear definition of orgasm - applicable to both sexes and to various clinical conditions -, before definite conclusions on its pathways and mechanisms can be ascertained.

The many recordings of climax in both women and men show that genital responses (pulsations, contractions of the perineal muscles) are very similar in both sexes and that signs of autonomic discharge, including hypertension, tachycardia, hyperventilation, sweating, piloerection, and red skin spots are also quite identical in both sexes (Bohlen et al. 1980; 1982; 1984; Carmichael et al. 1994; Gerstenberg et al, 1990; Hite, 1976; Levin 2004; 2006;

Littler et al, 1974; Masters & Johnson, 1966; Meston et al. 2004a; 2004b; Nemec, et al, 1976; Pollock & Schmidt 1995). These responses and physiological recordings in able bodied men and women have further been recorded in individuals with spinal cord injury (SCI), a finding which lead Courtois et al (2011; 2013) to propose that orgasm is a multisegmental reflex, modulated by brain influences, and perceived as a result of the transmission of these climactic genital and bodily responses. Adding Basson's circular model (2000) to this interpretation, it could be suggested that the brain during climax interprets incoming peripheral information, with additional emotional and cognitive attributes that have been associated these responses upon previously positive or negative reinforcing experiences.

At the peripheral level, Courtois et al (2004; 2008a; 2008b; 2011; 2013) suggest that orgasm is an autonomic hyperreflexia normally submitted to supraspinal inhibition. In men, this autonomic hyperreflexia can be visually observed (and confirmed/reinforced) with emission, where the internal reproductive organs contract, distend the urethra, and trigger a new reflex to induce ejaculation. Accompanying physiological responses can also be perceived and recorded. Neurologically, the process described in chapter 1 involves the splanchnic nerves exiting the spinal cord from the thoracolumbar segments T11 to L2, and synapsing with the hypogastric nerve to trigger emission in men; followed by a reflex loop triggering ejaculation through the sacral segments S2 to S4. As the splanchnic nerves trigger emission, they can also stimulate the entire sympathetic chain and explain the overall response characterizing orgasm (i.e., hypertension, tachycardia, hyperventilation and the like). In women, although ejaculation seldom occurs and seldom provides a visual feedback for the perceptual experience of climax, the process activating the splanchnic nerves along with stimulation of the entire sympathetic chain, can still be activated upon the threshold of climax. As for men, women could therefore perceive orgasm through the same neurophysiological transmission and pathways but without the objective visual confirmation of ejaculation (Courtois et al 2001).

The neural transmission of orgasm could therefore be reconciliated with this multisegmental hypothesis, which would explain the similarities between men and women's physiological responses at climax (despite the varying subjective and perceptual experiences described). The sensory transmission of these physiological responses has also been subject to much controversy. Sensory transmission is a neurological process that is usually attributed to the somatic nervous system, while the autonomic nervous system is usually attributed to efferent pathways only. Yet, studies on individuals with SCI suggest that autonomic nerves could mediate sensory information from the genitals, a conclusion that has been open to debate. Several studies on men (Courtois et al 2009; 2012; Sipski et al 2006; Soler et al 2008) and women (Bérard 1989; Courtois et al 2011b; Komisaruk et al 2004; Sipski et al 1995; 2001; Whipple et al 1996; 2002) with SCI have described orgasm despite complete lesions to the spinal cord. Whipple et al (2002) and Komisaruk et al (2004) further recorded brain activity from fMRI studies on women with SCI, while demonstrating that the lesions were complete. Altogether, these findings argued for a possible autonomic transmission of genital and climactic responses. Rees et al (2007) in the latest article on the neural control of sexuality in women has summarized these various transmissions. Accordingly, sensory information arising from stimulation, or from erection, of the clitoris can be mediated through the dorsal clitoral nerve, as well as from afferent fibres of the perineal nerves, to which could be added the afferent fibres of the pelvic (parasympathetic) nerve. Vulvar and vaginal vasocongestion, along with stretching of the vaginal tissues during penetration, can also be mediated by the dorsal clitoral and perineal afferent nerves, to which could be added afferent inputs from the pelvic (parasympathetic) nerve for the external portion of the vagina, and afferent inputs from the hypogastric (sympathetic) nerve for the deeper portion of the vagina and cervix. Cervix stimulation and uterine contractions could similarly be perceived by afferent inputs from the hypogastric (sympathetic) nerve, as well as afferent inputs from the Vagus (parasympathetic) nerve, which Whipple et al (2002) and Komisaruk et al (2004) suggested to convey the above mentioned climactic perception of women with SCI.

SUPRASPINAL MODULATION OF SEXUAL RESPONSES

The ascending perception of sexual arousal and climax, as well as the descending influence of sexual desire and arousal on sexual reflexes necessarily involve brain activity (Pfaus 2009). Recent studies on positron emission tomography (PET) and functional magnetic resonance imaging (fMRI) have shown that many structures are activated in the brain during sexual stimulation and orgasm (Bianchi-Demicheli & Ortigues, 2007; Georgiadis et al 2009; Hostege et al 2003). The problem is to distinguish the brain areas that modulate sexual reflexes, from those that are activated as a result of peripheral sensory transmission, and to differentiate the effect of sexual desire from that of arousal, or that of arousal from that of climax.

Studies have generally shown that the medial preoptic area (MPOA) of the hypothalamus, and the paraventricular nucleus (PVN) exert excitatory influences on sexual reflexes, while the paragigantocellularis nucleus (nPGI) in the lower brain stem (more specifically in the reticular formation) exert inhibitory influences on the spinal pathways mediating sexual responses. Pituitary hormones can also influence the production of genital reflexes, while the periacqueductral gray (PAG) exerts inhibition on the nPGI, itself inhibiting sexual reflexes. The PAG's inhibition of the inhibitory nPGI can therefore induce sexual responses. As these structures have interconnections between themselves, as well as interconnections with other brain areas, including the cortex (rational reasoning) and the limbic system (emotional responses, memories of past events), cognitive and emotional states can facilitate or inhibit sexual reflexes, or modulate the perceptual experience of genital reflexes as an arousing or climactic response, or conversely, as an aversive response.

The neural activity that is recorded during the various phases of the male or female sexual responses can therefore both suggest an initiation of genital responses as a result of direct brain activity, or mediate the perception of genital congestion through sensory feedback. In this context, sexual desire could be viewed as initiating genital congestion, or as removing the supraspinal inhibition normally keeping sexual reflexes quiet. Sexual arousal could similarly be viewed as the brain producing genital congestion or as the perceptual feedback of genital congestion from reflex activity. Studies on orgasm have shown that it could involve a generalized activation of many brain areas, but cannot differentiate what is activated by arousal, as opposed to orgasm or post-climatic resolution. Others to the contrary, which have compared "real" and "faked" orgasm, have shown that climax involved a transient but "complete shut off of the brain" (Georgiadis et al. 2009).

Definite advances have therefore been made in the neurophysiology of sexual responses and studies on brain imagery have offered a unique contribution to assess the various stimulation modes that can elicit brain activity (Bianchi-Demicheli & Ortigues, 2007; Georgiadis et al 2009; Hostege et al 2003; Komisaruk et al 2011). Yet, the interpretation of the findings remains open to debate as long as a proper definition of climax is not achieved and as long as a distinction between sexual arousal and sexual climax cannot be made specifically. In the meantime, brain activity is found to participate in the production and/or perception of genital responses, and conversely, genital reflexes are known to be elicited in the absence of any brain inputs, as suggested by the numerous studies on spinal transection (animal studies) and spinal injury (humans).

CONCLUSION

Normal sexual function in women involves a complex set of structures and stimulation sources and responses, with their anatomophysiological and neurological substrates helping us understanding the aetiology of many sexual dysfunctions, which are covered throughout the chapters of this book.

ACKNOWLEDGMENTS

The authors wish to thank Thomas Lefebvre (tal.illustrator@gmail.com) for his drawings of the figures.

REFERENCES

Alzate, H., Useche, B., & Villegas, M. Heart rate change as evidence for vaginally elicited orgasm and orgasm intensity. *Annals of Sex Research* 1989;2:345-357.

Barnas JL, Pierpaoli S, Ladd P, Valenzuela R, Aviv N, Parker M, Qaters WB, Flanigan RC, Mulhall JP. The prevalence and nature of orgasmic dysfunction after radical prostatectomy. *BJU Int.*, 2004; 94(4):603-5.

Basson R. The female sexual response: a different model. *J. Sex Marital Ther.* 2000;26(1):51-65. Review.

Battaglia C, Nappi RE, Mancini F, Alvisi S, Del Forno S, Battaglia B, Venturoli S. PCOS and urethrovaginal space: 3-D volumetric and vascular analysis. *J. Sex. Med.* 2010;7(8):2755-64.

Bérard E. The sexuality of spinal cord injured women: physiology and pathophysiology. A review. *Paraplegia* 1989;27(2): 99-112.

Bianchi-Demicheli F & Ortigue S. Toward an understanding of the cerebral substrates of womand's orgasm. *Neuropsychologia*, 2007;45:2645-2659.

Bohlen JG, Held JP, Sanderson MO, Ahlgren A. The female orgasm: pelvic contractions. *Arch. Sex. Behav.* 1982;11:367-386.

Bohlen JG, Held JP, Sanderson MO, Boyer CM. Development of a woman's multiple orgasm pattern : a research. Case report. *J. Sex Research*, 1982;18(2):130-145.

Bohlen JG, Held JP, Sanderson MO, Patterson RP. Heart rate, rate-pressure product, and oxygen uptake during four sexual activities. *Arch. Internal Med.* 1984;144:1745-1748.

Bohlen JG, Held JP, Sanderson MO. The male orgasm : Pelvic contractions measured by anal probe. *Arch. Sex. Behav.* 1980;9(6).

Buisson O, Foldes P, Paniel BJ. Sonography of the clitoris. *J. Sex. Med.* 2008;5(2):413-7.

Burnett AL, Calvin DC, Silver RI, Peppas DS, Docimo SG. Immunohistochemical descripton fo nitric oxide synthase isoforms in human clitoris. *J. Urol.* 1997;158:75-78.

Carmichael MS, Warburton VL, Dixen J, Davidson JM. Relationships among cardiovascular, muscular, and oxytocin responses during human sexual activity. *Arch. Sex. Behav.* 1994;23(1), 59-79.

Caruso S, Cianci A, Malandrino C, Cavallari L, Gambadoro O, Arena G, PispisaL, Agnello C, Romano M, Cavallari V. Ultrastructural and quantitative study of clitoral cavernous tissue from living subjects. *J. Sex. Med.* 2011;8(6):1675-85.

Courtois F, Carrier S, Charvier K, Guertin P, *Morel Journel N.* The control of male sexual responses. Current Pharm Design 2013, in press.

Courtois F, Charvier K, Bélanger D, Vézina J-G, Côté I, Boulet M, Carrier S, Jaquemin G. Clinical approach to anorgasmia in women with spinal cord injury. *Journal of Sexual Medicine* 2011b;8(suppl5):380.

Courtois F, Charvier K, Carrier S, Vézina J-G, Côté I, Dahan V, Morel Journel N. Sexual options for men and women with spinal cord injuries. AA Martin & JE Jones (Eds). Spinal cord injuries: Causes, risk factors and management. New York: Novapublishers. 2012.

Courtois F., Charvier K, Vézina J-G, Carrier S, Morel Journel N, Jacquemin G, Leriche A. Assessment of sexual potential and treatment of sexual dysfunctions in men and women with spinal cord injury. Ed Tanya C Berkovsky, Handbook of Spinal Cord Injuries: Types, Treatments and Progronis. New York: Novapublishers. 2009.

Courtois, F, Charvier, K., Leriche, A., Vézina, J.-G., Côté, I, Raymond, D, Jacquemin, G, Fournier, C & Bélanger, M. Perceived physiological and orgasmic sensations at ejaculation in spinal cord injured men. *J. Sex. Med.* 2008b, 5(10), 2419-2430.

Courtois, F, Charvier, K., Leriche, A., Vézina, J.-G., Côté, M & Bélanger, M. Blood pressure changes during sexual stimulation, ejaculation and midodrine treatment in spinal cord injured men. *BJU Int.* 2008a,101,331-337.

Courtois, F, Charvier, K., Vézina, J.-G., Morel-Journel N, Carrier S., Jacquemin, G, Côté, I. Assessing and conceptualizing orgasm following a spinal cord injury. *BJU Int.* 2011a, 108(10):1624-1633.

Courtois, F., Geoffrion, R., Landry, E. & Bélanger, M. H reflex and physiological measures of ejaculation in spinal cord injured men. *Arch. Phys. Med. Rehabil.* 2004, 85, 910-918.

Cuzin B. Anatomy and physiology of female sexual organs. In Porst J & Reisman Y. The ESSM Syllabus of Sexual Medicine. Amsterdam: MEDIX publishers, 2012.

Deliganis AV, Maravilla KR, Heiman JR, Carter WO, Garland PA, Peterson BR, Hackbert L, Cao Y, Weisskoff RM. Female genitalia: dynamic MR imaging with use of MS-325- initial experiences evaluating female sexual response. *Radiology* 2002;225(3):791-799.

Deng J, Crouch NS, Creighton SM, Linney AD, Todd-Pokropek A, Rodeck CH. Minimally-compressive, three- and four-dimensional ultrasound imaging of the clitoris: a feasibility study. *Ultrasound Med. Biol.* 2006;32(10):1479-84.

Dubbelman Y, Wildhagen M, Schröder F, Bangma C, Dohle G. Orgasmic dysfunction after open radical prostatectomy: Clinical correlates and prognostic factors. *J. Sex. Med.* 2009 Nov 13. [Epub ahead of print].

Foldes P, Buisson O. The clitoral complex: a dynamic sonographic study. *J. Sex. Med.* 2009;6(5):1223-31.

Georgiadis JR, Reinders AATS, PaansAMJ, Renken R, Dortekaas R. men versus women on sexual brain function: prominent differnces during tactile genital stimulation, but not during orgasm. *Human Brain Mapping*, 2009, 30:3089-3101.

Gerstenberg TC, Levin RJ, Wagner G. Erection and ejaculation in man. Assessment of the electromyographic activity of the bulbocavernosus and ischiocavernosus muscles. *BJU Int.* 1990;65:395-402.

Gillan P & Brindley GS. Vaginal and pelvic floor responses to sexual stimulation. *Psychophysiology* 1979;16(5):471-481.

Giuliano F, Rampin O, Allard J. Neurophysiology and pharmacology of female genital sexual response. *J. Sex Marital Ther.* 2002;28 Suppl 1:101-21.

Grafenberg, E. The role of the urethra in female orgasm. *International Journal of Sexology* 1950;3:145-148.

Gragasin FS, Michelakis ED, Hogan A, Moudgil R, Hashimoto K, Wu X, Bonnet S, Haromy A, Archer SL.The neurovascular mechanism of clitoral erection: nitric oxide and cGMP-stimulated activation of BKCa channels. *FASEB J.* 2004;18(12):1382-91.

Gravina GL, Brandetti F, Martini P, Carosa E, Di Stasi SM. Morano S, Lenzi A, Jannini EA. Measurement of the thickness of the urethrovaginal space in women with or without vaginal orgasm. *J. Sex. Med.* 2008;5(3):610-8.

Graziottin A. Introduction to female sexual disorders. In H Porst & J Buvat Standard Practice in Sexual Medicine. Oxford: Blackwell Publishing 2006

Hite, S. The Hite report: A nationwide study of female sexuality. New York, Macmillan, 1976.

Hostege G, Georgiadis JR, Paans AMJ, Meiners LC, van der Graaf FHCE, Reinders AATS. Brain activation during male ejaculation. *J. Neuroscience*, 2003, 23(27):9185-9193.

Jannini EA, Whipple B, Kingsberg SA, Buisson O, Foldès PE, Vardi Y.Who's afraid of the G-Sport?, *J. Sex. Med.* 2010;7: 25-34.

Kaplan, H.S. The new sex therapy. New York, Brunner/Mazel, 1974.

Kato M, Niikura J, Yaegashi N, Murakami G, Tatsumi H, Matsubara A. Histotopography of the female cavernous nerve: using donated fetuses and adult cadavers. *Int. Urogynecol. J.* 2008;19:1687-1695.

Khalifé S, Binik YM, Cohen DR, Amsel R. Evaluation of clitoral blood flow by color doppler ultrasonography. *J. Sex Marit. Ther.* al 2000; 26:187-189.

Kim SW, Jeong SJ, Munarriz R, Kim NN, Goldstein I, Traish AM. Role of the nitric oxide-cyclic GMP pathway in regulation of vaginal blood flow. *Int. J. Impot. Res.* 2003; 15(5):355-61.

Kinsey, A.C., Pomeroy, W.B., Martin, C.E., & Gebhard, P.H. Sexual behavior in the human female. Philadephia, Saunders, 1953.

Komisaruk BR, Whipple B, Crawford A, Liu WC, Kalnin A, & Mosier K. Brain activation during vaginocervical self-stimulation and orgasm in women with complete spinal cord injury: fMRI evidence of mediation by the vagus nerves. *Brain Res.*, 2004 1024(1-2), 77-88.

Komisaruk BR, Wise N, Frangos E, Wen-Ching L, Allen K, Brody S. Women's clitoris, vagina, and cervix mapped on the sensory cortex: fMRI evidence. *J. Sex. Med.* 2011;8(10):2822-2830.

Kukkonen TM, Paterson L, Binik YM, Amsel R, Bouvier F, Khalifé S. Convergent and discriminant validity of clitoral color doppler ultrasonography as a measure of female sexual arousal. *J. Sex Marit. Ther.* 2006;32:281-287.

Levin RJ. An orgasm is… who defines what an orgasm is? *Sexual Relationship Therapy*, 2004;19(1):101-107.

Levin RJ. Vocalised sounds and human sex. Science update. *Sexual Relationship Therapy* 2006;21(1):99-107.

Littler WA, Honour AJ, Sleight P. Direct arterial pressure, heart rate and electrocardiogram during human coitus. *J. Reprod. Fertil.* 1974;40:321-331.

Mah K & Binik YM. The nature of human orgasm: a critical review of major trends. *Clin. Psychol. Rev.* 2001;21(6):823-56.

Mah, K., & Binik, Y.M. (2002). Do all orgasms feel alike? Evaluating a two-dimensional model of the orgasm experience across gender and sexual context. *J. Sex Research*, 2002; 39(2): 104-113.

Masters, W. H., & Johnson, V. E. *Human Sexual Response.* Boston, Little Brown. 1966.

McMahon CG, Abdo C, Incrocci L, Perelman M, Rowland D, Studkey B, Waldinger M ChengXin Z. Disorders of orgasm and ejaculation in men. In T Lue, Basson R, Rosen R, Giuliano F, Khoury S, Montorsi F (Eds). Sexual Medicine: Sexual Dysfunctions in Men and Women. 2nd International consultation on Sexual dysfunctions, Paris: Editions 21, 2004.

Meston CM, Hull E, Levin RJ, Sipski M. Women's orgasm. In T Lue, Basson R, Rosen R, Giuliano F, Khoury S, Montorsi F (Eds). Sexual Medicine: Sexual Dysfunctions in Men and Women. 2nd International consultation on Sexual dysfunctions, Paris: Editions 21, 2004a.

Meston, C., Levin, R., Sipski, M., Hull, E. & Heiman, *J. Women's orgasm*, review. Annual Review of Sex Research, 2004b;15:173-257.

Musicki B, Liu T, Lagoda GA, Bivalacqua TJ, Strong TD, Burnett AL.Endothelial nitric oxide synthase regulation in female genital tract structures. *J. Sex. Med.* 2009;6 Suppl 3:247-53.

Nemec ED, Mansfield L, Kennedy JW. Heart rate and blood pressure responses during sexual activity in normal males. *Am. Heart J.*, 1976;92:274-277.

Netter FH. Reproductive System. The CIBA Collection of Medical Illustrations (Vol 2). New York: CIBA Pharmaceutical Company (7th ed), 1984.

Newman HF, Reiss H, Northup JD. Physical basis of emission, ejaculation, and orgasm in the male. Urology 1982;19(4):341-350.

O'Connell HE & DeLancey JOL. Clitoral anatomy in nulliparous, healthy, premenopausal volunteers using unenhanced magnetic resonance imaging. *J. Urol.* 2005;173:2060-2063.

O'Connell HE, Eizenberg N, Rahman M, Cleeve J. The anatomy of the distal vagina: towards unity. *J. Sex. Med.* 2008;5(8):1883-91.

Perelman MA. Post-prostatectomy orgasmic response. *J. Sex. Med.*, 2008, 5(1)248-9.

Pfaus JG. Pathways of sexual desire. *J. Sex. Med.* 2009;6(6):1506-33.

Pollock ML, Schmidt DH. Heart Disease and Rehabilation. Champaign, IL: Human Kinetics, 1995;372.

Rees PM, Fowler CJ, Paas, CP. Sexual function in men and women with neurological disorders. *The Lancet* 2007;369:512-525.

Sipski LM, Alexander CJ, Rosen R. Orgasm in women with spinal cord injuries: A laboratory-based assessment. *Arch. Phys. Med. Rehabil.* 1995;76:1097-1102.

Sipski LM, Alexander CJ, Rosen R. Sexual arousal and orgasm in Women: effects of spinal cord injury. *Ann. Neurol.* 2001;49:35-44.

Sipski M, Alexander CJ, Gómez-Marín O. Effects of level and degree of spinal cord injury on male orgasm. *Spinal Cord.* 2006;44:798-804.

Soler JM, Previnaire JG, Plante P, Denys P, Chartier-Kastler E. Midodrine improves orgasm in spinal cord-injured men: the effects of autonomic stimulation. *J. Sex. Med.* 2008; 5(12):2935-41.

Suh DD, Yang CC, Cao Y, Garland PA, Maravilla KR. Magnetic resonance imaging anatomy of the female genitalia in premenopausal and postmenopausal women. *J. Urol.* 2003; 170:138-144.

Whipple B, Gerdes CA, Komisaruk BR. Sexual response to self-stimulation in women with complete spinal cord injury. *J. Sex Research* 1996;33(3):231-40.

Whipple B, Komisaruk BR. Brain (PETG) responses to vaginal-cervical self-stimulation in women with complete spinal cord injury: preliminary findings. *J. Sex Marital Ther.* 2002;28:79-86.

In: Sexual Dysfunctions
Editor: Frédérique Courtois

ISBN: 978-1-62808-765-9
© 2013 Nova Science Publishers, Inc.

Chapter 11

FEMALE SEXUAL DYSFUNCTIONS AND UROGYNECOLOGICAL DISORDERS

Emilio Sacco[1,] and Daniele Tienforti[2]*

[1]Urologic Clinic, Department of Surgical Sciences, "Agostino Gemelli" Hospital,
Catholic University School of Medicine of Rome, Rome, Italy
[2]Urologic Surgery, Columbus Integrated Complex,
Catholic University Medical School of Rome, Rome, Italy

ABSTRACT

Female sexual function represents a very important dimension of a woman's quality of life and female sexual dyfunctions have been recognized as a highly prevalent, age-related health problem among women affected by lower urinary tract disorders such as urinary incontinence, overactive bladder syndrome and bladder pain syndrome/interstitial cystitis. These observations are of utmost importance for physicians dealing with women's health, especially because these disorders are an exceedingly common and increasing health problem worldwide. Reportedly, female sexual dysfunctions affect 26-64% of women with lower urinary tract symptoms and women with urinary incontinence are twice as likely as women without urinary incontinence to experience diminished libido, vaginal dryness, and dyspareunia; up to 65% of women with urinary incontinence report loss of urine during sexual intercourse, and about two third of them report that the condition has a negative impact on sexual relationships. Herein we present a review of the research aimed to investigate the impact of urogynecological disorders on female sexual function and of the available treatment options for these disorders.

INTRODUCTION AND EPIDEMIOLOGY

Sexuality is one of the most important components of quality of life (QoL) in both sexes. Basic scientific research on this issue has been limited for many years. Recent advances in

---

* Corresponding author: Emilio Sacco MD., Urologic Clinic, Department of Surgical Sciences, "Agostino Gemelli" Hospital, Catholic University School of Medicine of Rome, Rome, Italy. E-mail: emilio.sacco@gmail.com.

our understanding of male sexual dysfunction and treatment options have facilitated the interest for women psychosexual well being that prompted studies on the anatomy and physiology of normal female sexual response and on female sexual dysfunctions (FSDs) [1].

Several epidemiological studies recognized FSDs as a common problem in women and found an association between FSDs and various demographic characteristics, including age, education and race throughout the world. Laumann et al. [2] analyzed data from the National Health and Social Life Survey (NHSLS), a probability study of sexual behavior on a sample of 1,749 women and 1,410 men aged 18 to 59 years from the USA, reporting a very high prevalence of sexual dysfunctions in both sexes, higher in women (43%) than men (31%). These data were confirmed by further studies like the Global Study of Sexual Attitudes and Behaviors (GSSAB) on 13,882 women and 13,618 men aged 40-80 years from 29 countries [3] and the National Social Life, Health, and Aging Project (NSHAP) on 1,550 women and 1,455 men aged 57-85 from USA [4], that showed a comparable prevalence of sexual problems in the analyzed populations.

Lower urinary tract symptoms (LUTS) and pelvic floor disorders (PFDs) are exceedingly common health problems and increasing in incidence worldwide. According to Irwin et al. [5] 45.2%, 10.7%, 8.2% and 21.5% of the 2008 worldwide population (4.3 billion) was affected by at least one LUTS, overactive bladder syndrome (OAB), urinary incontinence (UI) and LUTS suggestive of bladder outlet obstruction (LUTS/BOO), respectively. By 2018, an estimated 2.3 billion individuals will be affected by at least one LUTS (18.4% increase), 546 million by OAB (20.1%), 423 million by UI (21.6%) and 1.1 billion by LUTS/BOO (18.5%). The study of Nygaard et al. [6] represents the first nationwide, population-based estimates of the three primary pelvic floor disorders in women in the United States derived from a single source. Overall, 23.7% of women had symptoms of at least one pelvic floor disorder. Of these, 15.7% experienced urinary incontinence, 9.0% experienced fecal incontinence and 2.9% experienced symptomatic pelvic organ prolapse. The proportion of women that reported at least one pelvic floor disorder increased incrementally with age: 9.7% in women aged 20 to 39 years, 26.5% in women aged 40 to 59 years, 36.8% in women aged 60 to 79 years, and 49.7% in women aged 80 years or older. Other characteristics that were significantly associated with at least one pelvic floor disorder were family poverty income ratio, body mass index and parity.

Female sexual function (FSF) is intuitively influenced by LUTS and PFDs and several observational studies confirmed that FSDs are a highly prevalent health problem among women affected by LUTS [7-13]. However, data on the relative impairment of female sexuality in women with different types of LUTS/PFDs are deficient [11], and the consistency of studies is often limited by several biases such as use of non-condition-specific instruments and lack of a control group or of a comprehensive urodynamic evaluation [12]. Herein we reviewed the available data on the epidemiological, clinical and biological relationships linking FSDs with LUTS and PFDs, including OAB, UI, urinary tract infections (UTIs), pelvic organ prolapse (POP), bladder pain syndrome/interstitial cystitis (BPS/IC).

DEFINITIONS

In the past years, FSF was described using linear-type models. Masters and Johnson [14] first characterized the female sexual cycle as four consecutive phases: excitement, plateau, orgasm, and resolution. Kaplan [15] proposed a three-phase model, which included desire, arousal, and orgasm. In these models sexual desire is described as a force that spontaneously "per se" stimulates sexual arousal. Recently, Basson [16] has developed a circular model of female sexuality, which introduces the association of the physiological stage of resolution with a process of subjective evaluation of the experience in terms of satisfaction / dissatisfaction. The circularity of the model showed a new dynamic relationship between the dimensions of sexual function: a frustrating experience can take to progressive inhibition of sexual desire (negative feedback), while a satisfactory experience can improve it (positive feedback). This model underlines the strong reciprocity between desire and arousal and helps to understand the frequent co-presence of sexual dysfunctions considering the close interdependence between the different phases of sexual response [17].

The second International Conference of Consensus on Women's Sexual Disorders [18] classified FSDs in 4 categories: sexual desire disorders, sexual arousal disorders, orgasmic disorders and sexual pain disorders. It has been estimated that 40–50% of women report at least one sexual complaint related to these aspects of sexual function [19].

The Diagnostic and Statistical Manual of Mental Disorders (DSM) IV-TR defines FSD as "disturbances in sexual desire and in the psycho-physiological changes that characterize the sexual response cycle and cause marked distress and interpersonal difficulty" [20], as a result both sexual function and sexually related personal distress should be considered when assessing FSD. In fact, not all sexual complaints lead to dissatisfaction or sexual distress and, until recently, most research on FSF has focused on sexual complaints but has not considered the quality of life (QoL) impact of these complaints in relation to sexual distress [21]. In this regard, focusing on sexual distress and using the Female Sexual Distress Scale (FSDS), Knoepp et al. [22] assessed sexual complaints among 305 women seeking outpatient gynecologic care because of LUTS and PFDs. Twenty-six percent of the scores reflected distress, and distressed women were more likely to be younger, have higher depression scores and report decreased arousal, infrequent orgasm, and dyspareunia. Women with sexual distress were also more likely to report sexual difficulty related to pelvic floor symptoms, including UI with sexual activity, sexual avoidance due to vaginal prolapse, or sexual activity restriction due to fear of UI.

DIAGNOSIS AND EVALUATION

The diagnosis of sexual dysfunction requires a complete anamnesis with regard to the medical and psycho-sexual history. Many medical conditions may negatively affect sexual life, including hormonal factors (low estrogens or androgens level, thyroid dysfunctions, high prolactin level, adrenal alterations), chronic diseases (diabetes, chronic renal failure, cardiovascular or autoimmune diseases), vascular alterations, neurological or psychiatric conditions and drug treatments. The role of LUTS and PFDs in contributing to and maintaining FSDs is often neglected in female patients, while a complete physical exam, including an external and internal gynecological exam, is essential to avoid both a systematical medical omission and a gender bias [23].

Regarding sexual anamnesis, some studies have shown that physicians are reluctant to address sexual matters, citing many reasons including "embarrassment in sexual language", "fear of offending the patient", "feeling uncomfortable with the topic", "not knowing the exact questions to ask or how to ask" [24-26] but data show that patients believe that sexual function is a relevant topic and are relieved when they discuss it with their doctor [27]. Many men and women demand to know where are located in the continuum from normality to malfunction. Direct and open-ended interview can help the doctor and patient to better understand the patient's sexual dysfunction. As reported by Graziottin et al. [28], the so-called "descriptors" of the disorders, as defined by the International Consensus Conferences held in 1998 and 2003, include the etiology, further detailed in predisposing, precipitating and maintaining factors, the presence of a generalized (in every situation) or situational (precipitated by contextual factors) disorder, the disorder being lifelong or acquired after previous satisfying sexual experiences and the level of distress, defined as the impact of the FSD on personal life.

The self-administered questionnaires are a reliable and inexpensive standardized method for data collection as well as a clinical evaluation of the objective QoL in these patients. Several self-report validated or not validated questionnaires are available for assessing different aspects of sexual function in women [29-41] and may be divided into generalized or condition-specific. Generalized questionnaires were designed to evaluate sexual function in a general population and not specifically in women with LUTS and PFDs. These types of questionnaires may not be sensitive enough to detect differences due to the disease process of UI, OAB and/or POP in this specialized population. Most of the published studies in this specific population have investigated FSF using the Female Sexual Function Index (FSFI) [39] or the POP/UI Sexual Questionnaire (PISQ) [42]. The FSFI is a 19-item questionnaire that features six areas of sexual function in general population: desire, arousal, lubrication, orgasm, satisfaction and pain. The PISQ assesses sexual function in women with POP and/or UI. The original long form of the PISQ has 31 questions and contains three domains: behavioral-emotive, physical, and partner-related. The behavioral-emotive domain measures the frequency of sexual activity, the desired frequency, orgasm rates, and satisfaction with one's sexual relationship. The physical domain examines episodes of pain, incontinence, sensation of prolapse, and fear of fecal and/or urinary incontinence during sexual activity. The partner-related domain includes any difficulty with erectile dysfunction, premature ejaculation, vaginal attenuation, vaginal tightness, or the patient's perception of a partner's avoidance of intercourse. Their abbreviated forms (figure 1) have a wider applicability in the clinic to minimize the time of administration [43, 44].

Among other most used sexual questionnaire, the Brief Index of Sexual Function in Women (BISF-W) [36] is a self-administered validated questionnaire with 21 items related to sexual interest, activity, satisfaction, and preference that can be used to differentiate between patients with depression, sexual dysfunction and healthy patients.

The McCoy Female Sexuality Questionnaire (MFSQ) [45] was developed from the questionnaire used in a longitudinal study of the menopausal transition and designed to measure aspects of female sexuality likely to be affected by changing sex hormone levels. The original questionnaire was revised to insure that questions were easy to understand and that labels for the Likert scales described a continuum. The revised MFSQ contains 19 questions, 18 items using 7-point Likert scales with labels at the center and endpoints and one item requesting a frequency of activity. Seven studies involving both clinical and convenience samples and two with double blind randomized controlled trials used 7, 9, 10 or 17 MFSQ items and demonstrated acceptable reliability, internal consistency, apparent face and content validity as well as considerable evidence of construct validity.

The International Continence Society (ICS) provided a validated questionnaire, the ICIQ-Female Sexual Matters associated with Lower Urinary Tract Symptoms (ICIQ-FLUTSsex) [46], which is useful for researchers and clinicians in both primary and secondary care institutions to obtain a brief, yet comprehensive, summary of female sexual matters and the impact of urinary symptoms on this.

Up until now there have been no reported standardized values for what should be considered a "normal" sexual function and the majority of studies shows the changes in the overall score over time. However, average values of the women with and without LUTS and UI have been reported for the FSFI [44] and for the PISQ [42].

LUTS and Overactive Bladder

The ICS divides LUTS into three groups based on the phases of the micturition cycle: storage, voiding, and postmicturition LUTS [47]. However, the ICS also recognizes a number of pain syndromes that are poorly defined and cannot be easily classified. Storage symptoms include increased daytime frequency, urgency, incontinence and nocturia. Increased daytime frequency is the complaint by the patient who considers that he/she voids too often by day. Nocturia is the complaint that the individual has to wake at night one or more times to void. Urgency is the complaint of a sudden compelling desire to pass urine, which is difficult to defer. Voiding symptoms are experienced during the voiding phase and include slow stream, splitting or spraying of the stream, intermittent stream, hesitancy, straining to void and terminal dribble. Postmicturition symptoms are experienced immediately after micturition and include a feeling of incomplete emptying and postmicturition dribble. Urinary urgency, often associated with urinary frequency and nocturia, characterized OAB. OAB with urgency, frequency and nocturia is referred to as OAB-dry, whereas OAB-wet is the term used when urgency urinary incontinence (UUI) is also present. Detrusor muscle overactivity is often, although not always, the urodynamic condition underlying the OAB [48].

Several studies showed that LUTS and OAB have a significant negative effect on patients' QoL, impairing not only physical well being but also emotional health, work productivity, social and personal relationships and sleep [49-51], but only a few studies have assessed the specific impact of OAB on sexual health [52-54]. Coyne et al. [53] performed a case-control study of 1, 434 OAB cases that were matched by age, gender and country, with 1, 434 participants designated as controls. Decreased enjoyment of sexual activity was reported by 15.4% of cases versus only 2.8% of controls. Patel et al. [55] found that a quarter of studied women with OAB reported difficulty with sexual arousal, orgasm and sexual enjoyment. These findings were confirmed in other studies, which reported that sexual activity and QoL were significantly impaired in women with OAB [49, 50].

Mechanisms associated with the impact of OAB on FSF can be the fear of leakage during stimulation and intercourse, coital UI during orgasm, the need to interrupt intercourse to void, urgency and frequency after coitus, dyspareunia and pelvic floor dysfunction.

Discordant data are reported on the impact of the type of OAB on sexual function. In a retrospective evaluation of 236 female patients with LUTS, Cohen et al [11] reported that patients with clinical diagnosis of OAB-dry had higher sexual function than patients with OAB-wet. In a cross-sectional studies, Sacco el at. [12] observed that among patients with LUTS or OAB, those with OAB-wet or urodynamically-proven detrusor overactivity incontinence reported the highest degree of FSD in all items of the PISQ-12 except for pain, according to other studies [13, 56]. Studies based on focus group also suggested that OAB continence status affects different areas of women's sexuality. Coyne et al. [52] studied sexual health of 34 sexually active women with OAB (11 continent and 23 incontinent) and reported that arousal and orgasm were found to be adversely affected in both groups, but continent women appeared to retain sexual desire, although pain, frequency and urgency reduced sexual pleasure and led to frustration with their sex lives, while incontinent women reported a decrease in sexual desire, pain with intercourse, and the need to interrupt intercourse to void. On the other hand, some studies did not confirm these data. In a national Korean telephone survey with 2, 005 subjects (1, 005 women and 1, 000 men) interviewed, Choo et al. [57] found that in female subjects the likelihood of the impact on sexual life and willingness to seek medical help was not related to urge incontinence, and in a study comparing FSFI score of 40 patients with OAB to 40 controls, all domains in the OAB group were found to be lower than in the control group but OAB-dry and OAB-wet group were similar to each other [58].

Controversial data are available about the relationship between voiding-LUTS suggesting of BOO and FSD. Salonia et al.[10] reported a significant association between sexual pain disorder and voiding dysfunctions, particularly when associated to recurrent cystitis. The study of Sacco et al [12] did not confirm this finding because voiding-LUTS did not significantly impair FSF in their cohort of women with LUTS.

URINARY INCONTINENCE

Urinary incontinence (UI) is defined as "any involuntary loss of urine" [47]. As reported by Blaivas and Sandha [59], it denotes a symptom, a sign, and a condition. It indicates the patient's (or caregiver's) statement of involuntary urine loss. The sign is the objective demonstration of urine loss. The condition is the pathophysiology underlying incontinence as demonstrated by clinical, cystoscopic, or urodynamic techniques. The symptoms of incontinence include stress, urge, mixed, unaware, continuous incontinence, and nocturnal enuresis [47]. Stress urinary incontinence (SUI) is the complaint of involuntary leakage on effort or exertion or on sneezing or coughing, and urgency incontinence (UUI) is the complaint of involuntary leakage accompanied by or immediately preceded by urgency. Mixed urinary incontinence (MUI) is the complaint of involuntary leakage associated with urgency and with exertion, effort, sneezing, or coughing. Enuresis means any involuntary loss of urine, and nocturnal enuresis is the complaint of loss of urine occurring during sleep.

Continuous UI is the complaint of continuous leakage. Other types of UI may be situational, such as the report of incontinence during sexual intercourse or giggle incontinence.

The loss of urine significantly impairs the QoL of women, who are forced to organize exhausting strategies to prevent or mask stains and/or odors [60]. At emotional and behavioral level a generalized apathy, feelings of guilt and depressive attitude may develop to different areas of life, especially when UUI is concerned because of the unpredictable nature of the symptoms [61]. Thus, several studies showed a correlation between UI and major depression, which has a three times higher incidence in patients with UI than in those continents [62]. Specifically, women with UI feel threatened in their femininity expressing feelings of shame, inadequacy and reduced self-esteem [63-65] and subsequently a communicative and emotional inability with a strong sense of isolation [66]. These psychological consequences together with the lack of libido and reduced level of self-esteem because of a fear of uncontrolled leakage are the main factors in women with UI and FSDs [67]. Dyspareunia secondary to urine dermatitis or UI surgery and uncontrollable leakage during intercourse may also contribute.

Prevalence rates of FSDs in women with UI are estimated to range between 26-47% [68-70]. All forms of UI are associated with FSD of all phases of the sexual cycle and studies have examined the impact of UI on individual domains of sexual function and satisfaction [11, 58, 71-74].

Salonia et al. [10] found in population of women with LUTS that 47% of patients who reported a hypoactive sexual desire had SUI, and 46% of those who reported orgasm problems also had significant symptoms of OAB with UUI. The study concluded that patients with UI or LUTS more frequently suffer from FSDs compared to healthy control patients. Accordingly, Yip et al. [13] found that patients with SUI or OAB have a decreased QoL measured with King's Health Questionnaire (KHQ) [75], less sexual satisfaction and worse marital relations than controls.

In the study of Coksuer et al. [76], patients with a diagnosis of MUI had significantly lower mean PISQ-12 scores than the ones with SUI and detrusor overactivity whereas patients with SUI had lower mean PISQ-12 scores than patients with detrusor overactivity, consequently they concluded that MUI has the greatest impact on sexual function when compared with SUI and detrusor overactivity alone. Sacco et al. [7] reported that, among women with UI and/or OAB, those with UUI and MUI reported worse FSD as compared with those with SUI or OAB-dry. Women with urodynamically-proven detrusor overactivity incontinence appeared in this and other studies to have the worst FSF [7, 12, 56].

Nilsson et al. [77] evaluated women with UI and/or urinary urgency and their partners and reported that 22% of the men and 43% of the women stated that the female urinary symptoms impaired their sexual life, 49% of the women expressed worries about having urinary leakage during sexual activity, but 94% of their men did not. Twenty-three percent of the men and 39% of the women reported that the woman leaked urine during sexual activity and the majority (84%) of women considered this a problem, but 65% of their partners did not.

The fear of urine leakage during intercourse was found in 11-45% of women with UI [78-83]. Moran et al. [82] found that 11% of 2, 153 women had UI during intercourse, most of which reported this symptom only in a questionnaire, 70% reported urine leakage during penetration, 20% only during orgasm and 11% during both penetration and orgasm. A SUI was present in 80% of women with UI during penetration, in 93% of women with UI during orgasm and in 92% of women with UI during both phases. The pathophysiology leading to UI during intercourse is not clear. During penetration, the displacement of the anterior wall of the vagina and bladder neck or the increase of the intra-abdominal pressure loss can cause SUI. Detrusorial simultaneous contractions and urethral relaxation were demonstrated in urodynamic studies during orgasm [80].

Recent studies evaluated the relationship between body mass index (BMI), UI and FSD among perimenopausal and postmenopausal [84] or overweight and obese women [85, 86] showing that UUI and SUI are more common and have greater impact on sexual function in obese women and increased BMI early in menopause represents a risk both for UI and for FSD, although the severity of the FSD may not be directly related to the severity of UI or obesity.

BLADDER PAIN SYNDROME/INTERSTITIAL CYSTITIS

According to ESSIC consensus criteria [87], bladder pain syndrome/interstitial cystitis (BPS/IC), also referred to as chronic pelvic pain (CPP), would be diagnosed on the basis of chronic (>6 months) pelvic pain, pressure or discomfort perceived to be related to the urinary bladder accompanied by at least one other urinary symptom like persistent urge to void or frequency, confusable diseases as the cause of the symptoms must be excluded, further documentation and classification of BPS might be performed according to findings at cystoscopy with hydrodistension and morphological findings in bladder biopsies. The presence of other organ symptoms as well as cognitive, behavioural, emotional and sexual symptoms should be addressed.

Sexual dysfunction issues have been reported among women with BPS/IC and can contribute to reduced QoL in these patients. Pelvic pain due to inflammation of the bladder wall and neuropathic dysfunction, dyspareunia, and fear of pain during intercourse are particularly frequent among these patients and may cause resistance to penetration and consequent pelvic floor overactivity, vulvodynia, and vaginismus [12].

Peters et al. [88] sent a mailed survey to 5, 000 randomly selected women from the United States (controls) and 407 women with IC (cases) from a large referral center, including the Female Sexual Distress Scale (FSDS) and questions about sexual function, desire, orgasm, and pain. A significantly greater proportion of cases reported fear of pain and pain with intercourse. In adulthood, a significantly greater proportion of cases reported having pelvic pain, fear of pain during intercourse, and dyspareunia. Furthermore, after the diagnosis of IC, the number of cases reporting moderate to high desire and orgasm frequently and very frequently declined significantly. Verit et al. [89] evaluated 112 women complaining of CPP with a comprehensive history, including FSFI, compared with a group of 108 healthy women without CPP. Among 112 CPP patients, 78 (69.6%) of them had FSD in this study. Among patients with FSD, 42 patients (53.8%) had hypoactive sexual desire disorder, 26 patients (33.3%) had sexual arousal disorder, 17 patients (21.7%) had orgasmic disorder and finally 58 patients (74.3%) had sexual pain disorder. In compliance with these findings, using FSFI to compare FSD in 75 patients affected by IC with 22 controls, Ottem et al. [90] reported that total adjusted FSFI scores differed between patients and controls and that 51 patients (68%) had an abnormal FSFI score versus 3 controls (14%), concluding that patients with IC have sexual dysfunction, including pain, dyspareunia, sexually related distress and significant declines in desire and orgasm frequency, more commonly than do controls. Accordingly, in their cross-sectional study Sacco et al. [12] showed that among women with several types of lower urinary tract disorders, those with BPS reported the greatest adverse impact on FSF (evaluated with the PISQ-1), mostly because of sexual pain, followed by those with UUI.

In a survey of 1, 469 women who met criteria for BPS/IC diagnosis, 88% of those with a sexual partner reported ≥1 general sexual dysfunction symptom and 90% reported ≥1 BPS/IC-specific sexual dysfunction symptom in the past 4 weeks [91]. In the multivariate models, BPS/IC-specific sexual dysfunction was significantly associated with more severe BPS/IC symptoms, younger age, worse depression symptoms, and worse perceived general health. Of note, only a small proportion (about 10–20%) of those women with sexual dysfunction seek medical help for the condition.

According to AUA Guidelines [92], sexual functioning is a primary predictor of mental QoL in women with long-standing BPS/IC and may be a salient therapeutic target in the multifaceted treatment of patients with this bothersome disease.

RECURRENT URINARY TRACT INFECTIONS

As reported by Cardozo [93], many women have an urge to void urine during or immediately after sexual intercourse. This has been associated with a rigid perineum and nulliparity causing the posterior wall of the bladder to be irritated with repeated penile thrusting. The resultant postcoital dysuria is sometimes followed by a urinary tract infection (UTI), usually uncomplicated acute cystitis. Organisms are massaged into the bladder during intercourse, and if they are not voided soon after they multiply and cause infection.

Some women are particularly susceptible to such UTIs. According to the European Association of Urology guidelines [94], recurrent UTIs are defined as at least three episodes of uncomplicated infection documented by urine culture with the isolation of greater than 10^3 colony-forming units/ml. It is estimated that approximately 20% of patients with UTI will develop a second infection within 6 months. As reported by Chung et al [95] the increased incidence of UTIs in women may be attributed to urethral length, which provides an effective barrier to bacterial ascent. Risk factors for UTIs include sexual intercourse in younger women, while mechanical and/or physiologic factors that affect bladder emptying, UI, cystocele and large postvoid residual volumes or atrophic vaginitis in postmenopausal women. Yoon et al [96] conducted a retrospective analysis of 254 patients with acute cystitis to evaluate the risk factors for recurrent cystitis patients following acute cystitis, compared with 90 healthy subjects. Women in the cystitis groups were more likely to have sexually transmitted infections (STIs), frequent sexual intercourse and to use contraception more frequently than the normal control group.

It could be supposed that recurrent UTI may have a negative impact on women's sexual life because of 1) fear of a cystitis episode after intercourse leading to avoiding sex, 2) dyspareunia due to chronic urethritis and frequent concomitant vaginal STIs in women with recurrent UTIs, 3) pelvic/sexual pain and pelvic floor overactivity causing chronic bladder inflammation, 4) vestibule and vaginal atrophy and reduction in vaginal lubrication during intercourse, often associated to recurrent UTIs especially in menopausal women with inadequate oestrogen supply [10]. Accordingly, Salonia et al. [10] found in a population of women with LUTS that 60% of the women with sexual arousal disorders and 61% of those with sexual pain disorders also complained of recurrent bacterial cystitis.

PELVIC ORGAN PROLAPSE

Several studies investigated the specific impact of POP on FSF, with conflicting results. Intuitively, POP would seem likely to have an adverse impact on sexual function, however, older age and postmenopausal status, common in women with prolapse, are also associated with sexual dysfunctions and may confound the association between POP and FSD [97, 98].

In a recent cross-sectional observational study, Athanasiou et al. [99] evaluated the effect of POP on FSF in 101 women compared with 70 women without POP, and found that FSF was worse in POP group than control group, but did not seem to worsen with an increasing grade of POP. Based on a linear regression model, they concluded that the presence of prolapse only partly explained impaired sexual functioning in women with POP. Investigating 495 women scheduled for hysterectomy with evidence of PFD, Handa et al. [9] found that UI was significantly associated with low libido, vaginal dryness, and dyspareunia and independent of age, educational attainment and race, but POP was not associated with any sexual complaint. Barber et al. [7] reported that 81% of sexually active patients described their sex as 'somewhat' or 'very' satisfactory, and that neither UI nor POP influenced significantly the answer to this question. Weber et al. [79] reported that women with POP and/or UI have a similar sexual function than women without these PFD. In this study, increasing age was the only significant factor predictive of FSD, and increasing grade of POP predicted interference with sexual activity, without affecting frequency of intercourse or description of satisfaction with the sexual relationship.

On the other hand, Novi et al. [100] compared sexual function of women with POP to that of women without POP using the PISQ, and reported that mean PISQ score in sexually active women with POP were significantly lower compared to controls, with significant difference in satisfaction with sexual relationship, actual frequency of intercourse and ability to achieve orgasm with masturbation, but no difference in the desired frequency of intercourse, initiation of sexual activity, rate of anorgasmia or subjective assessment of partner satisfaction. The study of Digesu et al [101] reported a comparison of prolapse symptoms and QoL with physical examination findings and urinary, bowel and sexual dysfunctions in symptomatic and asymptomatic women. They identified women as symptomatic from prolapse if they complained of any of the prolapse symptoms and/or on direct questioning the patients reported a "sensation of dragging" or "a lump or fullness in the vagina". These symptoms were correlated with anterior, posterior and apical compartment prolapse severity. For the symptomatic women only, sexual symptoms severity was correlated with apical and posterior wall prolapse, so they concluded that FSD was related to uterine displacement, likely leading cervix to obstruct penile penetration. Displacement of the uterus coming down, pulling the ligaments, pedicles and peritoneum may also lead to a sensation of heaviness or "dragging" vaginal feeling, which may interfere with sexual function.

THERAPY

In patients where an underlying medical condition has been diagnosed, treatment targeted to the cure is mandatory. However, patients should be aware that the treatment of their disease does not always guarantee the elimination of their sexual dysfunction. Consideration should also be given to withholding any medications suspected of contributing to sexual dysfunction or, if possible, switching to an alternative drug. For patients with a component of psychogenic dysfunction, the use of a psychologist or psychiatrist with experience in sexual dysfunction can be helpful.

HORMONE REPLACEMENT THERAPY

The medical management of sexual dysfunction in women has focused on hormonal treatment. Both estrogen and testosterone are used alone and in combination. In postmenopausal women, it has been reported that estrogen replacement can improve vaginal and clitoral sensitivity, increase libido, reset the thresholds of sensitivity to vibration and pressure, and decrease the symptoms of vaginal dryness and pain during intercourse [102, 103]. In 2003, the FDA stated that local estrogen therapy should be used for the treatment of moderate-to-severe symptoms of vulvar and vaginal atrophy. Estrogens are available in several forms, including oral pill, skin patch, vaginal ring, and cream. The vaginal ring is a therapeutic option for women with breast cancer who are not able to take estrogen orally or transdermally.

A decrease in testosterone levels can be seen in women with premature ovarian failure or after natural or surgical menopause or induced by chemotherapy. Testosterone supplementation has been shown to improve mood and well being in these patients [104-106]. Women treated with intramuscular testosterone and estradiol were found to have improvements in sexual desire, fantasy, arousal, and orgasm [107-109]. Benefits of testosterone therapy include improving libido, increased vaginal and clitoral sensitivity, increased vaginal lubrication, and increased arousal. For replacement therapy, testosterone is available in the form of pills, sublingual, dermal patch, and cream. The transdermal testosterone patch is under clinical study. The cream with testosterone has been approved for the treatment of vaginal lichen planus. Side effects of testosterone that should be monitored include weight gain, clitoral enlargement, increased facial hair, and hypercholesterolemia. The measurement of testosterone levels before and after therapy, lipid profile (cholesterol, triglycerides, HDL, LDL), and liver function tests are recommended [110, 111].

Recently some authors evaluated the efficacy of dehydroepiandrosterone (DHEA) in the treatment of hypoactive sexual desire disorder (HSDD). Twenty-seven postmenopausal women with HSDD were randomized by Bloch et al. [112] to receive either DHEA 100mg daily or placebo for 6 weeks in a controlled, double blind study. Primary outcome measures were sexual function questionnaires.. Participants on active treatment showed a significant increase in circulating serum levels of DHEAS, while bioavailable testosterone levels increased in women. For arousal, a significant improvement was observed for the DHEA treated group at 6 weeks. Significant correlations were observed between bioavailable testosterone and sexual cognitions, arousal and orgasm, while DHEAS was correlated with satisfaction. These positive results suggest that the neurosteroid DHEA may be effective as a treatment for women with HSDD if administered at a dose of at least 100mg per day.

To evaluate the effects of different types of hormonal replacement therapy (HRT) on sexual function, frequency of sexual intercourse, and quality of relationship in early postmenopausal women, Genazzani et al. [113] recruited 48 healthy postmenopausal women aged 50–60 years and randomized into three groups receiving either dehydroepiandrosterone (DHEA 10 mg) daily, or daily oral estradiol (1 mg) plus dihydrogesterone (5 mg), or daily oral tibolone (2.5 mg) for 12 months. Women who refused hormonal therapy were treated with oral vitamin D (400 IU). Efficacy was evaluated using the McCoy Female Sexuality Questionnaire before treatment and after 12 months. The groups receiving DHEA or HRT reported a significant improvement in sexual function compared to baseline. The quality of relationship was similar at baseline and after 3, 6 and 12 months of treatment. There were significant increases in the numbers of episodes of sexual intercourse in the previous 4 weeks in women treated with DHEA, HRT and tibolone in comparison with the baseline value, while no changes in the McCoy score occurred in women receiving vitamin D.

Many studies described the efficacy on several FSDs of other agents such as flibanserine [114, 115], bupropion [116, 117], topical alprostadil [118], sildenafil [119], yohimbine [120] and bremelanotide [121].

OVERACTIVE BLADDER TREATMENT

Pharmacotherapy with anticholinergic drugs is often the first line medical therapy, either alone or as an adjunct to various non-pharmacological therapies after conservative options such as reducing intake of caffeine drinks have been tried. Non-pharmacologic therapies consist of bladder training, pelvic floor muscle training with or without biofeedback, behavioral modification, electrical stimulation and surgical interventions.

Administration of anticholinergics for OAB results in statistically significant improvement in urinary symptoms compared with placebo [122]. Several studies investigated the impact of antimuscarinics on various aspects of QoL, but only few of these are particularly interested in FSF. The Multicenter Assessment of Transdermal Therapy in Overactive Bladder with Oxybutynin study [123] was an open-label, prospective trial of 2, 878 subjects with overactive bladder, treated with transdermal oxybutynin for 6 months or less. The impact of OAB on sexual function before and after treatment was assessed via item responses from the King's Health Questionnaire and Beck Depression Inventory-II. At baseline, 586 patients (23.1%) reported that OAB had an impact on their sexual life. After treatment, coital incontinence in 569 (22.8%) decreased to 438 (19.3%), effects of symptoms on subjects' sex lives improved in 19.1% (worsened in 11.2%), the effect on relationships with partners improved in 19.6% (worsened in 11.9%) and reduced interest in sex, reported by 52.1% at baseline, improved significantly. Therefore the authors concluded that treatment with transdermal oxybutynin improved sexual function and marital relationships. Rogers et al [124] evaluated sexual and emotional health in 411 sexually active women with OAB/UUI randomized to placebo or tolterodine extended release (ER), concluding that OAB symptoms improved with tolterodine ER as did the scores of sexual health and anxiety measures. Improvement in all domains of sexual function (libido, orgasm, sexual enjoyment, overall satisfaction and vaginal wetness) measured by a non-validated questionnaire is also confirmed by a study with tolterodine immediate release (IR) [125]. The main limitation of all these studies is the generally short-term period over which the studies were conducted, so a longer follow-up would give more valuable information on the real effect of anticholinergic drugs on sexual satisfaction of these patients.

Recently, mirabegron, a novel orally active, first-in-class, potent and selective β_3-AR agonist has been approved for the treatment of OAB [126]. Studies are expected to investigate also the potential beneficial effects of this new class of drug on FSF in the specific population of women with OAB.

There is little published on the effect of non-pharmacological therapy for refractory OAB on FSF. Sacral neuromodulation has been found to improve FSF in correlation with improvement in urinary symptoms. Pauls et al [127] evaluated sexual function in 7 sexually active female patients that underwent a sacral neuromodulator (SNM) implantation before and after placement. Three subjects felt the device impacted on their sexual function in a positive way by decreasing urgency and by increasing desire. Overall sexual frequency increased significantly after the surgery with significant increases in the FSFI total and domain scores for desire, lubrication, orgasm, satisfaction and pain. The authors found no correlation between patient report of urinary symptom improvement and FSFI scores. These results were confirmed by a recent study on 16 female patients with OAB undergoing the two-stage procedure of SNM [128]. Regarding sexuality, the mean improvement in the total FSFI score was 27.9% on midterm follow-up and 29.3% on final follow-up. Only 4 patients showed a >50% improvement in global FSFI score on midterm follow-up, and 3 on final follow-up. In this study a significant correlation was found between clinical improvement and improvement in sexual function, but no significant correlation was found between differences in FSFI and other QoL indexes. Yih et al. [129] also observed improved sexual function after neuromodulation in 167 women with voiding dysfunctions.

Peripheral percutaneous tibial nerve stimulation has also been shown to improve sexual function in women with OAB, in particular the overall satisfaction, libido and frequency of sexual activities [130].

Despite many studies have demonstrated the effectiveness and safety of onabotulinumtoxin-A for the treatment of neurogenic and refractory idiopathic OAB and a positive effect on several areas of QOL [131], until today there are no studies concerning the impact of this therapy on FSF.

STRESS URINARY INCONTINENCE TREATMENT

Management of women with SUI is initially conservative. Until recently, the next treatment option offered to women with persistent symptoms was a surgical procedure to correct the anatomical defect. This treatment escalation from conservative management directly to surgical management reveals a distinct gap for effective medical treatments. Medications such as estrogens and tricyclic antidepressants have been used off-label in the past for SUI with little or no evidence of efficacy and often significant side effects [132]. The introduction of the serotonin and noradrenaline reuptake inhibitor (SNRI) duloxetine as a drug therapy for stress incontinence was hailed as a significant step forward in terms of widening treatment options for women with SUI, being the first available pharmacological option for SUI which had proven efficacy in randomized controlled trials, thus filling the treatment void between conservative and surgical therapies. Several studies investigated the frequencies of treatment emergent sexual dysfunctions in patients treated with duloxetine for psychiatric disorders, in particular major depressive disorder [133, 134], but there are no studies evaluating the impact of duloxetine on sexual function in women with SUI.

Often, the initial approach for treatment of SUI and other PFDs is to start with the least invasive treatment modality, which entails strengthening the pelvic floor musculature in conjunction with behavioral modification. Since Arnold Kegel identified pelvic floor muscle weakness in women as a source of urinary and sexual dysfunction, pelvic floor hypotonus has been purported to impact negatively on sexual activity [135]. However, there are few studies evaluating the effect of pelvic floor muscle strengthening as an intervention on sexual function using validated research tools in women with specific PFDs. Bø et al. [136] evaluated the effect of pelvic floor muscle exercise on quality of life and sex-life variables in genuine stress incontinent women. Fifty-nine women with clinically and urodynamically proven SUI were randomized to either pelvic floor muscle exercise or an untreated control group. The results showed that general QoL measured by the generic QoL questionnaire was not much affected by UI, while the disease specific questionnaire demonstrated that ability to participate in physical activity and some sex-life variables were affected by the condition. There was a statistically significant reduction in number of women having problems with sex-life, social life, and physical activity in the exercise group after six months of pelvic floor muscle exercise. These results are confirmed by articles using validated questionnaires. Zahariou et al. [137] assessed the effect of a program of supervised pelvic floor muscle training (PFMT) on sexual function in a group of 70 women with SUI, using FSFI score. At the end of the study, all domains of the FSFI were also significantly improved with median total FSFI scores increasing from 20.3 to 26.8. Liebergall-Wischnitzer et al. [138] compared the effectiveness of two exercise methods (the Paula method of circular muscle exercises vs. pelvic floor muscle training) on sexual function with PISQ questionnaire, founding significant function score improvement with both methods with no significant difference between groups.

When the conservative treatments fail, surgical treatment options should be considered in these patients. Although SUI surgery is thought to improve sexual function [67, 139, 140], data reporting sexual function following surgical repair are limited and conflicting [141].

Moran et al. [142] evaluated 55 women with SUI and coital incontinence treated with Burch colposuspension. Before the procedure, 36 women (65%) had coital leakage only with penetration, 9 women (16%) had only with orgasm and 10 (18%) with both. After the procedure, 81% described no further coital incontinence. In Baessler [143] cohort of sexually active women affected by SUI with concomitant coital incontinence, this problem was cured in 70% of patient and improved in almost 7% after Burch colposuspension. Brubaker et al. [67] studied sexual function in 655 women randomized to Burch colposuspension or sling surgery and reported that patients with successful surgery had a greater improvement in PISQ-12 scores in both Burch and sling groups.

Berthier et al. [144] found no significant postoperative changes regarding frequency of sexual intercourse, satisfaction with sexual intercourse or personal importance of having an active sexual live in 66 women undergoing tension-free vaginal tape (TVT) procedure for SUI. These results are in agreement with those of previous studies [145-147]. Ghezzi et al.

[148] reported that 62.2% of women undergoing TVT procedure had no change in sexual function after surgery, no significant difference in the incidence of dyspareunia and two patients (3.8%) referred intercourse to be worse, one because of erosion and one for "de novo" anorgasmia.

Also studies on trans-obturatory slings (TOT) reported no impact of this procedure on FSF [149-151]. Filocamo et al. [149] included in their study women complaining of urodynamic SUI that were both sexually and non-sexually active at baseline. One hundred five women out of 133 underwent a TOT procedure, while 28 out of 133 had a retropubic procedure. Twelve months after surgery, 22 out of 54 non-sexually active women (40%) re-established sexual activity, whereas only 6 out of 79 (7.5%) patients, sexually active at baseline, were not sexually active 1 year after surgery. The authors concluded that after a sling procedure, FSF improves and a very relevant percentage of nonsexually active women can recover sexual activity after sling. Accordingly, Xu et al [151] evaluated sexual function before and 6 months after a TOT procedure in 55 sexually active women. More than half (54.5%) the women reported an improvement in sexual function after surgery and 45.5% reported no change, and no statistically significant difference was found between preoperative and postoperative total or domain scores on the FSFI, so they concluded that TOT procedure did not significantly affect sexual function. In a recent study, Zyczynski et al. [152] described an increase of mean PISQ-12 scores after mid-urethral sling surgery (TOT and TVT) and a reduction of dyspareunia, incontinence during sex and fear of UI during sex.

However, surgeons should know that vaginal sling procedures may have a potential negative effect on FSF due to damage to vascular and/or neural genital structures or to "de novo" dyspareunia. Baessler et al [153] reported that dyspareunia was a severe indication for removing the posterior intravaginal synthetic sling. Bekker et al. [154] described the autonomic and somatic pathways in relationship to sling surgery in 14 adult female dissected hemipelves, after TVT or TOT procedures have been performed. They concluded that the dorsal nerve of the clitoris was not disturbed during the placement of the TOT but the autonomic innervation of the vaginal wall was disrupted by the TVT procedure, which could lead to altered lubrication-swelling response.

BLADDER PAIN SYNDROME/INTERSTITIAL CYSTITIS TREATMENT

The published literature regarding the typical course of BPS/IC is conflicting, and there are insufficient publications to address BPS/IC diagnosis and overall management from an evidence basis. The limitations of the BPS/IC literature include: poorly-defined patient groups or heterogeneous groups, small sample sizes, lack of placebo controls for many studies, resulting in a likely over-estimation of efficacy, short follow-up durations and use of a variety of outcome measures. According to AUA guidelines [92], BPS/IC treatment strategies should proceed using more conservative therapies first, with less conservative therapies employed if symptom control is inadequate for acceptable quality of life. Treatments that may be offered are divided into first to sixth-line groups based on the balance between potential benefits to the patient, potential severity of adverse events and the reversibility of the treatment. Because the underlying pathophysiology of BPS/IC is unknown, treatment goals are to manage symptoms and optimize QoL. It includes self-care practices and behavioral modifications, stress management practices to improve coping techniques, manual physical therapy, oral pharmacotherapy (amitriptyline, cimetidine, hydroxyzine, pentosan polysulfate), intravesical treatments (dimethyl sulfoxide, heparin, or lidocaine), cystoscopy under anesthesia with hydrodistension and Hunner's lesions fulguration (with laser or electrocautery) and/or injection of triamcinolone, neuromodulation, oral cyclosporine A, intradetrusor botulinum toxin A or major surgery (substitution cystoplasty, urinary diversion with or without cystectomy) in carefully selected patients for whom all other therapies have failed.

Not surprisingly, few studies described the relationship between symptom reduction and sexual functioning of women with BPS/IC. Schmid et al [155] evaluated the effect of therapeutical management in 69 patients with IC on sexual function, QoL and bladder symptoms using validated tools (FSFI, King's Health Questionnaire and VAS). All patients were managed applying determined therapeutical steps including tetracycline, bladder instillation consisting of heparine, local anaesthetic and natrium-bicarbonate, prednisolon and antihistaminics or instillation with dimethyl sulfoxide, then FSFI improved significantly in all domains but orgasm, so the authors concluded that defined therapeutical steps including tetracycline, bladder instillation and anti-inflammatory agents significantly improved sexual function in these patients. Nickel et al [156] treated 128 patients with 300 mg/day pentosan polysulfate sodium for 32 weeks. These patients showed statistically significant improvement in symptom and sexual functioning scores at weeks 8, 16, 24, and 32, with a positive correlation between the mean change scores of sexual functioning score and physical and mental QoL components.

RECURRENT URINARY TRACT INFECTIONS MANAGEMENT

Behavioral changes can affect the frequency of UTIs recurrence. Managing recurrent infections should include modification of known risk factors. As reported by Kodner et al. [157] postcoital prophylaxis may be preferable in women with UTIs temporally related to intercourse. No marked difference in recurrent UTIs has been noted when using postcoital prophylaxis compared with daily prophylaxis [158], and depending on the frequency of sexual intercourse, postcoital prophylaxis usually results in less antibiotic use [158, 159]. Low-dose antimicrobial therapy may be used to prevent recurrent UTIs in affected women but it generates antimicrobial resistance and side effects like micotic infection due to the alteration of normal flora of healthy vaginal mucosa and acidic ph environment, which prevent the adherence of uropathogens. Thus, non-antimicrobial prevention strategies are welcomed.

Various bacterial lysates have been proposed with this indication. In a recent meta-analysis Naber et al [160] assess the efficacy and safety of bacterial lysates in the management of recurrent UTIs. Seven of the studies dealt with an oral immunostimulant (OM-89), of which about five (1, 000 adult patients) were retained for analysis with an observation period of 6–12 months. The mean number of UTIs was significantly lower in OM-89-treated patients in all the trials analysed (mean 39%), as was the use of antibacterials. Four of the studies dealt with a vaginal vaccine, of which three small studies were retained for analysis (220 adult patients). The results suggest that this vaginal vaccine is effective when administered with a booster cycle (no recurrent UTI in 50% vs. 14% with placebo). No blind controlled studies could be identified with other bacterial lysates claiming the same indication. So they concluded that among the various immunotherapeutic products, studies were published only for one product (OM-89) that are in accordance with current standards. This product was shown to be effective under conditions of daily practice. A second product (vaginal vaccine) also appears to be effective but adequate phase III studies are necessary.

Cranberry products seem to notably reduce the recurrence of symptomatic cystitis. Although there is no clear evidence about dosage or duration of use [161], small studies have reported that a daily intake of 150 to 750 mL of cranberry juice or concentrated equivalent is effective in preventing recurrent UTIs [162, 163].

Several studies of postmenopausal women have demonstrated the effectiveness of using topical estrogen, but adverse effects are common [164, 165].

Some evidence suggests that sodium hyaluronate and sodium chondroitin sulphate instillation can be recommended for women with recurrent UTIs [166], and a few studies showed how overall urinary symptoms and QoL significantly improved compared with placebo [167], but there are no studies on sexual function after these therapies.

POP SURGERY

Functional results are as important an outcome measure as anatomical results in the assessment of pelvic floor surgery [168]. Sexual function in particular has been overlooked and superficially assessed in the past and several studies of the impact of surgical intervention have also been limited by absence of baseline data [169].

Based on data from the Colpopexy and Urinary Reduction Efforts (CARE) study [170], Handa et al. [97] administered the PISQ-12 to 224 sexually active stress-continent women planning abdominal sacrocolpopexy for stage II-IV prolapse, before and one year after the intervention. In the CARE trial, concomitant Burch colposuspension was randomly assigned at the time of sacrocolpopexy, and posterior colporrhaphy was performed at the discretion of the surgeon, so the potential impact of those procedures on postoperative sexual function was assessed. One year after colposacropexy, the number of sexual active women rose significantly from 148 (66.1%) to 171 (76.3%), the number of women who avoided sex because of vaginal bulging decreased from 103 (47.3%) to 10 (4.6%) and the mean PISQ-12 score among women who were sexually active before and after surgery improved significantly. Fifty-eight percent of women with dyspareunia at baseline did not report pain during intercourse after surgery and 14.5% of women without dyspareunia reported pain 1 year after sacrocolpopexy, regardless of concomitant Burch colposuspension. The proportion of women with infrequent sexual desire, sexually excited during sexual activity and who reported orgasm with intercourse did not change substantially. Only 11 of 148 women who were sexually active before surgery became inactive after surgery. They did not differ in age or preoperative prolapse severity from women who continued sexual activity after surgery, reported no postoperative sexual interference from fear of incontinence, vaginal bulging or pain, however more of these women reported infrequent sexual desire after surgery. Comparing Burch colposuspension group versus non-Burch group, they did not find difference in proportion of sexually active women, dyspareunia and PISQ-12 scores 1 year after surgery, while more women who underwent posterior repair reported postoperative dyspareunia, although the difference did not reach statistical significance. These data are consistent with previous studies reporting a high percentage of dyspareunia after posterior repair, both with levator ani muscle plication narrowing of mid-vagina [171-173] and with posterior colporrhaphy [174, 175]. The authors concluded that most sexually active women can expect to continue sexual activity following sacrocolpopexy and experience less impact from pelvic floor symptoms [97].

Costantini et al [176] designed an observational prospective longitudinal cohort study in order to evaluate the impact of uterus preservation after POP repair on sexual function. Sixty-eight patients with POP underwent colposacropexy with or without hysterectomy: 32 underwent uterus-sparing surgery and 36 hysterectomy plus colposacropexy. After surgery both groups had significant improvements in the total FSFI score and in the domains of desire, arousal and orgasm. The median post-operative scores of desire, arousal, and orgasm domains showed significant improvements in the uterus-sparing group compared with the hysterectomy group, so they concluded that uterus sparing surgery is associated with a greater improvement in sexual function.

The presence of prosthetic material in the vagina may adversely affect sexual function, although several studies reported contradictory results. Wang et al [168] evaluated the short-term impact (6 months) of surgical repair with total transvaginal mesh (TVM) on FSF among 27 sexually active women with symptomatic POP. In these patients the TVM surgery corrected the pelvic anatomy and urinary symptoms successfully; while there were no significant changes in sexual desire, sexual arousal, orgasm, satisfaction, the mean postoperative score of the lubrication and dyspareunia domains worsened significantly, with two-thirds of all participants showing a lower total FSFI score postoperatively. The authors explained that changes in vaginal blood flow and ischemia, disruption of the dense nerve innervation of the anterior and lateral vaginal wall during dissection and the insertion of permanent mesh in the vagina might have contributed to the painful sensation and loss of lubrication postoperatively. Similar results were obtained by other studies [177, 178]. On the other hand, Hoda et al [179] reported an initial deterioration of sexual function during the first 3 months after transobturator mesh implants, followed by a steady improvement that reached a significant difference at 24 months postoperatively and Dwyer and O'Really [180] reported a significantly decreased dyspareunia in 97 women with recurrent or large POP undergoing polypropylene mesh repair to reinforce anterior and posterior compartment after 6, 12 and 24 months.

Lowestein et al. [181] evaluated sexual function, prolapse symptoms and self-perceived body image after treatment for POP to explore differences in body image perception and sexual function following conservative and surgical treatment for POP. At 6-month follow-up visits, the patients reported significant improvement in FSF from baseline in both groups and the improvement in FSF, as measured by PISQ-12, was not significant among sexually active patients treated with a pessary compared with those treated surgically. In this study, body mass index and changes in body image perception were the only independent factors associated with changes in PISQ-12 score following POP treatment.

PSYCHO-SEXOLOGICAL THERAPY

As underlined by Silverstein et al. [182], treatments of FSDs have been largely unsuccessful because they do not address the psychological factors that underlie female sexuality. Negative self-evaluative processes interfere with the ability to attend and register physiological changes (interoceptive awareness). Treatment for sexual dysfunction may be challenging and require a coordinated team of clinicians with expertise in urology, physical therapy, psychological and sexual therapy using an "integrated approach" [17]. When possible, treatment and counseling should involve the patients' sexual partner, so that couples can learn how to communicate openly about sexual issues and concerns about pain. In many cases, treatment consists of graded exercises to be done individually or in pairs [14, 15] whose final result depends on the motivation and commitment to change even mental and behavioral patterns, learned and become habitual, about self and other. Finally, for many disorders, a significant aspect constitutes proper scientific information and sex education to be administered in the form of bibliotherapy, scientific and educational films, as well as through some brief sexological counseling sessions for demystification of myths and widespread and rooted irrational beliefs about sex [183] or suggest coping strategies such as vaginal moisturizers and lubricants use for women who experience vaginal dryness and painful intercourse to enhance sexual intimacy or sexual devices such as vaginal dilators or self-stimulators that can help lengthen and widen the vagina and the scar tissue that may contribute to distress associated with vaginal intercourse. Ongoing supportive physical therapy is essential, and often behavioral therapy can be influential for continued compliance.

Clitoral stimulator is a battery-operated device with a suction cup that fits around the clitoris and facilitates engorgement approved by US Food and Drug Administration (FDA) for the treatment of female sexual complaints for patients who have had cervical cancer and for some with intravaginal radiation or other pelvic cancers, such as rectal and vaginal cancers [184].

Cognitive-behavioral therapy (CBT) can teach patients pain self-management, which enables them to alter unwanted thoughts, feelings, and behaviors in order to gain control over sexual experiences [185]. Some studies showed how CBT has been used effectively to reduce vulvar pain among women with vulvodynia (a disorder that has overlapping symptoms with BPS/IC) [186]. If the pain of intercourse is too severe and therapy is insufficient, couples could be taught non-coital ways to achieve sexual satisfaction and intimacy. Silverstein et al [182] described the effect of mindfulness meditation training on interoceptive awareness and the three categories of known barriers to healthy sexual functioning: attention, self-judgment, and clinical symptoms on 30 college students participated in either a 12-week course containing a "meditation laboratory" or an active control course with similar content or laboratory format. Interoceptive awareness was measured by reaction time in rating physiological response to sexual stimuli. Psychological barriers were assessed with self-reported measures of mindfulness and psychological well being. Women who participated in the meditation training became significantly faster at registering their physiological responses (interoceptive awareness) to sexual stimuli compared with active controls and also improved their scores on attention, self-judgment and symptoms of anxiety and depression. The authors concluded that improvements in interoceptive awareness were correlated with improvements in the psychological barriers to healthy sexual functioning, and highlight the potential of mindfulness training as a treatment of female sexual dysfunction.

CONCLUSION

Sexual dysfunctions are common health issues in women with urogynecological disorders. Although there is sufficient evidence on the detrimental impact on women's sexual function due to urinary incontinence, overactive bladder and bladder pain syndrome/interstitial cystitis, findings of published studies are often conflicting on the role of pelvic organ prolapse. These observations are of utmost importance for physicians dealing with women's health, especially because lower urinary tract dysfunctions are exceedingly common and increasing in incidence worldwide. Data on the relative impairment of sexual function in women with different types of urogynecological disorders are deficient, and the consistency of studies is often limited by several biases such as use of non-condition-specific instruments, and lack of a control group or urodynamic evaluation.

The diagnosis of FSD requires a complete anamnesis with regard to the sexual history and self-administered questionnaires represent useful tools not only for research but also for patient-clinician discussions on sexuality.

The pharmacological approach has been limited for many years to hormone replacement therapy, but in recent years new classes of drugs are being tested for the treatment of FSDs and of PFDs with promising results, and more space is given to the use of rehabilitation and behavioral therapies.

Although urogynecological surgery is thought to improve sexual well being, data reporting sexual function following surgical repair are still limited and often diverging. More research is needed using standardised assessment tools to define clear endpoints in this field.

REFERENCES

[1]   Walsh KE, Berman JR. Female Sexual Disfunction. In Vasavada SP, Rodney AA, Sand PK and Raz S eds, Female Urology, Urogynecology, and Voiding Dysfunction, Chapt 5. *CRC Press* 2004: 65-78.

[2]   Laumann EO, Paik A, Rosen RC. Sexual dysfunction in the United States: prevalence and predictors. *JAMA*. 1999 Feb 10;281(6):537-44.

[3]   Laumann EO, Nicolosi A, Glasser DB, Paik A, Gingell C, Moreira E, Wang T, GSSAB Investigators' Group. Sexual problems among women and men aged 40-80 y: prevalence and correlates identified in the Global Study of Sexual Attitudes and Behaviors. *Int. J. Impot. Res.* 2005 Jan-Feb;17(1):39-57.

[4]   Laumann EO, Waite LJ. Sexual dysfunction among older adults: prevalence and risk factors from a nationally representative U.S. probability sample of men and women 57-85 years of age. *J. Sex. Med.* 2008 Oct;5(10):2300-11.

[5]   Irwin DE, Kopp ZS, Agatep B, Milsom I, Abrams P. Worldwide prevalence estimates of lower urinary tract symptoms, overactive bladder, urinary incontinence and bladder outlet obstruction. *BJU Int.* 2011;108(7):1132–8.

[6]   Nygaard I, Barber MD, Burgio KL, Kenton K, Meikle S, Schaffer J, Spino C, Whitehead WE, Wu J, Brody DJ; Pelvic Floor Disorders Network. Prevalence of symptomatic pelvic floor disorders in US women. *J. Am. Med. Assoc.* 2008;300(11): 1311–6.

[7]   Barber MD, Visco AG, Wyman JF, Fantl JA, Bump RC. Sexual function in women with urinary incontinence and pelvic organ prolapse. *Obstet. Gynecol.* 2002;99(2): 281–9.

[8]   Pauls RN, Segal JL, SilvaWA, Kleeman SD, Karram MM. Sexual function in patients presenting to urogynecology practice. *Int. Urogynecol. J. Pelvic Floor Dysfunct.* 2006; 17(6):576–80.

[9]   Handa VL, Harvey L, Cundiff GW, Siddique SA, Kjerulff KH. Sexual function among women with urinary incontinence and pelvic organ prolapse. *Am. J. Obstet. Gynecol.* 2004;191(3):751–6.

[10] Salonia A, Zanni G, Nappi RE, Briganti A, Dehò F, Fabbri F, Colombo R, Guazzoni G, Di Girolamo V, Rigatti P, Montorsi F. Sexual dysfunction is common in women with lower urinary tract symptoms and urinary incontinence: results of a cross-sectional study. *Eur. Urol.* 2004;45(5):642–8.

[11] Cohen BL, Barboglio P, Gousse A. The impact of lower urinary tract symptoms and urinary incontinence on female sexual dysfunction using a validated instrument. *J. Sex. Med.* 2008;5(6):1418–23.

[12] Sacco E, D'Addessi A, Racioppi M, Pinto F, Totaro A, Bassi P. Bladder pain syndrome associated with highest impact on sexual function among women with lower urinary tract symptoms. *Int. J. Gynaecol. Obstet.* 2012 May;117(2):168-72.

[13] Yip SK, Chan A, Pang S, Leung P, Tang C, Shek D, Chung T. The impact of urodynamic stress incontinence and detrusor overactivity on marital relationship and sexual function. *Am. J. Obstet. Gynecol.* 2003;188(5):1244–8.

[14] Masters EH, Johnson VE. Human Sexual Response. Boston: Little Brown, 1966.

[15] Kaplan HS. The New Sex Therapy. London: Bailliere Tindall, 1974.

[16] Basson R. Using a different model for female sexual response to address women's problematic low sexual desire. *J. Sex Marital Ther.* 2001; 27(5):395–403.

[17] Simonelli C, Fabrizi A, Lenzi A, Jannini EA. I disturbi del desiderio maschili e femminili. In L'approccio integrato in sessuologia clinica, Chapt 2. Franco Angeli 2010: 30-60.

[18] Basson R, Leiblum S, Brotto L, Derogatis L, Fourcroy J, Fugl-Meyer K, Graziottin A, Heiman JR, Laan E, Meston C, Schover L, van Lankveld J, Schultz WW. Revised definitions of women's sexual dysfunction. *J. Sex. Med.* 2004 Jul;1(1):40-8.

[19] DeRogatis LR, Burnett AL. The epidemiology of sexual dysfunctions. *J. Sex. Med.* 2008;5:289–300.

[20] American Psychiatric Association (2000), *Diagnostic and Statistical Manual of Mental Disorders*, Fourth Edition, Text Revision, American Psychiatric Association, Washington DC.

[21] Aslan E, Fynes M. Female sexual dysfunction. *Int. Urogynecol. J. Pelvic Floor Dysfunct.* 2008;19:293–305.

[22] Knoepp LR, Shippey SH, Chen CC, Cundiff GW, Derogatis LR, Handa VL. Sexual complaints, pelvic floor symptoms, and sexual distress in women over forty. *J. Sex. Med.* 2010 Nov;7(11):3675-82.

[23] Graziottin A. Women's right to a better sexual life. In Graziottin A (guest ed) "Female sexual dysfunction: clinical approach." *Urodinamica* 2004;14:57-60.

[24] Bull SS, Rietmeijer C, Fortenberry JD, Stoner B, Malotte K, VanDevanter N. Middlestadt SE, Hook EW 3rd. Practice patterns for the elicitation of sexual history education and counseling among providers of STD services: results from the gonorrhea community action project (GCAP). *Sex Transm. Dis.* 1999;26:584–9.

[25] Moore LW, Amburgey LB. Older adults and HIV. *AORN J.* 2000;71:873–6.

[26] Merrill JM, Laux LF, Thornby JI. Why doctors have difficulty with sex histories. *South Med. J.* 1990;83:613–7.

[27] Nusbaum MR, Hamilton CD. The proactive sexual health history. *Am. Fam. Physician.* 2002 Nov 1;66(9):1705-12.

[28] Graziottin A, Dennerstein L, Alexander LA, Giraldi A, Whipple B. Classification, Etiology and Key Issues in Female Sexual Disorders. In Porst H, Buvat J eds, Standard Practice in Sexual Medicine, Chapt 20. Blackwell Publishing 2006: 305-14.

[29] Rust J, Golombok S. The Golombok–Rust Inventory of Sexual Satisfaction (GRISS). *Br. J. Clin. Psychol.* 1985; 24:63–4.

[30] Derogatis LR. The psychosocial adjustment to illness scale (PAIS). *J. Psychosom. Res.* 1986;30:77–91.

[31] Trudel G, Ravart M, Matte B. The use of the multiaxial diagnostic system for sexual dysfunctions in the assessment of hypoactive sexual desire. *J. Sex Marital Ther.* 1993; 19:123–30.

[32] Clayton AH, McGarvey EL, Clavet GJ. The Changes in Sexual Functioning Questionnaire (CSFQ): development, reliability, validity. *Psychopharmacol. Bull.* 1997; 33:731–45.

[33] Hudson WW. Methodological observations on applied behavioural science. A measurement package for clinical workers. *J. Appl. Behav. Sci.* 1982;18:229–38.

[34] Snell WE Jr, Fisher T, Walters AS. The Multidimensional Sexuality Questionnaire: an objective self-report measure of psychological tendencies associated with human sexuality. *Ann. Sex Res.* 1993;6:27–55

[35] Lowe FC. Treatment of lower urinary tract symptoms suggestive of benign prostatic hyperplasia: sexual function. *BJU Int.* 2005;95(Suppl. 4): 12–8.

[36] Taylor JF, Rosen RC, Leiblum SR. Selfreport assessment of female sexual function: psychometric evaluation of the Brief Index of Sexual Functioning for Women. *Arch. Sex Behav.* 1994;23: 627–43.

[37] Dennerstein L, Lehert P, Dudley E. Short scale to measure female sexuality: adapted from McCoy Female Sexuality Questionnaire. *J. Sex Marital Ther.* 2001; 27:339–51.

[38] Brookes ST, Donovan JL, Wright M, Jackson S, Abrams P. A scored form of the Bristol Female Lower Urinary Tract Symptoms questionnaire: data from a randomized controlled trial of surgery for women with stress incontinence. *Am. J. Obstet. Gynecol.* 2004;191:73–82.

[39] Rosen R, Brown C, Heiman J, Leiblum S, Meston C, Shabsigh R, Ferguson D, D'Agostino R Jr.. The Female Sexual Function Index (FSFI): a multidimensional self-report instrument for the assessment of female sexual function. *J. Sex Marital Ther.* 2000;26:191–208.

[40] Giberti C, Rovida S. Transvaginal boneanchored synthetic sling for the treatment of stress urinary incontinence: an outcomes analysis. *Urology* 2000;56:956–61.

[41] Walters MD, Taylor S, Schoenfeld LS. Psychosexual study of women with detrusor instability. *Obstet. Gynecol.* 1990;75: 22–6.

[42] Rogers RG, Kammerer-Doak D, Villarreal A, Coates K, Qualls C. A new instrument to measure sexual function in women with urinary incontinence or pelvic organ prolapse. *Am. J. Obstet. Gynecol.* 2001;184:552–8.

[43] Rogers RG, Coates KW, Kammerer-Doak D, Khalsa S, Qualls C. A short form of the Pelvic Organ Prolapse/Urinary Incontinence Sexual Questionnaire (PISQ-12). *Int. Urogynecol. J. Pelvic Floor Dysfunct.* 2004;15:219.

[44] Meyer-Bahlburg HF, Dolezal C. The female sexual function index: a methodological critique and suggestions for improvement. *J. Sex Marital Ther.* 2007;33: 217–24.

[45] McCoy ML. The McCoy female sexuality questionnaire. *Quality of life research* 2000;9:739-745.

[46] Jackson S, Donovan J, Brookes S, Eckford S, Swithinbank, L, Abrams P. The Bristol Female Lower Urinary Tract Symptoms questionnaire: development and psychometric testing. *BJU* 1996; 77:805-812.

[47] Abrams P, Cardozo L, Fall M, Griffiths D, Rosier P, Ulmsten U, van Kerrebroeck P, Victor A, Wein A; Standardisation Sub-committee of the International Continence Society. The standardisation of terminology of lower urinary tract function: report from the Standardisation Sub-committee of the International Continence Society. *Neurourol. Urodyn.* 2002;21(2):167-78.

[48] Sacco E. [Physiopathology of overactive bladder syndrome]. *Urologia.* 2012;79(1):24-35.

[49] Temml C, Haidinger G, Schmidbauer J, Schatzl G, Madersbacher S. Urinary incontinence in both sexes: Prevalence rates and impact on quality of life and sexual life. *Neurourol. Urodyn.* 2000; 19: 259–71.

[50] Lenderking WR, Nackley JF, Anderson RB, Testa MA. A review of the quality-of-life aspects of urinary urge incontinence. *Pharmacoeconomics* 1996; 9: 11–23.

[51] Wyman JF, Harkins SW, Choi SC, Taylor JR, Fantl JA. Psychosocial impact of urinary incontinence in women. *Obstet. Gynecol.* 1987; 70: 378–81.

[52] Coyne KS, Margolis MK, Jumadilova Z, Bavendam T, Mueller E, Rogers R. Overactive bladder and women's sexual health: what is the impact? *J. Sex. Med.* 2007 May;4(3):656-66.

[53] Coyne KS, Sexton CC, Thompson C, Kopp ZS, Milsom I, Kaplan SA. The impact of OAB on sexual health in men and women: results from EpiLUTS. *J. Sex. Med.* 2011 Jun;8(6):1603-15.

[54] Heidler S, Mert C, Wehrberger C, Temml C, Ponholzer A, Rauchenwald M, Madersbacher S. Impact of overactive bladder symptoms on sexuality in both sexes. *Urol. Int.* 2010;85(4):443-6.

[55] Patel AS, O'Leary ML, Stein RJ, Leng WW, Chancellor MB, Patel SG, Borello-France D. The relationship between overactive bladder and sexual activity in women. *Int. Braz. J. Urol.* 2006 Jan-Feb;32(1):77-87.

[56] KimYH, Seo JT, Yoon H. The effect of overactive bladder syndrome on the sexual quality of life in Korean young and middle aged women. *Int. J. Impot. Res.* 2005;17(2): 158–63.

[57]   Choo MS, Ku JH, Lee JB, Lee DH, Kim JC, Kim HJ, Lee JJ, Park WH. Cross-cultural differences for adapting overactive bladder symptoms: results of an epidemiologic survey in Korea. *World J. Urol.* 2007 Oct;25(5):505-11.

[58]   Sen I, Onaran M, Tan MO, Acar C, Camtosun A, Sozen S, Bozkirli I. Evaluation of sexual function in women with overactive bladder syndrome. *Urol. Int.* 2007;78(2):112-5.

[59]   Blaivas JG, Sandha J. Clinical evaluation of lower urinary tract symtoms. In Raz S and Rodriguez L eds, Female Urology, Chapt 7. *Saunders Elsevier* 2008: 77-85.

[60]   Simonelli C, Tripodi F, Vizzari V, Rossi R. Psycho-relational aspects of urinary incontinence in female sexuality. *Urologia.* 2008 January-March;75(1):14-19.

[61]   Rubini S. Incontinenza urinaria: un problema troppo spesso nascosto. *Rivista della Società Italiana di Medicina Generale* 2002; 2: 23-5.

[62]   Ko Y, Lin SJ, Salmon JW, Bron MS. The impact of Urinary Incontinence on Quality of Life of the Elderly. *The American Journal of Managed Care* 2005; 11: 103-11.

[63]   Robles JE. La incontinencia urinaria. *An Sist Sanit Navar* 2006; 29: 219-32.

[64]   Melville JL, Delaney K, Newton K, Katon W. Incontinence severity and major depression in incontinent women. *Obstetrics & Gynecology* 2005; 106: 585-92.

[65]   Klingele CJ. Advances in urogynecology. Int J Fertil Women Med 2005; 50: 18-23.

[66]   Salloum M. Self-esteem disturbance in patients with urinary diversions: assessing the void. *Ostomy Wound Manage* 2005 Dec;51(12):64-9.

[67]   Brubaker L, Chiang S, Zyczynski H, Norton P, Kalinoski DL, Stoddard A, Kusek JW, Steers W; Urinary Incontinence Treatment Network. The impact of stress incontinence surgery on female sexual function. *Am. J. Obstet. Gynecol.* 2009 May;200(5):562.

[68]   Ozel B, White T, Urwitz-Lane R, Minaglia S.. The impact of pelvic organ prolapse on sexual function in women with urinary incontinence. *Int. Urogynecol. J. Pelvic Floor Dysfunct.* 2006;17: 14–7.

[69]   Nusbaum MR, Gamble G. The prevalence and importance of sexual concerns among female military beneficiaries. *Mil. Med.* 2001 Mar;166(3):208-10.

[70]   Geiss IM, Umek WH, Dungl A, Sam C, Riss P, Hanzal E. Prevalence of female sexual dysfunction in gynecologic and urogynecologic patients according to the international consensus classification. *Urology.* 2003 Sep;62(3):514-8.

[71]   Aslan G, Köseoğlu H, Sadik Ö, Gimen S, Cihan A, Esen A.. Sexual function in women with urinary incontinence. *Int. J. Impot. Res.* 2005 May-Jun;17(3):248-51.

[72]   Norton P, Brubaker L. Urinary incontinence in women. *Lancet* 2006;367: 57–67.

[73]   Gordon D, Groutz A, Sinai T, Wiezman A, Lessing JB, David MP, Aizenberg D. Sexual Function in Women Attending a Urogynecology Clinic. *Int. Urogynecol. J.* (1999) 10:325-328.

[74]   Møller LA, Lose G. Sexual activity and lower urinary tract symptoms. *Int. Urogynecol. J.* (2005) 17: 18-21.

[75]   Kelleher CJ, Cardozo LD, Khullar V, Salvatore S. A new questionnaire to assess the quality of life of urinary incontinent women. *Br. J. Obstet. Gynaecol.* 1997; 104:1374-9.

[76]   Coksuer H, Ercan CM, Haliloğlu B, Yucel M, Cam C, Kabaca C, Karateke A. Does urinary incontinence subtype affect sexual function? *Eur. J. Obstet. Gynecol. Reprod. Biol.* 2011 Nov;159(1):213-7.

[77]   Nilsson M, Lalos O, Lindkvist H, Lalos A. Impact of female urinary incontinence and urgency on women's and their partners' sexual life. *Neurourol. Urodyn.* 2011 Sep; 30(7):1276-80.

[78]   Rogers GR, Villarreal A, Kammerer-Doak D, Qualls C. Sexual function in women with and without urinary incontinence and/or pelvic organ prolapse. *Int. Urogynecol. J. Pelvic Floor Dysfunct.* 2001;12(6):361-5.

[79]   Weber AM, Walters MD, Schover LR, Mitchinson A.. Sexual function in women with uterovaginal prolapse and urinary incontinence. *Obstet. Gynecol.* 1995 Apr;85(4):483-7.

[80]   Vierhout ME, Gianotten WL. Mechanisms of urine loss during sexual activity. *European Journal of Obstetrics, Gynecology and Reproductive Biology* 1993; 52(1): 45–47.

[81]   Hilton P. Urinary incontinence during sexual intercourse: a common, but rarely volunteered, symptom. *British Journal of Obstetrics and Gynaecology* 1988; 95(4): 377–381.

[82]   Moran PA, Dwyer PL, Ziccone SP. Urinary laekage during coitus in women. *J. Obstet. Gynaecol.* 1999; 19(3): 286–288.

[83]   Khan Z, Bhola A, Starer P. Urinary incontinence during orgasm. *Urology* 1988; 31(3): 279–282.

[84]   Pace G, Silvestri V, Gualá L, Vicentini C. Body mass index, urinary incontinence and female sexual dysfunction: how they affect female postmenopausal health. *Menopause.* 2009 Nov-Dec;16(6):1188-92.

[85]   Huang AJ, Stewart AL, Hernandez AL, Shen H, Subak LL; Program to Reduce Incontinence by Diet and Exercise. Sexual function among overweight and obese women with urinary incontinence in a randomized controlled trial of an intensive behavioral weight loss intervention. *J. Urol.* 2009 May;181(5):2235-42.

[86]   Melin I, Falconer C, Rössner S, Altman D. Sexual function in obese women: impact of lower urinary tract dysfunction. *Int. J. Obes.* (Lond). 2008 Aug;32(8):1312-8.

[87]   van de Merwe JP, Nordling J, Bouchelouche P, Bouchelouche K, Cervigni M, Daha LK, Elneil S, Fall M, Hohlbrugger G, Irwin P, Mortensen S, van Ophoven A, Osborne JL, Peeker R, Richter B, Riedl C, Sairanen J, Tinzl M, Wyndaele JJ. Diagnostic criteria, classification, and nomenclature for painful bladder syndrome/interstitial cystitis: an ESSIC proposal. *Eur. Urol.* 2008 Jan;53(1):60-7.

[88]   Peters KM, Killinger KA, Carrico DJ, Ibrahim IA, Diokno AC, Graziottin A. Sexual function and sexual distress in women with interstitial cystitis: a case-control study. *Urology.* 2007 Sep;70(3):543-7.

[89]   Verit FF, Verit A, Yeni E. The prevalence of sexual dysfunction and associated risk factors in women withchronic pelvic pain: a cross-sectional study. *Arch. Gynecol. Obstet.* 2006 Aug;274(5):297-302.

[90]   Ottem DP, Carr LK, Perks AE, Lee P, Teichman JM. Interstitial cystitis and female sexual dysfunction. *Urology.* 2007 Apr;69(4):608-10.

[91]   Bogart LM, Suttorp MJ, Elliott MN, Clemens JQ, Berry SH. Prevalence and correlates of sexual dysfunction among women with bladder painsyndrome/interstitial cystitis. *Urology.* 2011 Mar;77(3):576-80.

[92]   Hanno PM, Burks DA, Clemens JQ, Dmochowski RR, Erickson D, Fitzgerald MP, Forrest JB, Gordon B, Gray M, Mayer RD, Newman D, Nyberg L Jr, Payne CK,

Wesselmann U, Faraday MM; Interstitial Cystitis Guidelines Panel of the American Urological Association Education and Research, Inc. AUA guideline for the diagnosis and treatment of interstitial cystitis/bladder pain syndrome. *J. Urol.* 2011 Jun;185(6) 2162-70.

[93] Cardozo L. Sex and the bladder. *Br. Med. J.* (Clin Res Ed). 1988 Feb 27;296(6622): 587-8.

[94] Naber KG, Bergman B, Bishop MC, Bjerklund-Johansen TE, Botto H, Lobel B, Jinenez Cruz F, Selvaggi FP; Urinary Tract Infection (UTI) Working Group of the Health Care Office (HCO) of the European Association of Urology (EAU). EAU guidelines for the management of urinary and male genital tract infections. Urinary TractInfection (UTI) Working Group of the Health Care Office (HCO) of the European Association of Urology (EAU). *Eur. Urol.* 2001 Nov;40(5):576-88.

[95] Chung A, Arianayagam M, Rashid P. Bacterial cystitis in women. *Aust. Fam. Physician.* 2010 May;39(5):295-8.

[96] Yoon BI, Kim SW, Ha US, Sohn DW, Cho YH. Risk factors for recurrent cystitis following acute cystitis in female patients. *J. Infect. Chemother.* 2013 Feb 5.

[97] Handa VL, Zyczynski HM, Brubaker L, Nygaard I, Janz NK, Richter HE, Wren PA, Brown MB, Weber AM; Pelvic Floor Disorders Network. Sexual function before and after sacrocolpopexy for pelvic organ prolapse. *Am. J. Obstet. Gynecol.* 2007;197: 629.e1-629.e6.

[98] Dennerstein L, Alexander JL, Kotz K. The menopause and sexual functioning: a review of the population-based studies. *Annu. Rev. Sex Res.* 2003;14:64-82.

[99] Athanasiou S, Grigoriadis T, Chalabalaki A, Protopapas A, Antsaklis A. Pelvic organ prolapse contributes to sexual dysfunction: a cross-sectional study. *Acta Obstet. Gynecol. Scand.* 2012 Jun;91(6):704-9.

[100] Novi JM, Jeronis S, Morgan MA, Arya LA. Sexual function in women with pelvic organ prolapse compared to women without pelvic organ prolapse. *J. Urol.* 2005 May; 173:1669-72.

[101] Digesu GA, Chaliha C, Salvatore S. The relationship of vaginal prolapse severity to symptoms and quality of life. *BJOG* 2005 July; 112:971-6.

[102] Sarrel PM. Sexuality and menopause. *Obstet. Gynecol.* 1990; 75(suppl 4):26S–30S.

[103] Collins A. Landgren BM. Reproductive health, use of estrogen and experience of symptoms in postmenopausal women: a population based study. *Maturitas* 1994; 20(2):101–111.

[104] Sherwin BB, Gelfand MM, Brender W. Androgen enhances sexual motivation in females: a prospective, crossover study of sex steroid administration in the surgical menopause. *Psychosom. Med.* 1985; 47:339–351.

[105] Montgomery JC, Appleby L, Brincat M, Versi E, Tapp A, Fenwick PB, Studd JW. Effect of oestrogen and testosterone implants on psychological disorders in the climacteric. *Lancet* 1987; 1:297–299.

[106] Shifren JL, Braunstein GD, Simon JA, Casson PR, Buster JE, Redmond GP, Burki RE, Ginsburg ES, Rosen RC, Leiblum SR, Caramelli KE, Mazer NA. Transdermal testosterone treatment in women with impaired sexual function after oophorectomy. *N. Engl. J. Med.* 2000; 343:682–688.

[107] Sherwin BB, Gelfand MM. Differential symptom response to parental estrogen and androgen in the surgical menopause. *Am. J. Obstet. Gynecol.* 1985; 151:153–160.

[108] Sarrel P, Dobay B, Wiita B. Estrogen and estrogen-androgen replacement in postmenopausal women dissatifsfied with estrogen-only therapy. Sexual behavior and neuroendocrine response. *J. Reprod. Med.* 1998 43(10):847–856.

[109] Davis SR, Tran J. Testosterone influences libido and well being in women. *Trends Endocrinol. Metab.* 2001; 12:33–37.

[110] Berman LA, Berman JR, Chhabra S, Goldstein I. Novel approaches to female sexual dysfunction. *Expert Opin. Invest. Drugs* 2001; 10(1) 85–95.

[111] Rako S. Testosterone supplemental therapy after hysterectomy with or without concomitant oophorectomy: estrogen alone is not enough. *J. Womens Health Gend. Based Med.* 2000; 9:17–23.

[112] Bloch M, Meiboom H, Zaig I, Schreiber S, Abramov L. The use of dehydroepiandrosterone in the treatment of hypoactive sexual desire disorder: A report of gender differences. *Eur. Neuropsychopharmacol.* 2012 Oct 17.

[113] Genazzani AR, Stomati M, Valentino V, Pluchino N, Pot E, Casarosa E, Merlini S, Giannini A, Luisi M. Effect of 1-year, low-dose DHEA therapy on climacteric symptoms and female sexuality. *Climacteric.* 2011 Dec;14(6):661-8.

[114] Thorp J, Simon J, Dattani D, Taylor L, Kimura T, Garcia M Jr, Lesko L, Pyke R; DAISY trial investigators. Treatment of hypoactive sexual desire disorder in premenopausal women: efficacy of flibanserin in the DAISY study. *J. Sex. Med.* 2012 Mar; 9(3):793-804.

[115] Derogatis LR, Komer L, Katz M, Moreau M, Kimura T, Garcia M Jr, Wunderlich G, Pyke R; VIOLET Trial Investigators. Treatment of hypoactive sexual desire disorder in premenopausal women: efficacy of flibanserin in the VIOLET Study. *J. Sex. Med.* 2012 Apr;9(4):1074-85.

[116] Safarinejad MR, Hosseini SY, Asgari MA, Dadkhah F, Taghva A. A randomized, double-blind, placebo-controlled study of the efficacy and safety ofbupropion for treating hypoactive sexual desire disorder in ovulating women. *BJU Int.* 2010 Sep; 106(6):832-9.

[117] Sayuk GS, Gott BM, Nix BD, Lustman PJ. Improvement in sexual functioning in patients with type 2 diabetes and depression treated with bupropion. *Diabetes Care.* 2011 Feb;34(2):332-4.

[118] Liao Q, Zhang M, Geng L, Wang X, Song X, Xia P, Lu T, Lu M, Liu V. Efficacy and safety of alprostadil cream for the treatment of female sexual arousal disorder: a double-blind, placebo-controlled study in chinese population. *J. Sex. Med.* 2008 Aug; 5(8):1923-31.

[119] Leddy LS, Yang CC, Stuckey BG, Sudworth M, Haughie S, Sultana S, Maravilla KR. Influence of sildenafil on genital engorgement in women with female sexual arousal disorder. *J. Sex. Med.* 2012 Oct;9(10):2693-7.

[120] Meston CM, Worcel M. The effects of yohimbine plus L-arginine glutamate on sexual arousal in postmenopausal women with sexual arousal disorder. *Arch. Sex Behav.* 2002 Aug;31(4):323-32.

[121] Safarinejad MR. Evaluation of the safety and efficacy of bremelanotide, a melanocortin receptor agonist, in female subjects with arousal disorder: a double-blind placebo-controlled, fixed dose, randomized study. *J. Sex. Med.* 2008 Apr;5(4):887-97.

[122] Chapple CR, Khullar V, Gabriel Z, Muston D, Bitoun CE, Weinstein D. The effects of antimuscarinic treatments in overactive bladder: an update of a systematic review and meta-analysis. *Eur. Urol.* 2008 Sep;54(3):543-62.

[123] Sand PK, Goldberg RP, Dmochowski RR, McIlwain M, Dahl NV. The impact of the overactive bladder syndrome on sexual function: a preliminary report from the Multicenter Assessment of Transdermal Therapy in Overactive Bladder with Oxybutynin trial. *Am. J. Obstet. Gynecol.* 2006 Dec;195(6):1730-5.

[124] Rogers RG, Omotosho T, Bachmann G, Sun F, Morrow JD. Continued symptom improvement in sexually active women with overactive bladder and urgency urinary incontinence treated with tolterodine ER for 6 months. *Int. Urogynecol. J. Pelvic Floor Dysfunct.* 2009 Apr;20(4):381-5.

[125] Hajebrahimi S, Azaripour A, Sadeghi-Bazargani H. Tolterodine immediate release improves sexual function in women with overactive bladder. *J. Sex. Med.* 2008 Dec; 5(12):2880-5.

[126] Sacco E, Bientinesi R. Mirabegron: a review of recent data and its prospects in the management of overactive bladder. *Ther. Adv. Urol.* 2012;4(6):315-24127).

[127] Pauls RN, Marinkovic SP, Silva WA, Rooney CM, Kleeman SD, Karram MM. Effects of sacral neuromodulation on female sexual function. *Int. Urogynecol. J. Pelvic Floor Dysfunct.* 2007 Apr;18(4):391-5.

[128] Signorello D, Seitz CC, Berner L, Trenti E, Martini T, Galantini A, Lusuardi L, Lodde M, Pycha A. Impact of sacral neuromodulation on female sexual function and his correlation with clinical outcome and quality of life indexes: a monocentric experience. *J. Sex. Med.* 2011 Apr;8(4):1147-55.

[129] Yih JM, Killinger KA, Boura JA, Peters KM. Changes in Sexual Functioning in Women after Neuromodulation for Voiding Dysfunction. *J. Sex. Med.* 2013 Feb 27. doi: 10.1111/jsm.12085.

[130] van Balken MR, Vergunst H, Bemelmans BL. Sexual functioning in patients with lower urinary tract dysfunction improves after percutaneoustibial nerve stimulation. *Int. J. Impot. Res.* 2006 Sep-Oct;18(5):470-5.

[131] 131)Duthie JB, Vincent M, Herbison GP, Wilson DI, Wilson D.Botulinum toxin injections for adults with overactive bladder syndrome. *Cochrane Database Syst. Rev.* 2011 Dec 7;(12):CD005493.

[132] Basu M, Duckett JR. Update on duloxetine for the management of stress urinary incontinence. *Clin. Interv. Aging.* 2009;4:25-30.

[133] Dueñas H, Brnabic AJ, Lee A, Montejo AL, Prakash S, Casimiro-Querubin ML, Khaled M, Dossenbach M, Raskin J. Treatment-emergent sexual dysfunction with SSRIs and duloxetine: effectiveness and functional outcomes over a 6-month observational period. *Int. J. Psychiatry Clin. Pract.* 2011 Nov;15(4):242-54.

[134] Clayton A, Kornstein S, Prakash A, Mallinckrodt C, Wohlreich M. Changes in sexual functioning associated with duloxetine, escitalopram, and placebo in the treatment of patients with major depressive disorder. *J. Sex. Med.* 2007 Jul;4(4 Pt 1):917-29.

[135] Rosenbaum TY. Pelvic floor involvement in male and female sexual dysfunction and the role of pelvic floor rehabilitation in treatment: a literature review. *J. Sex. Med.* 2007 Jan;4(1):4-13.

[136] Bø K, Talseth T, Vinsnes A. Randomized controlled trial on the effect of pelvic floor muscle training on quality of life and sexual problems in genuine stress incontinent women. *Acta Obstet. Gynecol. Scand.* 2000 Jul;7 (7):598-603.

[137] Zahariou AG, Karamouti MV, Papaioannou PD. Pelvic floor muscle training improves sexual function of women with stress urinary incontinence. *Int. Urogynecol. J. Pelvic Floor Dysfunct.* 2008 Mar;19(3):401-6.

[138] Liebergall-Wischnitzer M, Paltiel O, Hochner Celnikier D, Lavy Y, Manor O, Woloski Wruble AC. Sexual function and quality of life of women with stress urinary incontinence: a randomized controlled trial comparing the Paula method (circular muscle exercises) to pelvic floor muscle training (PFMT) exercises. *J. Sex. Med.* 2012 Jun; 9(6):1613-23.

[139] Achtari C, Dwyer L. Sexual function and pelvic floor disorders. *Best Pract. Res. Clin. Obstet. Gynaecol.* 2005 Dec;19(6):993-1008.

[140] De Souza A, Dwyer PL, Rosamilia A, Hiscock R, Lim YN, Murray C, Thomas E, Conway C, Schierlitz L. Sexual functioning following retropubic TVT and transobturator Monarc sling in women with intrinsic sphincter deficiency: a multicenter prospective study. *Int. Urogyn. J.* July 2012;23:153-8.

[141] Srikrishna S, Robinson D, Cardozo L, Gonzalez J. Can sex survive pelvic floor surgery? *Int. Urogynecol. J.* (2010) 21:1313-1319.

[142] Moran PA, Dwyer PL, Ziccone SP. Burch colposuspension for the treatment of coital urinary leakage secondary to genuine stress incontinence. *Journal of Obstetrics and Gynaecology* 1999; 19(3): 289-91.

[143] Baessler K, Stanton SL. Does Burch colposuspension cure coital incontinence? *Am. J. Obstet. Gynecol.* 2004;190:1030-3.

[144] Berthier A, Sentilhes L, Taibi S, Loisel C, Grise P, Marpeau L. Sexual function in women following the transvaginal tension free tape procedure for incontinence. *Int. J. Gynaecol. Obstet.* 2008 Aug;102(2):105-9.

[145] Mazouni C, Karsenty G, Bretelle F, Bladou F, Gamerre M, Serment G. Urinary complications and sexual function after the tension-free vaginal tape procedure. *Acta Obstet. Gynecol. Scand.* 2004;83:955-61.

[146] Maaita M, Bhaumik J, Davies AE. Sexual function after using tension-free vaginal tape for the surgical treatment of genuine stress incontinence. *BJU Int.* 2002;90:540-3.

[147] Shah SM, Bukkapatnam R, Rodríguez LV. Impact of vaginal surgery for stress urinary incontinence on female sexual function: is the use of polypropylene mesh detrimental? *Urology* 2005;65:270-4.

[148] Ghezzi F, Serati M, Cromi A, Uccella S, Triacca P, Bolis P. Impact of tension-free vaginal tape on sexual function: result of a prospective study. *Int. Urogynecol. J. Pelvic Floor Dysfunct.* 2006;17:54-9.

[149] Filocamo MT, Serati M, Frumenzio E, Li arzi V, Cattoni E, Champagne A, Salvatore S, Nicita G, Costantini E. The impact of mid-urethral slings for the treatment of urodynamic stress incontinence on female sexual function: a multicenter prospective study. *J. Sex. Med.* 2011 Jul;8(7):2002- 8.

[150] Roumeguere T, Quackels T, Bollens R, de Groote A, Zlotta A, Bossche MV, Schulman C. Trans-obturator vaginal tape (TOT®) for female stress incontinence: one year follow-up in 120 patients. *Eur. Urol.* 2005;48:805-9.

[151] Xu Y, Song Y, Huang H. Impact of the tension-free vaginal tape obturator procedure on sexual function in women with stress urinary incontinence. *IJGO* 112 (2011) 187-9.

[152] Zyczynski HM, Rickey L, Dyer KY, Wilson T, Stoddard AM, Gormley EA, Hsu Y, Kusek JW, Brubaker L; Urinary Incontinence Treatment Network. Sexual activity and function in women more than 2 years after midurethral sling placement. *Am. J. Obstet. Gynecol.* 2012;207;421.e1-6.

[153] Baessler K, Hewson AD, Tunn R, Schuessler B, Maher CF. Severe mesh complications following intravaginal slingplasty. *Obstet. Gynecol.* 2005 Oct;106(4):713-6.

[154] Bekker MD, Hogewoning CR, Wallner C. The somatic and autonomic innervation of the clitoris; preliminary evidence of sexual dysfunction after minimally invasive slings. *J. Sex. Med.* 2012 Jun;9(6):1566-78.

[155] Schmid C, Berger K, Müller M, Silke J, Mueller MD, Kuhn A. Painful bladder syndrome: management and effect on sexual function and quality of life. *Ginekol. Pol.* 2011 Feb;82(2):96-101.

[156] Nickel JC, Parsons CL, Forrest J, Kaufman D, Evans R, Chen A, Wan G, Xiao X. Improvement in sexual functioning in patients with interstitial cystitis/painful bladder syndrome. *J. Sex. Med.* 2008 Feb;5(2):394-9.

[157] Kodner CM, Thomas Gupton EK. Recurrent urinary tract infections in women: diagnosis and management. *Am. Fam. Physician.* 2010 Sep 15;82(6):638-43.

[158] Albert X, Huertas I, Pereiró II, Sanfélix J, Gosalbes V, Perrota C. Antibiotics for preventing recurrent urinary tract infection in non-pregnant women. *Cochrane Database Syst. Rev.* 2004;(3): CD001209.

[159] Nicolle L; AMMI Canada Guidelines Committee. Complicated urinary tract infection in adults *Can. J. Infect. Dis. Med. Microbiol.* 2005;16(6):349–360.

[160] Naber KG, Cho YH, Matsumoto T, Schaeffer AJ. Immunoactive prophylaxis of recurrent urinary tract infections: a meta-analysis. *Int. J. Antimicrob. Agents.* 2009 Feb;33(2):111-9.

[161] Sen A. Recurrent cystitis in non-pregnant women. *Clin. Evid.* 2006;(15): 2558–2564.

[162] Sheffield JS, Cunningham FG. Urinary tract infection in women. *Obstet. Gynecol.* 2005;106(5 pt 1):1085–1092.

[163] Kontiokari T, Sundqvist K, Nuutinen M, Pokka T, Koskela M, Uhari M. Randomised trial of cranberry-lingonberry juice and Lactobacillus GG drink for the prevention of urinary tract infections in women. *BMJ.* 2001;322(7302):1571.

[164] Raz R, Stamm WE. A controlled trial of intravaginal estriol in postmenopausal women with recurrent urinary tract infections. *N. Engl. J. Med.* 1993;329(11):753–756.

[165] Perrotta C, Perrotta C, Aznar M, Mejia R, Albert X, Ng CW. Oestrogens for preventing recurrent urinary tract infection in postmenopausal women. *Cochrane Database Syst. Rev.* 2008;(2):CD005131.

[166] Damiano R, Cicione A. The role of sodium hyaluronate and sodium chondroitin sulphate in the management of bladder disease. *Ther. Adv. Urol.* 2011 Oct;3(5):223-32.

[167] Damiano R, Quarto G, Bava I, Ucciero G, De Domenico R, Palumbo MI, Autorino R. Prevention of recurrent urinary tract infections by intravesical administration of hyaluronic acidand chondroitin sulphate: a placebo-controlled randomised trial. *Eur. Urol.* 2011 Apr;59(4):645-51.

[168] Wang CL, Long CY, Juan YS, Liu CM, Hsu CS. Impact of total vaginal mesh surgery for pelvic organ prolapse on female sexual function. *IJOG* 2011 (115):167-70.

[169] Silva WA, Pauls RN, Segal JL, Rooney CM, Kleeman SD, Karram MM. Uterosacral ligament vault suspension: five years outcomes. *Obstet. Gynecol.* 2006;108:255-63.

[170] Brubaker L, Cundiff G, Fine P, Nygaard I, Richter H, Visco A, Zyczynski H, Brown MB, Weber A; Pelvic Floor Disorders Network.. A randomized trial of colpopexy and urinary reduction efforts (CARE): design and methods. *Control Clin. Trials* 2003; 24:629-42.

[171] Jeffcoate TN. Posterior colpoperineorrhaphy. *American Journal of Obstetric and Gynecology* 1959;77(3):490-502.

[172] Haase P, Skibsted L. Influence of operations for stress incontinence and/or genital descensus on sexual life. *Acta Obstetrica et Gynecologica Scandinavica* 1988;67(7):659-61.

[173] Amias AG. Sexual life after gynaecological operations-II. *British Medical Journal* 1975; 2(5972): 680-1.

[174] Kahn MA, Stanton S. Posterior colporrhaphy: its effect on bowel and sexual function. *Br. J. Obstet. Gynecol.* 1997;104:82-6.

[175] Weber AM, Walters MD, Piedmonte MR. Sexual function and vaginal anatomy in women before and after surgery for pelvic organ prolapse and urinary incontinence. *Am. J. Obstet. Gynecol.* 2000;182:1610-5.

[176] Costantini E, Porena M, Lazzeri M, Mearini L, Bini V, Zucchi A. Changes in female sexual function after pelvic organ prolapse repair: role of hysterectomy. *Int. Urogynecol. J.* 2013 Jan 30.

[177] Su TH, Lau HH, Huang WC, Chen SS, Lin TY, Hsieh CH, Yeh CY. Short term impact on female sexual function of pelvic floor reconstruction with the Prolift procedure. *J. Sex. Med.* 2009;6(11):3201–7.

[178] Altman D, Elmér C, Kiilholma P, Kinne I, Tegerstedt G, Falconer C; Nordic Transvaginal Mesh Group. Sexual dysfunction after trocar-guided transvaginal mesh repair of pelvic organ prolapse.

[179] Hoda MR, Wagner S, Greco F, Heynemann H, Fornara P. Prospective follow-up of female sexual function after vaginal surgery for pelvic organ prolapse using transobturator mesh implants. *J. Sex. Med.* 2011;8(3):914–22.

[180] Dwyer PL, O'Reilly BA. Transvaginal repair of anterior and posterior compartment prolapse with atrium polypropylene mesh. *British Journal of Obstetrics and Gynaecology* 2004; 111(8): 831–836.

[181] Lowenstein L, Gamble T, Sanses TV, van Raalte H, Carberry C, Jakus S, Pham T, Nguyen A, Hoskey K, Kenton K; Fellow's Pelvic Research Network. Changes in sexual function after treatment for prolapse are related to the improvement in body image perception. *J. Sex. Med.* 2010 Feb;7(2 Pt 2):1023-8.

[182] Silverstein RG, Brown AC, Roth HD, Britton WB. Effects of mindfulness training on body awareness to sexual stimuli: implications forfemale sexual dysfunction. *Psychosom. Med.* 2011 Nov-Dec;73(9):817-25.

[183] Michael L. Krychman. Female Sexual Dysfunction: A Clinical Update. Online on: http://www.medscape.org/viewarticle/575789

[184] Schroder M, Mell LK, Hurteau JA, Collins YC, Rotmensch J, Waggoner SE, Yamada SD, Small W Jr, Mundt AJ. Clitoral therapy device for treatment of sexual dysfunction in irradiated cervical cancer patients. *Int. J. Radiat. Oncol. Biol. Phys.* 2005 Mar 15;61(4):1078-86.

[185] Stephenson KR, Rellini AH, Meston CM. Relationship satisfaction as a predictor of treatment response during cognitive behavioral sex therapy. Arch. Sex. Behav. 2013 Jan; 42(1):143-52.

[186] Masheb RM, Kerns RD, Lozano C, Minkin MJ, Richman S. A randomized clinical trial for women with vulvodynia: Cognitive-behavioral therapy vs. supportive psychotherapy. *Pain.* 2009 Jan;141(1-2):31-40.

In: Sexual Dysfunctions
Editor: Frédérique Courtois

ISBN: 978-1-62808-765-9
© 2013 Nova Science Publishers, Inc.

Chapter 12

SEXUAL DYSFUNCTION IN MIDDLE-AGED WOMEN: A REVIEW

Patricia Uchoa Leitão Cabral[1]
and Ana Katherine da Silveira Gonçalves[2,]*
[1]Universidade Federal do Rio Grande do Norte – UFRN,
Natal, Rio Grande do Norte, Brazil
[2]Universidade Estadual do Piaui – UESPI, Brazil

ABSTRACT

Female sexual dysfunction is highly prevalent among women of all ages and is frequently undetected, since complaints are often stifled by inhibition or not investigated because of embarrassment. Pharmacotherapy for female sexual dysfunction is quite restricted. Even though estrogen replacement therapy has been found to improve genital dryness complaints in perimenopausal women and to have a positive impact on sexual response, androgen therapy is still controversial. Gynecologists can address sexual health using their professional authority based on knowledge of anatomy, pharmacology and human behavior. In this way, female sexual dysfunction can be successfully treated when caused by a lack of knowledge concerning genital anatomy and human sexual response, coital pain caused by diseases of the genital tract, depression, and other systemic diseases such as diabetes, hypothyroidism, and hyperprolactinaemia. It is recommended that for cases associated with strong sexual repression and sexual violence, as well as those that do not respond to medical intervention, sexual therapy and psychotherapy be administered jointly.

[*] Corresponding author: Ana Katherine da Silveira Gonçalves, Universidade Estadual do Piaui – UESPI. Email: anakatherine@ufrnet.br.

INTRODUCTION

Sexual satisfaction is considered an integral component of overall well-being in middle-aged women [1], since higher levels of sexual activity have been correlated with better physical and mental health [1, 2, 3, 4]. Sexual pleasure has also been associated with a healthier dynamic within the married couple [4] and general psychological wellbeing [5].

Sexuality has a multidimensional character; it is not only influenced by physiologica., psychosocial and cultural factors, but also by interpersonal relationships and life experiences [6, 7]. Thus, sexual dysfunction is less likely to occur in women in good physical and emotional health [5].

Sexual dysfunction is defined as any disorder, which includes manifestations spannirg from unresponsiveness to stimuli to changes in the phases of desire, arousal and orgasm [8]. The American Psychiatric Association classifies sexual dysfunction as hypoactive sexual desire, arousal dysfunction, anorgasmia, dyspareunia and vaginismus [9]. Sexual dysfunctions are further classified as primary when the sexual response never reaches satisfactory levels during a lifetime, and secondary when it is singular, or only in specific circumstances [10].

Female sexual dysfunction (FSD) is highly prevalent, and affects 20 to 50% of the population [9, 11]. An American study found that 43% of American women have some sort of sexual dysfunction [12], while a Brazilian study showed that 30% of women suffered from sexual problems. Lack of desire was the most prevalent symptom (34,6%), followed by difficulties in reaching orgasm (29.3%) [13].

Many studies suggest that FSD increases with age [10, 14, 15], and state several contributing factors: loss of vigor and youth, changes in family structure "empty nest" syndrome, the inability to become pregnant and loss of sexual partner among others [13].

Another determinant of FSD is related to emotional factors such as sorrow, revenge, depression, sexual abuse, and rape to name a few. However, the latter have been shown to improve significantly with appropriate treatment [10].

Other variables such as poor health, any chronic disease, quality of relationship, sociodemographic and behavioral conditions such as low family income, low education, smoking, as well as stress, appear to significantly affect sexual function [10, 16, 17, 18]. Studies have also associated low sexual activity to feelings of guilt or embarrassment caused by sexual desire or marital difficulties, as well as the use of drugs that interfere with libido or sexual potency [7]. However, according to Kaiser [19], changes in sexual function due to the aging process should be analyzed separately from diseases that often arise at this stage of life.

This being considered, it seems that ageing alone is not responsible for decreased sexual function. Research has shown that sex steroids (estrogen, progesterone and androgen) causes major changes in female sexual function and decreased secretion of these hormones are inversely proportional to sexual complaints at this stage of life [10, 13, 20]. As a result, it is unclear if increase in FSD at this age is due to the reduction in hormone levels or advancing age [21].

Advancing age results in falling levels of estrogen, progesterone and the absence of peripheral conversion of androgens to estrone, can cause hot flashes, night sweats, vaginal dryness, dyspareunia, insomnia, mood swings, anxiety, depression and increased risk of chronic diseases [10, 20, 22]. Lower levels of testosterone are associated with less sexual interest during the climacteric period [23]. In older women with long-term relationships, there is a significant increase in sexual complaints such as hypoactive sexual desire (HSD), orgasmic dysfunction and dyspareunia [24]. Another study, the Assessment of Ageing in Women (AAW), investigated the sexual behavior of Australian women ranging between 40 to 49 and 70 to 79 years, and noted that the demand for sexual intercourse decreased markedly with age [25].

The fact that aging changes hormone levels, reduces the action of neurotransmitters and neuropeptides, and reduces tissue growth factors and the efficiency of other biological functions [26] causes serious biological and psychological repercussions unfavorable to normal sexual response [10, 27, 28].

Even though FSD is extremely prevalent in middle-aged women, doctors rarely ask about their patients' sexual life, because they feel uncomfortable or because they lack sufficient training in investigation techniques [10].

Over the past decade, women have generally resorted to medical care in search of a solution for decreased sexual function. However, less than 10% of doctors take the initiative, inquire and try to solve the complaints of these patients [29, 30]. In a study conducted in Brazil, 4753 gynecologists claimed that decreased sexual desire was one of the main reasons for patient consultation [31]. Most women admit that their gynecologist is key to the diagnosis and management of their sexual difficulties, and wish they were more skilled in this area [30].

Despite the high rates of FSD, a large portion of affected women do not seek medical help because of shame, frustration or failed attempts at treatment [31]. It is possible that some gynecologist have personal difficulties regarding their own sexuality, resulting in difficult discourse concerning the sexuality of their patients [32].

Other limiting factors include the lack of clinical trials concerning sexual dysfunction interventions of organic origin, the absence of approved drugs for treatment, and insufficient evidence showing the efficacy or effectiveness of drugs and psychological intervention [33].

Many physiological, psychological, interpersonal, and sociocultural factors contribute to FSD (Table 1) [34]. These range from age or illness related causes to results of surgical or therapeutic interventions. In addition, sexual motivation and performance can also be affected by psychosexual issues [10].

Table 1. General causes of female sexual dysfunction

Physiological	Psychological	Interpersonal	Sociocultural
• Aging and menopause	• Defective physical or mental status	• Lack of partner	• Inadequate sex education
• Endocrine changes	• Physical or sexual abuse	• Perceived unattractiveness	• Antagonistic religious or family values
• Illness, injury, or disability	• Poor self-esteem or self-image	• Fastidiousness with nonsexual aspects	• Cultural taboos
• Surgical therapies	• Unrealistic goals	• Interpersonal conflicts	• Gender discrimination
• Medications	• Stress and performance anxiety	• Lack of desire	
	• Sexual inexperience or inadequacy	• Inadequate foreplay or poor technical skill	
	• Conflicting gender or sexual orientation	• Obsession with intercourse	
		• Rushing toward orgasm	
		• Communication problem	
		• Sexual dysfunctions of the partner	
		• Routine	

CLINICAL ASSESSMENT OF FEMALE SEXUAL DYSFUNCTION

The Sexual History

Investigation begins with careful identification and description of the patient, since this is often the most important clue to the cause of the sexual pathology. Increasing age may be associated with varying degrees of self-esteem, especially concerning the phases of desire and orgasm [35]. Other factors such as work can cause stress and interfere with sexual desire, whereas socioeconomic status and culture often modulate sexual expression [36].

Generally, the patient complains of having no desire to have sex. The professional must identify the affected phase of sexual response, establish the time of occurrence of the disorder, and verify if the complaint is associated with a specific event. It is also important to evaluate sexual history such to compare sexual expression from prior relationships, as well as determine the use of any drugs (antidepressants, contraceptives and other) that may affect actual sexual response [37]. Diseases such as diabetes mellitus, hypothyroidism and hyperprolactinaemias may also cause problems.

It is important to remember that the clinical sexual interrogation can be embarrassing, and may bring out negative feelings concerning sexuality, and may require the intervention of a psychotherapist [38]. It is also important to know why the patient is seeking treatment. Patients do not always seek help to improve the quality of their sexual life: sometimes it is an imposition on behalf of the partner, or results from fear of separation. Consideration of patient motivation is fundamental for successful treatment as well as to evaluate the impact of the intervention [39, 40]. Generally, when sexual problems diminish the patient goes through positive changes in physical appearance, attitude and facial expression [41, 42].

Physical Examination for FSD

General assessment should include thyroid status, cardiovascular, musculoskeletal, and neurologic parameters, breast examination for further hyperprolactinaemia, and signs of anemia. A complete gynecological assessment should encompass these possible sources of sexual difficulties (Table 2).

The diagnosis of FSD is mainly clinical. However, hyperprolactinaemia may also be associated with sexual dysfunction and mainly affects desire [10]. This is why testing prolactin levels can also be useful when FSD is not thought to be related to drug use or psychological factors [10]. Testing free testosterone levels is not recommended because the use of testosterone in the treatment of FSD still remains controversial.

Treatment

The treatment of sexual complaints involves the consideration of several factors such as physical, and psychological variables, as well as problems within the couple and/or concerning the individual in question (Table 3) [43].

Table 2. Vulvovaginal causes of female sexual dysfunction

Vulvovaginal estratrophy
Abnormal discharge (bubbly, cheesy, foul-smelling)
Vaginal or perineal lesions (for example, condylomata acuminata, herpes, trauma)
Size and elasticity of introitus (any atrophy, lesions, scarring, or strictures)
Discharge or evidence of infection, vulvodynia, and deep tenderness
Sparse hair of the mons pubis (may suggest low androgen levels)
Vulvar skin lesions indicating possible infection (Candida, herpes), dermatitis (eczema, psoriasis, allergic reaction), or dermatoses (lichens)
Atrophy, lesions, or adhesions of the labia majora and minora
Phimosis and adhesions of the clitoris and female genital surgery (including circumcision)
Infection or prolapse of the urethra
Vaginal or perineal lesions (for example, condylomata acuminata, herpes, trauma)
Size and elasticity of introitus (any atrophy, lesions, scarring, or strictures)
Discharge or evidence of infection, vulvodynia, and deep tenderness
Sparse hair of the mons pubis (may suggest low androgen levels)
Vulvar skin lesions indicating possible infection (Candida, herpes), dermatitis (eczema, psoriasis, allergic reaction), or dermatoses (lichens)
Atrophy, lesions, or adhesions of the labia majora and minora
Phimosis and adhesions of the clitoris and female genital surgery (including circumcision)
Infection or prolapse of the urethra
Vuvovestibulitis of the vulva and bulbourethral glands (by swab)
Cystocele, rectocele, uterine prolapse, or urinary incontinence
Pain or masses impaired vaginal and rectal muscle tone, pelvic floor

Table 3. Female sexual dysfunction: options of treatment

Hormonal Therapy Replacement • Oral estrogen replacement • Topical estrogen • Promestriene • Androgens • Tibolone
Psychotherapy - Sexual orientation for the patient and his partner
Treatment of genital infections
Treatment of vulvodynea and Vuvovestibulitis
Chirurgical treatment
Non-drug alternatives - physical activity

The first strategies for intervention [43] include guidance on the anatomy of the genitalia and clarification about the human sexual response, prescription of vaginal lubricants, inviting the partner to programs concerning both female and male sexual function [18], sexual orientation for the patient and his partner, modification of reversible causes through counseling, and change of lifestyle among other [43].

Additionally, the doctor is also responsible for the treatment of any general health problems which might lead to FSD such as infectious diseases of the genital tract, as well as surgical procedures correcting urinary incontinence, pelvic organ prolapse, vaginal laxity, and any other condition providing cause for complaint [44, 45, 46]. It also includes the replacement of drugs that interfere with sexual response and prescribe specific exercises to strengthen the pelvic muscles [43].

Although the role of sex steroids in sexual function has not yet been clearly defined, oral replacement seems to favor sexual response in women going through menopause, improving symptoms such as irritability and insomnia [47, 48, 49]. Vaginal lubrication seems to be decreased when women complain of coital pain, and is generally improved in all layers of the vaginal wall when estrogen is administered orally [50]. However, if complaints of vaginal dryness persist, local application of estrogen may be necessary [51]. Women complaining about discomfort during intercourse, who have been discouraged from using oral estrogen replacement, greatly benefit from topical estrogen use since it improves vaginal trophism [52]. Daily treatment restores normal pH, normalizing the flora, and greatly reduces vaginal dryness, burning and urinary symptoms as a result [53]. Although there is no consensus on the duration of the results acquired through topical estrogen replacement, there is evidence that repeated short term use (intervals) is most effective, since constant exposure to estrogen saturates its receptors, resulting in inadequate response [54, 55, 56]. Oral hormone replacement is never prescribed solely to improve genital symptoms since local application is so effectiveness [57]. When trying to improve sexual response, the use of oral estrogen therapy is restricted to dysfunctional cases especially those with an inadequate excitement phase [58].

The treatment for hormone-dependent cancer causes major changes in sexual life and quality of life for women [59]. However, estrogen replacement, is not recommended in these cases [60]. Women being treated for breast and endometrial cancer must use vaginal lubricants regularly [61]. Another option is promestriene, which stimulates vaginal epithelial proliferation with no apparent effect on the endometrium [62].

Androgen replacement therapy remains controversial for the treatment of sexual dysfunctions, both in terms of safety and effectiveness [63, 64]. Some authors recommend prescribing androgens to women with androgen deficiency syndrome and for women undergoing ophorectomy [49, 57]. However, the Endocrine Society Clinical Practice Guideline advises that there is no evidence to support the recommendation of androgen use and can not attest to their safety for the control of female sexual dysfunction in geral [65]. However, in cases where the estrogen replacement did not show results, some authors recommend to consider administration of androgen as well [66, 67]. For oral replacement, the gynecologist should start by prescribing 1.5 mg/day of methyltestosterone. The dosage should be personalized and should not exceed 2.5 mg/dia [66] to avoid side effects. For topical use, 2% testosterone propionate may be used daily or on alternate days for a short period of time, since there is no consensus on duration of treatment. The risks of androgen therapy in women are known due the potential increase in serum cholesterol [68]. Levels of serum lipids need to be regularly monitored before the start of treatment and during the follow up.

Tibolone has a positive impact on sexual response and appears to be more effective in patients complaining of hypoactive sexual desire and for patients complaining of orgasmic dysfunction [58].

Psychotherapy should be suggested whenever psychological factors point to problems such as sexual abuse, conflicting relationships, behavior disorders, lowered self-esteem and depression.

Treatment of Specific Situations

Sexual Repression can cause FSD which usually stems from religious beliefs of the family or partner. The patient should be treated in psychotherapy or sex therapy, however, the gynecologist can discuss basic concepts involving the moral ideas that limit sexual expression. For example, self-eroticism: there seems to be a "collective truth" that men and women cannot masturbate. Religious sexual repression is secular and requires a careful inquiry which does not put religious beliefs into question [69]. Topics such as how rational the punitive image of God is towards sexual expression are important in these cases [38].

Low libido can result in relationship problems wherein one of the partners feels lonely, or needy, and often results in FSD. Conflict and strife can be caused by aggression, grief, and other negative emotions. Daily life, routine, stress, as well as male sexual dysfunction (eg, rapid ejaculation) can reduce desire significantly. The suggested treatment is to first provide information on gender differences (male and female sexual response). Highlight the importance of focusing on the partner's positive aspects since women with FSD often tend to focus on the negative. Encouraging the use of sexual fantasies in sexual play (psychotherapy or couples therapy) has also been found to have positive results [38].

Primary anorgasmia is one manifestation of FSD which is often caused by difficulty in letting go, as well as unawareness concerning anatomy, partner's inability, difficulty concentrating and lack of auto-eroticism. Possible treatments involve self-manipulation associated with sexual fantasy, rhythmic contraction of pelvic and perivaginal muscles, as well as manual stimulation by the partner [73, 74]. Morbidity and drugs are very frequently causes of hypoactive sexual desire. In such cases, use alternative medications for the following if possible: hypotensive, cimetidine, oral contraceptives, antidepressants, neuroleptics. The gynecologist should also treat recurrent vaginitis, correct hormone levels and treat depressive states when applicable. Bupropion has been used in cases of hypoactive sexual desire with depression since it seems to interfere less or at least improve FSD [70]. In cases of libido lowered by the use of hormonal contraceptive, it is suggested to replace pills for those containing derivatives of 19-nortestosterone or consider using a non-hormonal method [71, 72].

Vaginismus is a syndrome involving recurrent or persistent involuntary contraction of muscles surrounding the lower third of the vagina. The contraction can range from mild, causing stress and discomfort on penetration, to severe, preventing penetration altogether. This manifestation of FSD often results from sexual repression by the family, as well as social and religious cults of virginity, fear of pain, deep psychological conflict, anticipation of a negative sexual experience, and sexual abuse during childhood [74, 75, 76]. When a virgin is trying to have sexual intercourse for the first time and suffers from this condition, if the cause is not related to sexual trauma in general, muscle relaxation and penetration techniques are usually effective vectors. Treatment involves the gynecologist talking the patient through slow and gradual desensitization, by touching the perianal muscles and relaxing the muscles as they are touched. After achieving relaxation, muscles should be forced toward the anus. At home, the patient will do this exercise in the morning and evening. The patient should hold the partner's penis and control penetration. Botulinum toxin is suggested only in cases with unfavorable outcomes, but this should be a last resort [77]. If these guidelines are insufficient, the patient must be referred to both sex therapy and psychotherapy. It is essential to check whether the partner has sexual dysfunction or not, a situation commonly associated with women suffering from vaginismus.

Cases with a history of sexual abuse should be referred to psychotherapy. These cases are often accompanied by other psychological disorders [78].

In general, sexual dysfunction is not related to deep conflicts (grief, revenge, depression, sexual abuse, rape, etc.), and generally improve with proper sexual orientation. If the complaints continue, the gynecologist should refer the patient to a specialized service.

The uncertainty which can be conveyed by the physical and psychological problems of middle-aged menopausal women can easily interfere with family relationships, sexual adjustment and social integration [20]. Easing symptoms by using non-drug alternatives such as physical activity can improve quality of life for such women [79]. Studies have shown that menopausal symptoms seem to be less severe in women who exercise regularly [79, 80], and according to Nelson et al. [79], physically active women tend to have fewer menopausal symptoms, better sexuality and well-being.

REFERENCES

[1]   Lindau ST, Gavrilova N. Sex, health, and years of sexually active life gained due to good health: Evidence from two US population based cross sectional surveys of ageing. *BMJ* 2010; 340:c810.

[2]   Lindau ST, Schumm LP, Laumann EO et al. A study of sexuality and health among older adults in the United States. *N. Engl. J. Med.* 2007; 357:762–774.

[3]   Hawton K, Gath D, Day A. Sexual function in a community sample of middleaged women with partners: Effects of age, marital, socioeconomic, psychiatric, gynecological, and menopausal factors. *Arch. Sex. Behav.* 1994; 23:375–395.

[4]   Addis IB, Van Den Eeden SK,Wassel-Fyr CL et al. Sexual activity and function in middle-aged and older women. *Obstet. Gynecol.* 2006; 107:755–764.

[5]   Davison SL, Bell RJ, LaChina M et al. The relationship between self-reported sexual satisfaction and general well-being in women. *J. Sex. Med.* 2009; 6:2690–2697.

[6]   Bagherzadeh R, Zahmatkeshan N, Gharibi T, Akaberian S, Mirzaei K, Kamali F, et al. Prevalence of female sexual dysfunction and related factors for under treatment in Bushehrian women of Iran. *Sex Dis.* 2010; 28(1):39-49.

[7]   De Lorenzi DRS, Saciloto B. Sexual activity frequency in menopausal women. *Rev. Assoc. Med. Bras.* 2006; 52(4): 256-60.

[8]   Clayton AH. Epidemiology and neurobiology of female sexual dysfunction. *J. Sex. Med.* 2007; 4 Suppl 4:260-8.

[9]   Basson R, Berman J, Burnett A, Derogatis L, Ferguson D, Fourcroy J, et al. Report of the international consensus development conference on female sexual dysfunction: definitions and classifications. *J. Urol.* 2000; 163(3):888-93.

[10] Bancroft J, Loftus J, Long JS. Distress about sex: a national survey of women in heterosexual relationships. *Arch. Sex. Behav.* 2003; 32(3):192-208.

Lara LAS, Silva ACJSR, Romão APMS, Junqueira FRR. Manegement of female sexual dysfunction. *Rev. Bras. Ginecol. Obstet.* 2008; 30(6): 312-21.

[11] Bancroft J, Loftus J, Long JS. Distress about sex: a national survey of women in heterosexual relationships. *Arch. Sex. Behav.* 2003; 32(3):192-208.

[12] Laumann EO, Paik A, Rosen RC. Sexual dysfunction in the United States: prevalence and predictors. *JAMA.* 1999; 281(6):537-44.

[13] Abdo CHN, Oliveira Junior WM, Moreira Junior ED, Fittipaldi JAS. Sexual profile of the Brazilian population: results of the Brazilian sexual behavior study.. *Rev. Bras. Med.* 2002; 59(4):250-7.

[14] Hays RD. Bennett CM, Fairley CK, Dennerstein L. What can prevalence studies tell us about female sexual difficulty and dysfunction? *J. Sex. Med.* 2006; 3(4):589-95.

[15] DeRogatis LR, Burnett AL. The Epidemiology of Sexual Dysfunctions. *J. Sex. Med.* 2008; 5(2):289-300.

[16] Avis NE, Zhao X, Johannes CB, Ory M, Brockwell S, Greendale GA. Correlates of sexual function among multi-ethnic middle-aged women: results from the Study of Women's Health Across the Nation (SWAN). *Menopause* 2005; 12: 385-398.

[17] Abdo CH, Oliveira WM Jr, Moreira ED Jr, Fittipaldi JA. Prevalence of sexual dysfunctions and correlated conditions in a sample of Brazilian women-results of the Brazilian study on sexual behavior (BSSB). *Int. J. Impot. Res.* 2004;16 (2):160-6.

[18] González M, Viáfara G, Caba F, Molina T, Ortiz C. Libido and orgasm in middle-aged woman. *Maturitas* 2006; 53:1–10.

[19] Kaiser FE. Sexual function and the older woman. *Clin. Geriatr. Med.* 2003; 19:463-72.

[20] Bulcão CB, Carange E, Carvalho HP, Ferreira-França JB, Kligerman- Antunes J, Backkes J, et al. Physiological, cognitive, psychic and social aspects of sexual senescence Ciências Cognição 2004; 1(1):54-75.

[21] Bretschneider JG, McCoy NL. Sexual interest and behavior in healthy 80- to 102-year-olds. *Arch. Sex. Behav.* 1988; 17(2):109-29.

[22] Valadares AL, Pinto-Neto AM, Osis MJ, Conde DM, Sousa MH, Costa-Paiva L. Sexuality in Brazilian women aged 40 to 65 years with 11 years or more of formal education: associated factors. *Menopause* 2008; 15(2) 264-269.

[23] Kinsberg, 2007. Testosterone treatment for hypoactive sexual desire disorder in postmenopausal women. *J. Sex. Med.* 2007; 4(3):227-34.

[24] Hisasue S, Kumamoto Y, Sato Y, Masumori N, Horita H, Kato R, et al. Prevalence of female sexual dysfunction symptoms and its relationship to quality of life: a Japanese female cohort study. Urology. 2005;65(1):143-8.

[25] Howard JR, O'Neill S, Travers C. Factors affecting sexuality in older Australian women: sexual interest, sexual arousal, relationships and sexual distress in older Australian women. *Climacteric.* 2006;9(5):355-67.

[26] Garcia-Segura LM, Diz-Chaves Y, Perez-Martin M, Darnaudéry M. Estradiol, insulin-like growth factor-I and brain aging. *Psychoneuroendocrinology.* 2007; 32 Suppl 1:S57-61.

[27] Rosa e Silva ACJS, Sá MFS. Efeitos dos esteróides sexuais sobre o humor e a cognição. *Rev. Psiquiatr. Clin.* (São Paulo). 2006;33(2):60-7.

[28]   Stotland NL. Menopause: social expectations, women's realities. *Arch. Womens Ment Health.* 2002; 5(1):5-8.

[29]   Smith LJ, Mulhall JP, Deveci S, Monaghan N, Reid MC. Sex after seventy: a pilot study of sexual function in older persons. *J. Sex. Med.* 2007; 4(5):1247-53.

[30]   Martinez L. More education in the diagnosis and management of sexual dysfunction is needed. *Fertil. Steril.* 2008; 89(4):1035.

[31]   Abdo CHN, Oliveira Junior WM. The Brazilian gynecologist and female sexual complaints: a preliminary study. *RBM Rev. Bras. Med.* 2002; 59(3):179-86.

[32]   Berman L, Berman J, Felder S, Pollets D, Chhabra S, Miles M, et al. Seeking help for sexual function complaints: what gynecologists need to know about the female patient's experience. *Fertil. Steril.* 2003; 79(3):572-6.

[33]   Heiman JR, Guess MK, Connell K, Melman A, Hyde JS, Segraves RT, et al. Standards for clinical trials in sexual dysfunctions of women: research designs and outcomes assessment. *J. Sex. Med.* 2004;1(1):92-7.

[34]   Potter JE. A 60-year-old woman with sexual difficulties. *JAMA* 2007; 297:620–33.

[35]   Goldstein I. Current management strategies of the postmenopausal patient with sexual health problems. *J. Sex. Med.* 2007; 4 Suppl 3:235-53.

[36]   Abdo CH, Oliveira WM Jr, Moreira ED Jr, Fittipaldi JA. Prevalence of sexual dysfunctions and correlated conditions in a sample of Brazilian women-results of the Brazilian study on sexual behavior (BSSB). *Int. J. Impot. Res.* 2004;16(2):160-6.

[37]   DeLamater J, Friedrich WN. Human sexual development. *J. Sex. Res.* 2002; 39(1):10-4.

[38]   Junqueira FRR, Lara LAS, Romão APMS, Rosa e Silva ACJS, Romão GS, Ferriani RA. Implementation of outpatient sexuality in a gynecology service of a university hospital: results after one year. *Reprod. Clim.* 2005; 20:13-6.

[39]   Smith WJ, Beadle K, Shuster EJ. The impact of a group psychoeducational appointment on women with sexual dysfunction. *Am. J. Obstet. Gynecol.* 2008; 198(6): 697.e1-6.

[40]   Althof SE, Leiblum SR, Chevret-Measson M, Hartmann U, Levine SB, McCabe M, et al. Psychological and interpersonal dimensions of sexual function and dysfunction. *J. Sex. Med.* 2005; 2(6):793-800.

[41]   Hartman LM. Effects of sex and marital therapy on sexual interaction and marital happiness. *J. Sex. Marital. Ther.* 1983; 9(2):137-51.

[42]   Goldstein I. Current management strategies of the postmenopausal patient with sexual health problems. *J. Sex. Med.* 2007;4 Suppl 3:235-53.

[43]   Mishra G, Kuh D. Sexual functioning throughout menopause: the perceptions of women in a British cohort. *Menopause.* 2006;13(6):880-90.

[44]   Goldstein I. Current management strategies of the postmenopausal patient with sexual health problems. *J. Sex. Med.* 2007;4 Suppl 3:235-53.

[45]   Cohen BL, Barboglio P, Gousse A. The impact of lower urinary tract symptoms and urinary incontinence on female sexual dysfunction using a validated instrument. *J. Sex. Med.* 2008;5(6):1418-23.

[46]   Bradway C, Strumpf N. Seeking care: women's narratives concerning long-term urinary incontinence. *Urol. Nurs.* 2008;28(2):123-9.

[47]   Voorham-van der Zalm PJ, Lycklama A Nijeholt GA, Elzevier HW, Putter H, Pelger RC. "Diagnostic investigation of the pelvic floor": a helpful tool in the approach in patients with complaints of micturition, defecation, and/or sexual dysfunction. *J. Sex. Med.* 2008;5(4):864-71.

[48]   Kingsberg S, Shifren J, Wekselman K, Rodenberg C, Koochaki P, Derogatis L. Evaluation of the clinical relevance of benefits associated with transdermal testosterone treatment in postmenopausal women with hypoactive sexual desire disorder. *J. Sex. Med.* 2007;4(4 Pt 1):1001-8.

[49]   Gregersen N, Jensen PT, Giraldi AE. Sexual dysfunction in the peri- and postmenopause. Status of incidence, pharmacological treatment and possible risks. A secondary publication. *Dan Med. Bull.* 2006;53(3):349-53.

[50]   Nelson HD. Menopause. *Lancet.* 2008; 371(9614):760-70.
       Tourgeman DE, Slater CC, Stanczyk FZ, Paulson RJ. Endocrine and clinical effects of micronized estradiol administered vaginally or orally. *Fertil. Steril.* 2001;75(1):200-2.

[51]   Suckling J, Lethaby A, Kennedy R. Local oestrogen for vaginal atrophy in postmenopaus.

[52]   Barentsen R, van de Weijer PH, Schram JH. Continuous low dose estradiol released from a vaginal ring versus estriol vaginal cream for urogenital atrophy. *Eur. J. Obstet. Gynecol. Reprod. Biol.* 1997; 71(1):73-80.

[53]   Galhardo CL, Soares JM Jr, Simões RS, Haidar MA, Rodrigues de Lima G, Baracat EC. Estrogen effects on the vaginal pH, flora and cytology in late postmenopause after a long period without hormone therapy. *Clin. Exp. Obstet. Gynecol.* 2006;33(2):85-9.

[54]   Gorodeski GI. Aging and estrogen effects on transcervical-transvaginal epithelial permeability. *J. Clin. Endocrinol. Metab.* 2005; 90(1):345-51.

[55]   Gorodeski GI, Pal D. Involvement of estrogen receptors alpha and beta in the regulation of cervical permeability. *Am. J. Physiol. Cell Physiol.* 2000;278(4):C689-96.

[56]   Gorodeski GI. Vaginal-cervical epithelial permeability decreases after menopause. *Fertil. Steril.* 2001;76(4):753-61.

[57]   North American Menopause Society. The role of local vaginal estrogen for treatment of vaginal atrophy in postmenopausal women: 2007 position statement of The North American Menopause Society. *Menopause.* 2007;14(3 Pt 1):355-69.

[58]   Cayan F, Dilek U, Pata O, Dilek S. Comparison of the effects of hormone therapy regimens, oral and vaginal estradiol, estradiol + drospirenone and tibolone, on sexual function in healthy postmenopausal women. *J. Sex. Med.* 2008;5(1):132-8.

[59]   Conde DM, Pinto-Neto AM, Freitas Júnior R, Aldrighi JM. Quality of life in women with breast cancer. *Rev. Bras. Ginecol. Obstet.* 2006; 28(3):195-204.

[60]   Derzko C, Elliott S, Lam W. Management of sexual dysfunction in postmenopausal breast cancer patients taking adjuvant aromatase inhibitor therapy. *Curr. Oncol.* 2007;14 Suppl 1:S20-40.

[61]   Johnston SL, Farrell SA, Bouchard C, Farrell SA, Beckerson LA, Comeau M; SOGC Joint Committee-Clinical Practice Gynaecology and Urogynaecology. The detection and management of vaginal atrophy. *J. Obstet. Gynaecol. Can.* 2004; 26(5):503-15.

[62]   Borrelli AL, Casolaro AM, Esposito G, Berlingieri D. Biologic action of promestriene on the genital tract of the castrated rat. *Minerva Ginecol.* 1990;42(11):467-72.

[63]   Traish A, Guay AT, Spark RF; Testosterone Therapy in Women Study Group. Are the Endocrine Society's Clinical Practice Guidelines on Androgen Therapy in Women misguided? A commentary. *J. Sex. Med.* 2007;4(5):1223-34.

[64]   Braunstein GD. Management of female sexual dysfunction in postmenopausal women by testosterone administration: safety issues and controversies. *J. Sex. Med.* 2007;4(4 Pt 1):859-66.

[65] Wierman ME, Basson R, Davis SR, Khosla S, Miller KK, Rosner W, et al. Androgen therapy in women: an Endocrine Society Clinical Practice guideline. *J. Clin. Endocrinol. Metab.* 2006;91(10):3697-710.

[66] de Paula FJ, Soares JM Jr, Haidar MA, de Lima GR, Baracat EC. The benefits of androgens combined with hormone replacement therapy regarding to patients with postmenopausal sexual symptoms. *Maturitas.* 2007;56(1):69-77.

[67] Basson R. Hormones and sexuality: current complexities and future. directions. *Maturitas.* 2007;57(1):66-70.

[68] Alexanderson C, Eriksson E, Stener-Victorin E, Lystig T, Gabrielsson B, Lönn M, et al. Postnatal testosterone exposure results in insulin resistance, enlarged mesenteric adipocytes, and an atherogenic lipid profile in adult female rats: comparisons with estradiol and dihydrotestosterone. *Endocrinology.* 2007;148(11):5369-76.

[69] Hanly MA. Submission, inhibition and sexuality: masochistic character and psychic change in Austen's Mansfield Park. *Int. J. Psychoanal.* 2005; 86(Pt 2):483-501.

[70] Clayton AH, Croft HA, Horrigan JP, Wightman DS, Krishen A, Richard NE, et al. Bupropion extended release compared with escitalopram: effects on sexual functioning and antidepressant efficacy in 2 randomized, double-blind, placebo-controlled studies. *J. Clin. Psychiatry.* 2006;67(5):736-46.

[71] Caruso S, Agnello C, Intelisano G, Farina M, Di Mari L, Cianci A. Sexual behavior of women taking low-dose oral contraceptive containing 15 microg ethinylestradiol/60 microg gestodene. *Contraception.* 2004;69(3):237-40.

[72] Bancroft J, Sartorius N. The effects of oral contraceptives on well-being and sexuality. *Oxf. Rev. Reprod. Biol.* 1990;12:57-92.

[73] Buffat J. Why women consult sexologists: an approach for practicing physicians. *Rev. Med. Suisse.* 2005;1(11):754-6, 759-61.

[74] Meston CM, Levin RJ, Sipski ML, Hull EM, Heiman JR. Women's orgasm. *Annu. Rev. Sex. Res.* 2004;15:173-257.

[75] Badran W, Moamen N, Fahmy I, El-Karaksy A, Abdel-Nasser TM, 96. Ghanem H. Etiological factors of unconsummated marriage. *Int. J. Impot. Res.* 2006;18(5):458-63.

[76] Reissing ED, Binik YM, Khalifé S, Cohen D, Amsel R. Etiological correlates of vaginismus: sexual and physical abuse, sexual knowledge, sexual self-schema, and relationship adjustment. *J. Sex. Marital Ther.* 2003;29(1):47-59.

[77] Ghazizadeh S, Nikzad M. Botulinum toxin in the treatment of refractory vaginismus. *Obstet. Gynecol.* 2004;104(5 Pt 1):922-5.

[78] Fitzgerald MM, Schneider RA, Salstrom S, Zinzow HM, Jackson J, Fossel RV. Child sexual abuse, early family risk, and childhood parentification: pathways to current psychosocial adjustment. *J. Fam. Psychol.* 2008;22(2):320-4.

[79] Nelson DB, Sammel MD, Freeman EW, Lin H, Gracia CR, Schmitz KH. Effects of physical activity on menopausal symptoms among urban women. *Med. Sci. Sports Exerc.* 2008;40(1):50-8.

[80] Skrzypulec V, Dabrowska J, Drosdzol A. The influence of physical activity level on climacteric symptoms in menopausal women. *Climacteric.* 2010; 13(4):355-61.

In: Sexual Dysfunctions
Editor: Frédérique Courtois

ISBN: 978-1-62808-765-9
© 2013 Nova Science Publishers, Inc.

Chapter 13

LIMITATIONS OF THE FEMALE SEXUAL FUNCTION INDEX TOTAL SCORE IN HEALTHY COMMUNITY-DWELLING OLDER WOMEN

Susan E. Trompeter,[1,2] Ricki Bettencourt[3] and Elizabeth Barrett-Connor[3,]*

[1]Division of General Internal Medicine, Department of Medicine,
University of California, San Diego School of Medicine, La Jolla, CA, US
[2]Veterans Affairs San Diego Health Care System, San Diego, CA, US
[3]Division of Epidemiology, Department of Family and Preventive Medicine,
University of California, San Diego School of Medicine, La Jolla, CA, US

ABSTRACT

The Female Sexual Function Index (FSFI) is the most widely used instrument to measure female sexual function worldwide. Differentiation between women with and without sexual dysfunction is made by applying a full scale validated FSFI cut-off point. The majority of FSFI questions pertain to sexual activity, and the calculated FSFI full-scale score was originally applied to sexually active women. Today, however, a FSFI full scale or Total Score is being calculated in both sexually active and sexually inactive women to identify the population prevalence of sexual distress. Few studies have reported a full-scale score (FSFI Total Score) in healthy community-dwelling older women with or without an intimate partner. A total of 1303 older women were mailed a questionnaire about general health, past month sexual activity with or without a partner, and the Female Sexual Function Index. Of the 806 responders who answered the question about recent sexual activity, an FSFI Total Score could be calculated in 427; data showed a bimodal distribution of scores. For sexually active women with a partner (N = 302), the mean FSFI Total Score was 27.5 with a standard deviation of 5.7. Using the recommended cut-off score of 26.55, one-third (33.4%) met the criteria for sexual

* Corresponding author: Elizabeth Barrett-Connor, MD. Distinguished Professor and Chief, Division of Epidemiology, Department of Family and Preventive Medicine, University of California, San Diego, 9500 Gilman Drive, Mail Code 0607, La Jolla, CA 92093-0607. Ph: 858.534.0511; Fax: 858.534.8625; E-mail: ebarrettconnor@ucsd.edu.

dysfunction. All the 125 sexually inactive women who responded to the mailer met the criteria for sexual dysfunction because the FSFI Total score asks sexually inactive women to answer questions about behaviors that they have not had within the past month. These women all scored as having sexual dysfunction because a FSFI Total Score could not be calculated in sexually inactive women or those without a partner due to the design of the instrument. Conclusion: In general, the FSFI is a valuable instrument to screen for sexual distress in sexually active women. Sexually inactive women cannot be scored above zero in questions pertaining to sexual activity, and sexually active women without a partner could not complete the questionnaire as defined. Used as a general screening instrument, the FSFI Total Score creates the false impression that a high percentage of older women have sexual dysfunction, when in fact they are sexually inactive or without a partner. The FSFI Total Score should not be calculated in sexually inactive women or sexually active women without a partner.

INTRODUCTION

The most widely used instrument to quantify sexual distress is the Female Sexual Function Index (FSFI) which was developed by analyzing responses from normal controls and age matched subjects with Female Sexual Arousal Disorder (Rosen, 2000). Although case control clinical studies have used FSFI domain and total score results to evaluate sexual function in women with diabetes (Dimitropoulos, 2012; Enzlin, 2009; Esposito, 2010; Nowosielski, 2011), the metabolic syndrome (Martelli, 2012), breast reconstruction (Archangelo, 2012), coronary artery disease (Kaya, 2007) and other medical conditions, few studies have measured FSFI Total Score in healthy community-dwelling older women.

The FSFI has been widely adopted worldwide to identify Female Sexual Dysfunction due to brevity, clarity, validity, and ease of translation into other languages. Most responses to FSFI questions consist of a five point Likert response scale with a zero coding for "no sexual activity" in 12 items pertaining to arousal, lubrication, orgasm and emotional closeness. A zero is also assigned to questions pertaining to discomfort with the description "did not attempt intercourse" in sexually inactive women (Rosen, 2000). An FSFI Total Score of 26.55 has been proposed to be the optimal cut off score for differentiating women with and without sexual dysfunction (Wiegel, 2005). Because the FSFI is considered a general screening instrument, it is often applied to both sexually active and sexually inactive women.

We report here FSFI Total Score as reported by older community-dwelling women from the Rancho Bernardo Study cohort, as a total population and by presence or absence of sexual activity.

METHODS

Study Population

The Rancho Bernardo Study (RBS) included 82% of community-dwelling adult residents of Rancho Bernardo, a suburb of San Diego, California. Since inception in 1972-4, participants have been followed annually by mail for vital status and morbidity, and every other year for specific conditions or behaviors potentially related to healthy aging.

The Study was approved by the Institutional Review Board of the University of California, San Diego. Mailed questionnaires reminded participants that responses were voluntary and they did not need to answer any questions that they preferred not to answer.

MEASURES

Measures including the Female Sexual Function Index applied to surviving members of the Rancho Bernardo Study have been reported previously (Trompeter, 2012). In October 2002, 1303 surviving Rancho Bernardo Study women known to be alive and not institutionalized were mailed a questionnaire about physical and emotional health, menopause, hysterectomy status, current estrogen use, the presence or absence of an intimate partner, and the presence or absence of recent (past month) sexual activity with or without a partner.

Standard 5-point scales with the responses "excellent," "very good," "good," "fair," or "poor" were used to assess self-rated physical and emotional health. The Female Sexual Function Index (FSFI) was mailed in the same envelope, which included the participant's RBS identifier but no personal identifiers.

The FSFI multidimensional scale for assessing sexual dysfunction in women includes 19 questions developed by Rosen and colleagues(Rosen, 2000). The FSFI has demonstrated reliability and validity in women with or without sexual dysfunction, has good test-retest reliability for each of its individual domains ($r = .79 - .86$) and overall (Cronbach's alpha $\geq .82$). FSFI estimates the extent of difficulty in six domains of sexual function: desire, arousal, lubrication, orgasm, pain, and satisfaction.

The FSFI Total Score is obtained by adding the scores of the individual items that comprise a domain and multiplying the sum by the domain factor. The full-scale score is obtained by adding the six domain scores (Table 1) (Rosen, 2000).

Table 1. Scoring System (Rosen, 2000)
(Modified to include inserted sexual activity question 3)

Domain	Questions	Score Range	Factor	Minimum Score	Maximum Score
Desire	1,2	1 – 5	0.6	1.2	6.0
Arousal	4,5,6,7	0 – 5	0.3	0	6.0
Lubrication	8,9,10,11	0 – 5	0.3	0	6.0
Orgasm	12,13,14	0 – 5	0.4	0	6.0
Satisfaction	15,19,20	0 (or 1) – 5	0.4	0	6.0
Pain	16,17,18	0 – 5	0.4	0	6.0
Full Scale Score Range				2.0	36.0

Note: The individual domain scores and full-scale score of the FSFI are derived by the computation formula outlined here. Individual domain scores are obtained by adding the scores of the individual items that compose the domain and multiplying the sum by the domain factor. The full-scale score is obtained by adding the six domain scores. It should be noted that within the individual domains, a domain score of zero indicates that no sexual activity was reported during the past month.

The first two FSFI questions were answered independent of partner status or recent sexual activity and relate to sexual desire. We inserted the next question "Over the past 4 weeks, have you engaged in any sexual activity or intercourse?" Women who answered "no" were instructed to skip to the second to last question, "Over the past 4 weeks, how satisfied have you been with your sexual relationship with your partner?" followed by the last question, "Over the past 4 weeks, how satisfied have you been with your overall sexual life?" for a total of 20 questions (Table 2). The eleven questions pertaining to arousal, lubrication, and orgasm were answered by sexually active women only; sexually inactive women received a zero response to these questions. An FSFI Total Score was not calculated in sexually active women without a partner.

The FSFI questionnaire specifies that sexual activity could include caressing, foreplay, masturbation, and intercourse. Intercourse was defined as penile penetration (entry) of the vagina. The questionnaire specifically stated, "You do not need to have a partner to answer this questionnaire."

Statistical Analysis

The 427 of the 921 women (46.4%) who returned the questionnaire and answered each FSFI question required to calculate the FSFI Total Score are the basis of this report. Data are analyzed using SAS (version 9.3; SAS Institute, Cary, NC) and SPSS (version 17.0; SPSS Inc., Chicago, IL).

RESULTS

Table 3 shows the characteristics of the 427 women overall and separately by the presence or absence of recent sexual activity. The median age of the responders was 60.6 years (range 40 – 94), 54.8% (234/427) were postmenopausal, the mean number of years post menopause was 18.9 years, mean age at menopause based on last menses was 47.7 years, 20.6 % of women reported a bilateral oophorectomy. Overall, 61.8% reported using estrogen therapy at the time of the survey. More than half of these women had at least begun a college education; more than 90% of the heads of household were white-collar workers. The majority of women reported good or better physical and emotional health.

An FSFI Total Score was calculated in the 427 respondents (sexually active N = 302, sexually inactive N = 125) who completed the Female Sexual Function Index questions plus the added question about sexual activity. Using the zero category as part of the response scale, the mean FSFI total score was 20.8 with a standard deviation of 11.5. As Figure 1 shows, scores range from 2 to 36, with a bimodal distribution due to the inclusion of scores from women with zero responses due to sexual inactivity. Based on a recommended clinical cut off score of 26.55 (Wiegel, 2005) for differentiating women with and without Female Sexual Dysfunction (FSD), more than half (52.9 %) of all women met the criteria for FSD. For sexually active women (N = 302), the mean FSFI Total Score was 27.5 with a standard deviation of 5.7; one third (33.4%) of sexually active women met the criteria of FSD; all of the sexually inactive women (N = 125) met the criteria for FSD.

Table 2. Modified FSFI questions

1. Over the past 4 weeks, how often did you feel sexual desire or interest?
2. Over the past 4 weeks, how would you rate your level (degree) of sexual desire or interest?
3. Over the past 4 weeks, have you engaged in any sexual activity or intercourse? *Respondents who answered no were instructed to skip to #19.*
4. Over the past 4 weeks, how often did you feel sexually aroused during sexual activity or intercourse?
5. Over the past 4 weeks, how would you rate your level of sexual arousal during sexual activity or intercourse?
6. Over the past 4 weeks, how confident were you about becoming sexually aroused during sexual activity or intercourse?
7. Over the past 4 weeks, how often have you been satisfied with your arousal during sexual activity or intercourse?
8. Over the past 4 weeks, how often did you become lubricated during sexual activity or intercourse?
9. Over the past 4 weeks, how difficult was it to become lubricated during sexual activity or intercourse?
10. Over the past 4 weeks, how often did you maintain your lubrication until completion of sexual activity or intercourse?
11. Over the past 4 weeks, how difficult was it to maintain your lubrication until completion of sexual activity or intercourse?
12. Over the past 4 weeks, when you had sexual stimulation or intercourse, how often did you reach orgasm?
13. Over the past 4 weeks, when you had sexual stimulation or intercourse, how difficult was it for you to reach orgasm?
14 Over the past 4 weeks, how satisfied were you with your ability to reach orgasm during sexual activity or intercourse? *The following questions related to sexual activity with a partner. If you do not have a partner, please skip to question #20.*
15. Over the past 4 weeks, how satisfied have you been with the amount of emotional closeness during sexual activity between you and your partner?
16. Over the past 4 weeks, how would you rate your level (degree) of discomfort or pain during or following vaginal penetration?
17. Over the past 4 weeks, how often did you experience discomfort or pain during vaginal penetration?
18. Over the past 4 weeks, how often did you experience discomfort or pain following vaginal penetration?
19. Over the past 4 weeks, how satisfied have you been with your sexual relationship with your partner?
20. Over the past 4 weeks, how satisfied have you been with your overall sexual life?

DISCUSSION

Sexual medicine research relies primarily on self-reported questionnaires due to the challenges posed by evaluation of physiological sexual response in the laboratory. Instruments used to analyze sexual function include the Female Sexual Function Index (FSFI), the Brief Index of Sexual Functioning for Women (BISF-W) (Taylor, 1994), the Changes in Sexual Functioning Questionnaire (CSFQ) (Keller, 2006) (Clayton, 1997), the Derogates Interview of Sexual Functioning (DISF) (Derogatis, 1997), the Golombok-Rust Inventory of Sexual Satisfaction (GRISS) (Rust, 1986), the McCoy Female Sexuality Questionnaire (Rellini, 2005), The Relationship Assessment Scale and the Dyadic Adjustment Scale (Spanier, 1979).

Table 3. Characteristics of the 427 Rancho Bernardo Study women overall and separately according to the presence or absence of recent sexual activity

Characteristics	Total Respondents (n=427)			Sexual activity in last 4 weeks						
				No (n=125)			Yes (n=302)			
	n	Mean	SD	n	Mean	SD	n	Mean	SD	p-value
Age at Mailer	427	59.7	13.1	125	67.8	12.5	302	56.3	11.8	<.0001
Yrs post-menopausal	234	18.9	10.3	92	22.5	10.6	142	16.6	9.5	<.0001
BMI [**]	176	26.3	5.1	77	26.9	5.6	99	25.8	4.7	n.s.
	n	%		n	%		n	%		
Over age 65	150	35.1		79	63.2		71	23.5		<.0001
Marital Status [**]										
living w/spouse partner	158	89.8		75	97.4		83	83.8		Cells
widowed	12	6.8		1	1.3		11	5.1		too
other	6	3.4		1	1.3		5	11.1		small
Some college	216	52.8		71	60.7		145	49.7		.0435
Occupation										
executives/professionals	375	91.7		106	90.6		269	92.1		Missing
skilled/semi-skilled	28	6.9		11	9.4		17	5.8		cell
other	6	1.5		0	0.0		6	2.1		
Bilateral oopherectomy	88	20.6		27	21.6		61	20.2		n.s.
Ever HRT	245	57.7		79	63.7		166	55.2		n.s.
Current HRT	147	61.8		32	41.0		115	71.9		<.0001
Self-Reported Physical Health										
excellent	97	22.9		22	17.7		75	25.0		.0036
very good	179	42.2		43	34.7		136	45.3		
good	121	28.5		46	37.1		75	25.0		
fair/poor	27	6.4		13	10.5		14	4.7		
Self-Reported Emotional Health										
excellent	100	23.6		21	16.9		79	26.3		.0259
very good	182	42.9		55	44.4		127	42.3		
good	109	25.7		32	25.8		77	25.7		
fair/poor	33	7.8		16	12.9		17	5.7		
Satisfaction w/ current sex life										
very satisfied	151	35.4		38	30.4		113	37.4		<.0001
moderately satisfied	116	27.2		18	14.4		98	32.5		
equal satis/dissatisfied	67	15.7		27	21.6		40	13.2		
moderately dissatisfied	48	11.2		16	12.8		32	10.6		
very dissatisfed	45	10.5		26	20.8		19	6.3		

[**] Obtained from a sub-sample of women who attended a clinic visit in 1999-2002.

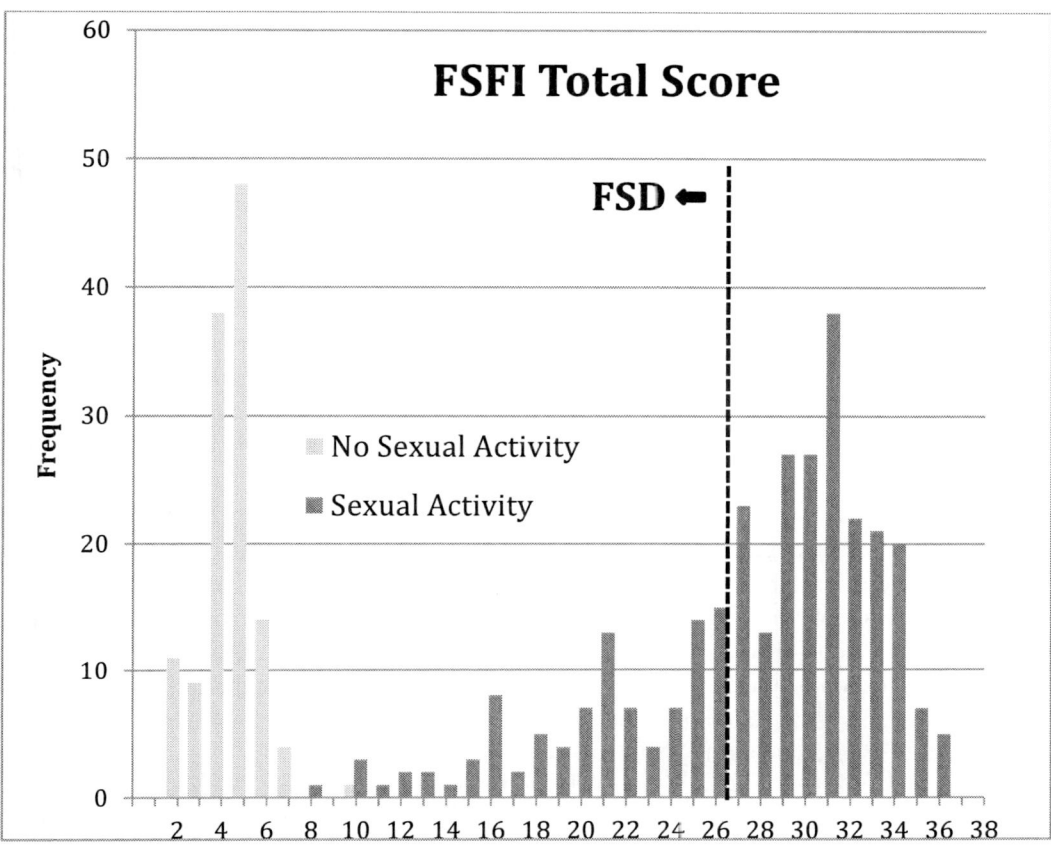

Figure 1. Distribution of FSFI Total Score when zero-responses are included.

The Rosen FSFI is the most widely used screening instrument worldwide for the identification of sexual dysfunction, with clearly worded questions that translate easily into other cultures and languages and have demonstrated statistical validity. Clinical studies identify women with Female Sexual Dysfunction on the basis of the FSFI Total Score.

Many sexuality concepts are abstract. Quantification of an abstract concept such as *the feelings people experience which lead them to want to have sexual intercourse* depends upon the creation of an operational definition known as "sexual desire." Conceptually, sexual desire is not uniform and will vary between individuals and within the same person at different times. Caution must be exercised during interpretation of sexual medicine questionnaires that use operational definitions to identify a norm, explore a trend, or define a disease state. The use of operational definitions and the application of ordinal scales assume homogeneity of results, but inexact measurements coupled with intra- and inter-user variability in effect result in a diagnostic mosaic (De Rogatis, 2007). Cumulative errors will likely result when imprecise measurements are used in the calculation of a total score.

Application of the FSFI Total Score to a population of both sexually active and inactive women introduces a bias because sexually inactive women are asked about behaviors that they have not had within the past month. As a screening tool the Rosen FSFI has been criticized when applied to sexually inactive populations (Meyer-Bahlburg, 2007) because a zero is applied for the 12 questions pertaining to sexual activity in sexually inactive women (Rosen, 2000), lowering their FSFI Total Score.

In fact, the authors state that a score of zero (in a domain total) conveys no meaningful information because the FSFI Total Score is most appropriately used only for women who have had some sexual activity (Rosen, 2000). A bimodal distribution will always result when sexually inactive women are assigned a zero for those questions pertaining to sexual activity, and most if not all sexually inactive women will meet the cut-off for sexual dysfunction (Meyer-Bahlburg, 2007). Female Sexual Dysfunction is only one of many possible reasons why women have not engaged in sexual activity during the previous month.

The FSFI structure requires that sexually inactive women skip to the end of the questionnaire to answer the final question regarding overall sexual satisfaction. Only about half of the sexually inactive women responded to this last question. Placing all questions that can be answered by sexually inactive women together in the questionnaire may avoid this problem.

The FSFI Total Score cannot be calculated in sexually active women without a partner because they cannot complete the questionnaire as defined. Two out of the three sexual satisfaction questions can only be answered by women with a heterosexual partner and there is no provision to calculate an FSFI Total Score in sexually active women without a partner. Using the FSFI in conjunction with brief questions concerning availability of a sexual partner or adding a question to the FSFI regarding specific sexual activity, including sexual activity with a partner only, sexual activity alone, or sexual activity both with a partner and alone has been proposed (Meyer-Bahlburg, 2007).

Calculating the FSFI Total Score in healthy community-dwelling sexually active older women with a partner identified one-third as having sexual dysfunction using the cut off of 26.55 (Wiegel, 2005), a group previously reported to maintain arousal, lubrication, and orgasm into old age with a high level of sexual satisfaction (Trompeter, 2012). The FSFI cut-off score has been validated for women with sexual dysfunction but appears to be inapplicable to many healthy community-dwelling older women.

The applicability of the FSFI as an instrument could be enhanced by using domain scoring to make comparisons between groups instead of calculating a Total Score. FSFI-desire subscale analysis has been used for comparison between groups instead of computation of a FSFI Total Score in women who do not report recent sexual activity (Brotto, 2010). FSFI-domain or subscale analysis as opposed to reliance on FSFI Total Score calculation may provide a more accurate means to compare like-groups to further identify Female Sexual Dysfunction without introducing a dysfunction bias . A mean score for FSFI-desire, FSFI-arousal, FSFI-lubrication, FSFI-orgasm, FSFI-satisfaction, and FSFI-pain have been used to compare sexual function between like groups. A FSFI-satisfaction subscale score can only be calculated in sexually active women with a partner.

In conclusion, the FSFI is a valuable instrument to screen for sexual distress in sexually active women with a partner; the FSFI Total Score as written should not be used in sexually inactive women or those without a partner because it gives a false impression that a high percentage of women are sexually dysfunctional when in fact they are sexually inactive. We endorse the original recommendation by Rosen that the FSFI Total Score be reserved for those who have some sexual activity. Otherwise the FSFI Total Score as a tool to identify Female Sexual Dysfunction will introduce a dysfunction bias when applied to sexually inactive women or sexually active women without a partner.

ACKNOWLEDGMENTS

The Rancho Bernardo Study was funded by the National Institutes of Health/National Institute on Aging grants AG07181 and AG028507 and the National Institute of Diabetes and Digestive and Kidney Diseases, grant DK31801.

REFERENCES

Archangelo, S. S.-N. (2012, April). Sexuality, body image and depression after breast reconstruction (Abstract). *Journal of Women's Health,* 21(4), 12.

Brotto, L. K. (2010). Asexuality: A Mixed-Methods Approach. *Arch. Sex Behavior,* 39, 599 - 618.

Clayton, A. M. (1997). The Changes in Sexual Functioning Questionnaire (CSFQ): development, reliability, and validity. *Psychopharmacology Bulletin,* 33(4), 731-45.

Derogatis, L. (1997). The Derogatis Interview of Sexual Functioning (DISF/DISF-SR): an introductory report. *J. Sex Marital Ther.,* 23(4), 291-304.

DeRogatis, P. L. (2007). Key Methodoloigcal Issues in Sexual Medicine Research. *Journal of Sexual Medicine,* 4, 527 - 537.

Dimitropoulos, K. B. (2012). Seuxal Functioning and Distress among Premenopausal Women with Uncomplicated Type 1 Diabetes. *Journal of Sexual Medicine.*

Enzlin, P. R. (2009). DCCT/EDIT Research Group. Sexual dysfunction in women with type iI diabetes: Long-term findings from the DCCT/EDIC study cohort. *Diabetes Care,* 32, 780-8.

Esposito, K. M. (2010). Determinants of female sexual dysfunction in type 2 diabetes. *International Journal of Impotence Research,* 22, 179-84.

Gerstenberger, E. R. (2010). Sexual Desire and the Female Sexual Function INdex (FSFI): A Sexual Desire Cutpoint for Clinical INterpretation of the FSFI in Women with and without Hypoactive Sexual Desire Disorder. *Journal of Sexual Medicine.*

Jimenez-Garcia, R. M.-H.-B.-T.-G. (2012). Sexuality among Spanish adults with diabetes: A population-based case control study. *Primary Care Diabetes.*

Kaya, C. Y. (2007). Sexual function in women with coronary artery disease: a preliminary study. *International Journal of Impotence Research,* 19, 326-329.

Keller, A. M. (2006). Reliability and Construct Validity of the Changes in Sexual Functioning Questionnaire Short-Form (CSFQ-14). *Journal of Sex and Marital Therapy,* 32(1), 43-52.

Martelli, V. V. (2012). Prevalence of sexual dysfunction among postmenopusal women with and without metabolic syndrome. *Journal of Sexual Medicine,* 2, 434 - 441.

Meyer-Bahlburg, H. F. (2007). The Female Sexual Function Index: A Methodological Critique and Suggestions for Improvement. *Journal of Sex and Marital Therapy,* 33, 217 - 223.

Nowosielski, K. S.-P. (2011). Mediators of sexual functions in women with diabetes. *Journal of Sexual Medicine,* 8 (9), 2532 - 2545.

Rellini, R. V. (2005). Validation of the McCoy Female Sexuality Questionnaire in an Italian Sample. *Arch. Sex Behavior,* 34(6), 641-7.

Rosen, R. B. (2000). The Female Sexual Function Index (FSFI): A Multidimensional Self-Report Instrument for the Assessment of Female Sexual Function. *Journal of Sex and Marital Therapy,* 26, 191-208.

Rust, J. G. (1986, Apr). The GRISS: a psychometric instrument of the assessment of sexual dysfunction. *Arch. Sex Behav.,* 15(2), 157-65.

Spanier, G. (1979). The measurement of marital quality. *J. Sex Marital Therapy,* 5(3), 288-300.

Taylor, J. R. (1994, Dec). Self-report assessment of female sexual function: psychometric evaluation of the Brief Index of Sexual Functioning for Women. *Arch. Sex Behav.,* 23(6), 627-43.

Trompeter, S. B.-C. (2012). Sexual Activity and Satisfaction in Healthy Community-dwelling Older Women. *American Journal of Medicine,* 125(1), 37-43.

Wiegel, M. M. (2005). The female sexual function index (FSFI): cross-validation and development of clinical cutoff scores. *Journal of Sex and Marital Therapy* (31), 1 - 20.

In: Sexual Dysfunctions
Editor: Frédérique Courtois

ISBN: 978-1-62808-765-9
© 2013 Nova Science Publishers, Inc.

Chapter 14

CONDITIONING FACTORS AMONG PALLIATIVE CARE PROFESSIONALS IN THE ASSESSMENT OF SEXUAL DYSFUNCTIONS

Claudio Calvo Espinós[1], and Estefanía Ruiz de Gaona Lana[2]*

[1]Palliative Care Service, Hospital San Juan de Dios, Navarra, Spain
[2]Hematology and Hemotherapy Service. Fundación Hospital Calahorra, Rioja, Spain

ABSTRACT

The prevalence of sexual dysfunctions in patients attended by palliative care services is high, as shown in previous work. It is also known that they wish to be able to talk about it with their caretakers. Our practice, however, lacks in this respect. We asked ourselves if it was possible to detect conditioning factors regarding this, from our opinion, experience and perception of our own competence. In order to answer these questions, we first reviewed the literature concerning sexuality, sexual dysfunction and palliative care. With this information, we designed a prospective study using an anonymous survey consisting of 10 questions. We addressed the questions to almost all health care professionals in the inpatient unit and the homecare settings of palliative cares in our hospital, using a closed question technique. Sex, age and profession were treated as independent variables. We found that the majority (100%) felt that the illness affected the patient's sexual experience and quality of life, however only half (48%) felt that they should ask about it. The whole sample agreed that they needed more professional development (78%) in order to provide good assessment. The agreement on the need of professional development in this area increased with age (18% in <30 year old, 72% in >41). Those who asked for more help were those who felt less qualified (0% psychologists, 30% nurses and 72% doctors). Finally, professionals did not see their own life experience as a conditioning factor (78%). These results suggest that there is a lack of consensus over the need of asking about the sexual sphere as a conditioning factor from our clinical practice. The study suggests that those who are less qualified see the need for support, which surely contributes to the way in which they deal with the issue.

---

* Corresponding author: Claudio Calvo Espinós MD, Palliative Care Service, Hospital San Juan de Dios (Navarra), Calle Beloso Alto, 3. 31006 Pamplona. Navarra. E-mail: ccalvo@ohsjd.es.

Good professional development could change this diverging dynamic to satisfy the needs of our patients and improve our skills in managing the issue.

Introduction

Issues related to sexuality are increasingly accepted as a factor that weighs heavily on the quality of life of our patients in palliative care units [1, 9]. In recent times, this issue has gained recognition from the fields of oncology and palliative care as perhaps one of the most forgotten [1, 8, 9]. It is well known that the impact of cancer and its different treatments affect sexual functioning [1, 2, 3, 11], sexual living [2, 3], and sexual identity [3]. The impact is variable depending on the stage of the disease, being greater when it is more advanced [5]. Not as well known is the impact of the role changes experienced by our patients in the eyes of their caregivers, from being a "sexual partner" to a "sick" partner, and subject to care. The resulting mismatch is a generator of guilt, rejection, sadness and anger, especially with regard to the companions and caregivers of our patients [1]. Patients (and their partners) affirm that the frequency and satisfaction in their sexual relationships are quite poor [1, 9] with a clear influence, in addition to the above, of age, functional status and the sense of well-being [9]. Within the overall experience in this area, the emotional component, the connection and interaction with others, appear to be most valued, even above the more physical aspects of the sexuality [4, 9, 11].

In turn, there are more and more studies demonstrating that our patients wish to express their experience with professionals that are taken care of them [1-9], especially if these professionals skilled and trained in this assessment [9]. However, despite the high incidence of sexual dysfunctions, and the clear need to talk about them, the assessment of sexual dysfunction is an area that usually escapes from our symptom control, and that it is rarely reported in our medical histories [10, 11].

There is even some controversy as to whether addressing sexual issues should be something concerning health professionals [11]. The literature shows that it is infrequently adressed, with little thoughts, and with a strategy that is basically pharmacological [2, 11]. We questioned why we managed this way, what professionals thought about the experience of their patients, how many times we have been asked for help on this issue and what we should do about it.

Study

To answer these questions, we conducted a survey in 2009 among the hospital's hospice professionals and home care settings of our unit (Table 1). The survey was designed to identify the possible constraints that professionals perceived regarding the assesment of sexuality in their patients. Our work presented several interesting results (Table 2 and 3):

- 60% of respondents suspected a sexual dysfunction in their patients (including 100% of physicians), and 100% believed it was the disease (particularly cancer in advanced stages) which affected them on this issue. However, only half of the professionals

(48%) believed that they should inquire about it (100% of physicians said so, but only 20% of nursing assistants).

- Asked about their perception of their qualification to assess and advise patients in this regard, more than half (57%) considered themselves as unqualified, and a majority (78%) manifested the need for training. Stratifying the results by occupation, 100% of psychologists perceived themselves as qualified, compared to only 20% of nursing assistants, 23% of nurses and 14% of physicians (figure 1). The perception of qualification increased with age (18% of professionals below the age of 30, 22% in the range of 31 to 40 years, and 58% older than 41, figure 2), and with the conviction that it is necessary to talk about these issues (36% of professionals younger 30, 50% in the range of 31 to 40 years, and 72% older than 41).

- With regard to the expression or the request of patients for help from palliative care professionals (figure 3), 46% of the respondents declared having discussed the issue of sexual living of their patients on at least one occasion. Analyzing separately affirmative responses, 100% said that they had a problem discussing this issue, but only two-thirds (67%) asked for help (0% of psychologists, 30% of nurses and 72% of physicians). The expression and ask for help appeared decreasing as the age of the professional grows (figure 4).

- Finally, exploring the possible influence of their own experience with sexuality related to in their management of their patients (figure 5), two-thirds of professionals (66%) thought that they treated this matter naturally (44% of physicians responded negatively). The data presented a clear downward curve with increasing age of the respondent (80% of professionals younger than 30, 65% in the group of 31-40 years, and 42% older than 41). A similar percentage (78%) said that they did not consider their own experience as a conditioning factor to address this issue with their patients (42% of physicians and 66% of psychologists). The data showed no significant variation with the age of the respondent.

Table 1. Survey about possible conditioning factors in our assesment

	YES	NO	OTHER
1. Do you think that your patients have any problems with their sexual living?			
2. Do you think that cancer affects their sexual living?			
3. Do you think that you should ask about it?			
4. Do you consider yourself as qualified for assessing this issue with them?			
5. Do you think that it is important to be qualified for it?			
6. Has anybody ever talked to you about his/her sexuality?			
7. Has anybody ever told you any problem in his/her living?			
8. Have you ever been asked for aid in this matter?			
9. Do you think that you talk about this sphere naturally?			
10. Do you think that your own living could condition your assessment of this sphere with your patients in any way?			

Table 2. Total results and stratified by occupation

%	TOT	TOT	TOT	NURS	NURS	NURS	AUX	AUX	AUX	PHYS	PHYS	PHYS	PSI	PSI	PSI
	YES	NO	NA	YES	NO	NA	YES	NO	NA	YES	NO	NA	YES	NO	NA
1	60	9	30	53	7.9	38	50	10	40	100	-	-	66	34	-
2	100	-	-	100	-	-	100	-	-	100	-	-	100	-	-
3	48	36	15	46	30	23	20	70	10	100	-	-	66	34	-
4	24	57	18	23	61	15	20	60	20	14	58	28	100	-	-
5	78	9	12	70	15	15	70	10	20	100	-	-	100	-	-
6	46	54	-	30	70	-	30	70	-	80	20	-	66	34	-
7	46	54	-	30	70	-	30	60	10	80	20	-	66	34	-
8	31	69	-	30	70	-	10	90	-	72	28	-	-	100	-
9	66	15	18	84	8	8	60	10	30	28	44	28	100	-	-
10	18	78	4	8	92	-	-	90	10	42	58	-	66	34	-

CONDITIONING FACTORS

The results of our study (table 4) were complementary to the literature on the wishes and problems revealed by patients and their families on this issue of sexuality. There is a majority consensus in the literature about the desire of our patients to talk about their experience in this matter [1-11]. In our study, it appears established that the professionals are convinced about the impact of the disease in this area.

However, the opinion was divided about the need to make it part of our daily practice. The age and occupation of professionals appeared to be a slight modulator of opinion, the most experienced physicians and psychologists being the most convinced of the need to assess this area.

The hospital is also generally perceived as a barrier to our patients in their sexual experience, mainly due to structural problems that make intimacy difficult (shared rooms, staff intrusions, beds, etc.) [4]. Perhaps this is why home care teams (both medical and nursing) are rated as more suitable by patients to address these issues [4].

In our research, we found that patients ask for help to the same professionals (physicians and nurses). Again, older age and psychologists were associated with an increased perception of qualification. However, these professionals were also the less requested for help according to our data.

Table 3. Results stratified by age

%	<30 Y YES	<30 Y NO	<30 Y OTHER	31-40 Y YES	31-40 Y NO	31-40 Y OTHER	>41 Y YES	>41 Y NO	>41 Y OTHER
1	54	-	46	72	14	14	58	14	28
2	100	-	-	100	-	-	100	-	-
3	36	45	18	50	35	15	72	14	14
4	18	72	-	22	50	28	58	28	14
5	81	9	9	79	7	14	86	14	-
6	46	54	-	57	43	-	28	72	-
7	45	55	-	57	43	-	28	72	-
8	36	64	-	36	64	-	14	86	-
9	81	9	10	65	14	21	42	28	28
10	10	81	9	22	78	-	28	72	-

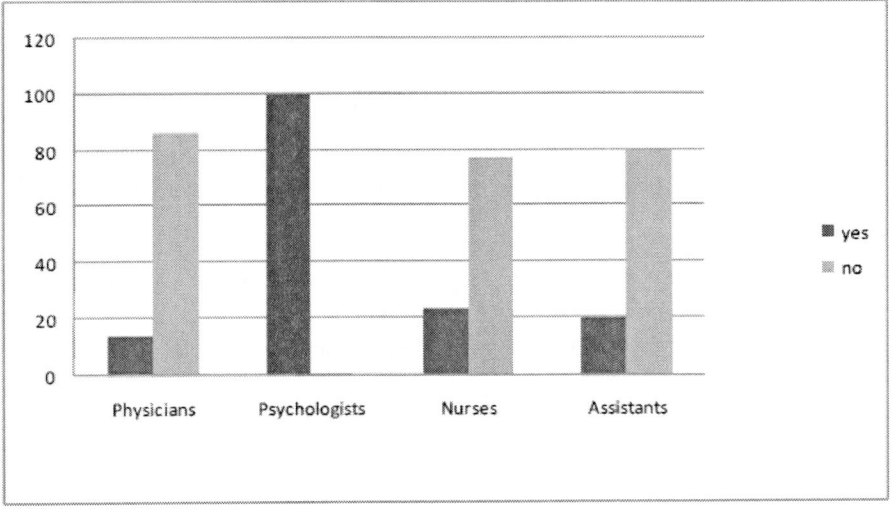

Figure 1. Perception of qualification to asses sexual dysfunction according to occupation.

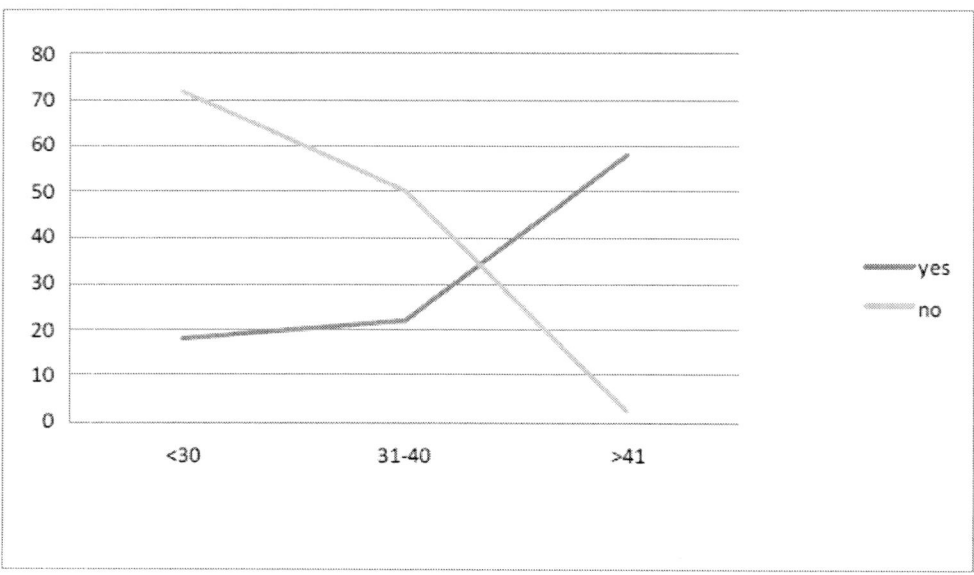

Figure 2. Perception of qualification according to age.

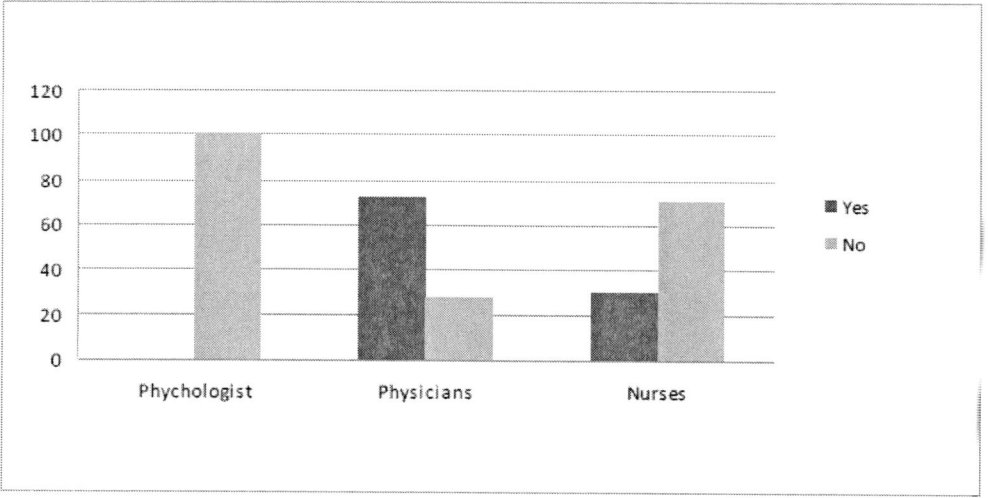

Figure 3. Askfot help according to accupation.

The literature indicates that our practice in palliative care is deficient in the assesment of this area of sexuality [2, 11], but does not suggest factors that may influence it. In our study, the vast majority of professionals suspected that their patients suffered some kind of sexual dysfunction, but there was no consensus on the need to include it in our medical records. This may be related to our infrequent approach.

Besides, the perception of most professionals surveyed that they were not skilled enough to adress the issue could also be a clear conditioning factor, as well as the fact that aid requests are made, according to our data, to the less qualified professionals (nursing and assistant as opposed to psychologists and/or physicians).

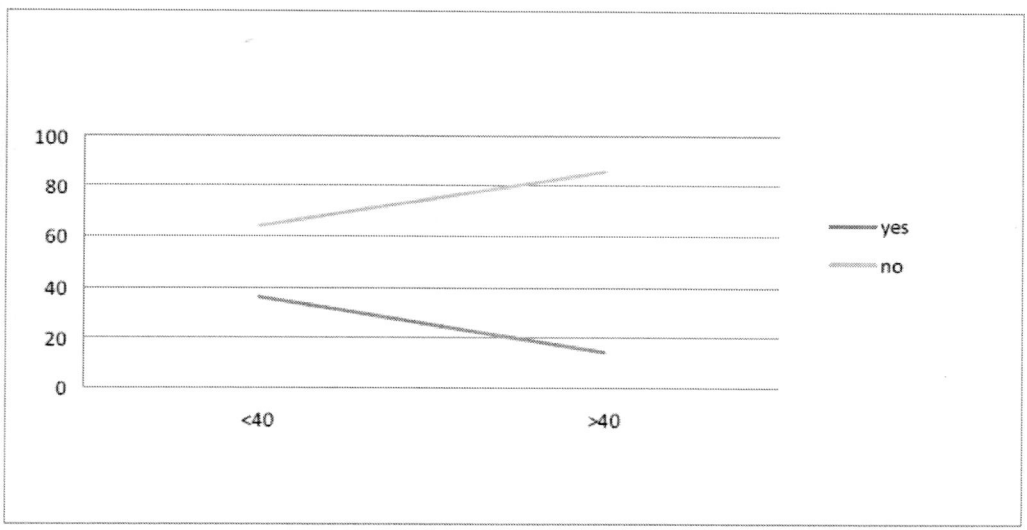

Figure 4. Ask for help according to age.

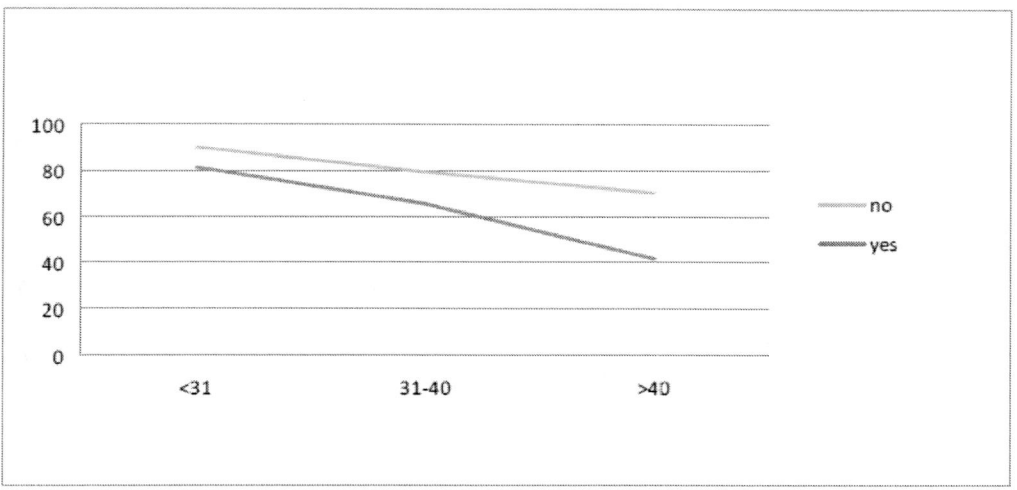

Figure 5. Influence of own sexual experience.

CONCLUSION

We believe that the divergence between the needs of our patients and the little or inadequate response on our part, is related to both our considerations of what is necessary or not for our patients for our good practice, and to the skill that we perceive possessing to manage these issues.

Perhaps an adequate training and a greater awareness of the magnitude of this problem for our patients, as well as developing communication skills in this particular area, could change the divergent dynamic detected, and improve the quality of life and satisfaction of our patients.

Table 4. Conditioning factors for sexual disfunction assesment

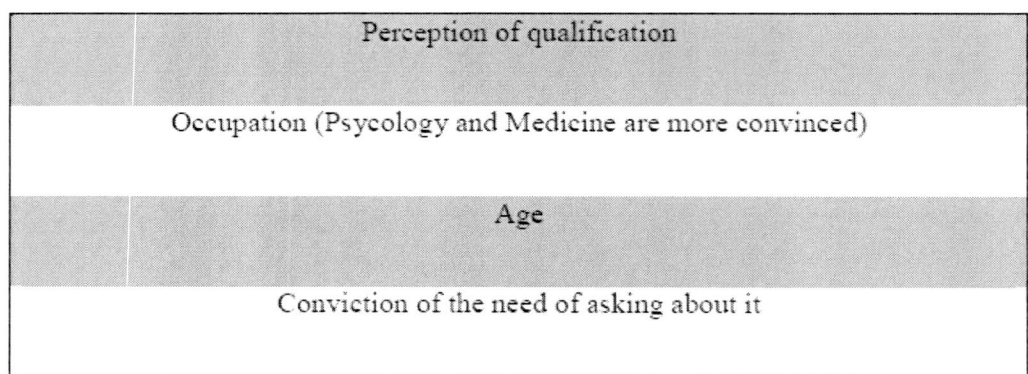

| Perception of qualification |
| Occupation (Psycology and Medicine are more convinced) |
| Age |
| Conviction of the need of asking about it |

REFERENCES

[1]   Mercadante, S., Vitrano, V., Catania, V. Sexual issues in early and late stage cancer: a review. *Support Care Cancer*. 2010 Jun.; 18(6):659-65.

[2]   Hordern, A. J., Street, A. F. Constructions of sexuality and intimacy after cancer: patient and health professional perspectives. *Soc. Sci. Med.* 2007 Apr.; 64(8):1704-18.

[3]   Yaniv, H. Sexuality of cancer patients – a palliative approach. *Eur. Journal of Pall. Care* 1995; 2(2): 69-72.

[4]   Lemieux, L., et al. Sexuality in palliative care: patient perspectives. *Palliat Med.* 2004; 18: 630-637.

[5]   Ananth, H., et al. The impact of cancer on sexual function: a controlled study. *Palliat Med.* 2003 Mar.;17(2):202-5.

[6]   Wells, P. Please: not-sex, I am dying. Exploring a common myth. *Eur. Journal of Pall. Care* 2002; 9(3): 119-122.

[7]   Ferrandino, M. A., Hernandez, M. Sexuality in cáncer patients. *Med. Paliat.* 2004, Vol. 11: nº3; 194-197.

[8]   Redelman, M. J. Is There a Place for Sexuality in the holistic Care of Patients in the Palliative Care Phase of Life? *Am. J. Hosp. Palliat Care.* 2008 Oct.-Nov.; 25(5): 366-71.

[9]   Vitrano, V., Catania, V., Mercadante, S. Sexuality in patients with advanced cáncer: a prospective study in a population admitted to an acute pain relief and palliative care unit. *Am. J. Hosp. Palliat Care.* 2001; 28: 198-202.

[10] Blagbrough, J. Importance of sexual needs assessment in palliative care. *Nurs. Stand.* 2010; 24: 35-9.

[11] Hawkins, Y., Ussher, J., Gilbert, E., Perz, J., Sandoval, M., Sundquist, K. Changes in sexuality and intimacy after the diagnosis and treatment of cancer: the experience of partners in a sexual relationship with a person with cancer. *Cancer Nurs.* 2009; 32: 271-280.

In: Sexual Dysfunctions
Editor: Frédérique Courtois

ISBN: 978-1-62808-765-9
© 2013 Nova Science Publishers, Inc.

Chapter 15

THE RELATION OF MENTAL HEALTH AND LOCUS OF CONTROL TO SEXUAL FUNCTIONING IN PATIENTS WITH MULTIPLE SCLEROSIS

Paraskevi Theofilou[1,2,] and Sophia Zyga[3]*

[1]Centre for Research and Technology, Department of Kinesiology,
Health and Quality of Life Research Group, Trikala, Thessaly, Greece
[2]General Hospital "Sotiria", Athens, Greece
[3]Nursing Department, University of Peloponnese,
Sparta, Greece

ABSTRACT

Sexual functioning is composed of both physiological and psychological factors among patients with multiple sclerosis (MS). However, the role of mental health and locus of control has not yet been studied extensively. This study was aimed to investigate the relationship between mental health and health locus of control and sexual functioning among patients with multiple sclerosis (MS). A sample of 90 individuals was recruited from three General Hospitals in the broader area of Athens, consisting of patients diagnosed with MS. Measurements were conducted with the following instruments: the World Health Organization Quality of Life instrument (WHOQOL-BREF), the General Health Questionnaire (GHQ-28) and the Multidimensional Health Locus of Control (MHLC). The results indicated that satisfaction with sexual life was negative associated with all sub-scales of GHQ-28 questionnaire (somatic symptoms, anxiety/insomnia, social dysfunction, severe depression). Sexual functioning was also positively related to internal health locus of control. Conclusion. The findings provide evidence that mental health and locus of control relate significantly to the evaluation of sexual functioning in patients with MS.

---

* Corresponding author: Paraskevi Theofilou. Eratous 12, 14568, Athens, Greece. Tel: +30 6977 441502, +30 210 6221435; Fax: +30 210 6221435; E-mail: theofi@otenet.gr.

INTRODUCTION

Multiple Sclerosis (MS) is a neurodegenerative disease characterized by chronic inflammation, demyelination, and scarring of the central nervous system. Symptoms include weakness, fatigue, sensory loss, vertigo, lack of coordination, impotence or sexual dysfunction, urinary incontinence, optic atrophy, dysarthria, and mental problems (Moller, Weidemann and Rohde, 1994; Weinshenker, 1995). The average age at onset of MS is 30 years, and the disease runs its course for the remainder of the patient's life frequently causing disability of varying degrees (Weinshenker, 1995). The prevalence of MS varies with both geography and ethnic background with women twice as likely to be afflicted as men (Hauser, 1994).

MS has a major impact on the lives of patients. The disease substantially interferes with daily activities and family, social and working life, disturbs emotional well-being, and reduces quality of life (QOL) (Brunet, Hopman, Singer, Edgar and MacKenzie, 1996; Fruewald, Loeffler-Stastka, Eher, Saletu and Baumhacki, 2001; Kroencke, Denney and Lynch, 2001; Murphy, Confavreux, Haas, Konig, Roullet and Sailer, 1998; Nortvedt, Riise, Myhr and Nyland, 1999; Rothwell, McDowell, Wong and Dorman, 1997; Solari and Radice, 2001; The Canadian Burden of Illness Study Group, 1998). Similar negative consequences on well-being, QOL and employment have also been found in partners of MS patients (Aronson, 1997; Hakim, Bakheit, Bryant, Roberts, McIntosh-Michaelis and Spackman, 2000; Knight, Devereux and Godfrey, 1997). This psychosocial impact of the disease in patients and partners was found to be significantly associated with the patients' severity of disability (Aronson, 1997; Hakim et al., 2000; Kroencke et al., 2001). A very important area that MS influences negatively is patients' sexual functioning (Theofilou, 2013).

Sexual dysfunction is a set of disorders characterized by physical and psychologic changes that result in the inability to perform satisfactory sexual activities. This condition has been found to be significantly more common in men and women with MS than in the general population (Foley and Werner, 2000).

Sexual dysfunction in MS has many causes. Primary causes may be the direct result of demyelinating lesions in the CNS (central nervous system) that can affect sexual response and sexual feelings (Foley and Werner, 2000). Primary sexual dysfunction includes decreased or loss in libido, painful or uncomfortable genital sensations (burning, tingling, numbness), and /or altered orgasmic response in both women and men (Campagnolo, Foley, Sipski et al., 2005; Demirkiran, Sarica, Uguz et al., 2006). Women may experience decreased vaginal lubrication and dryness, inorgasmia, and low sex drive (Demirkiran, Sarica, Uguz et al., 2006). Men may experience difficulty achieving and/or maintaining an erection, and diminished frequency of ejaculation (Seidman, Roose, Menza et al., 2001).

Secondary sexual dysfunction problems arise as a consequence of disability caused by MS. Examples of secondary symptoms include poor bladder and bowel control, fatigue, muscle weakness, spasticity, immobility, tremor, cognitive impairment, and sensory problems (Griswold, Foley, Helper et al., 2003). Secondary sexual dysfunction can also be a result of non MS health conditions such as hypertension, diabetes, depression, hypercholesterolemia, obesity, and smoking. In addition, medications that are used for MS (spasticity, urinary frequency, sensory pain) and non MS diseases (hypertension, diabetes, depression) can further contribute to secondary sexual dysfunction (Braun, Wassmer, Klotz et al., 2000).

Tertiary sexual dysfunction in MS occurs as a result of disability related psychological, social and cultural issues that affect sexual response (Braun, Wassmer, Klotz et al., 2000; Landtblom, 2006). These variables can include anxiety, low self esteem, altered marital and family roles, changes in body image, and fear of rejection by one's partner.

Although sexual dysfunction is a prevalent problem, in the MS population, and can be caused by a host of variables, for both men and women, it is a topic that is frequently overlooked, rarely discussed, and often left untreated (Campagnolo et al., 2005; Griswold, Foley, Zemon et al., 2003).

In Greece, there has been a great interest in investigating MS patients' QOL as well as sexual functioning during the past decades. Despite this scientific interest, few studies have been conducted so far related to this topic. Further, there is no study concerning the association of health locus of control and mental health with sexual functioning in Greek patients with MS. The purpose of this study is to examine the relation of mental health as well as health locus of control to sexual functioning in MS patients. We mainly hypothesize that a compromised mental health is related to a lower level of satisfaction regarding sexual life.

METHOD

Participants

A sample of 90 patients was recruited from three General Hospitals in the broader area of Athens. Selection criteria included:

1   > 18 years of age
2   Ability to communicate in Greek
3   Diagnosed with MS
4   Satisfying level of cooperation and perceived ability

The rate of response was very high, reaching 100%. Thus, the total sample includes all patients of these three hospitals, consisting of 45 males (50.0%) and 45 females (50.0%), with a mean age of 49.1 years ± 8.05. The values of the sample were found to fall within a normal distribution using Kolmogorov-Smirnov tests.

After the approval of the clinics' directors, two health psychologists selected the data using the relevant psychometric tools in the context of an interview at clinic. Concerning the selection of the patients, we were mainly based on the medical staff's advice about the level of cooperation of each patient. The participants were Greek adults having signed a consent form for participation.

All subjects had been informed of their rights to refuse or discontinue participation in the study according to the ethical standards of the Helsinki Declaration. Ethical permission for the study was obtained from the scientific committees of the participating hospitals. The study took place between September 2009 and December 2009. A sociodemographic questionnaire was used to collect information on the respondent's age, gender, education and marital status. There were also two questions related to patients' clinical characteristics, like duration of treatment and duration of diagnosis.

Table 1. Sociodemographic and clinical characteristics of the sample (N= 90)

	MS patients
Age (years) Mean (SD)	49.10 (8.05)
Gender Male	45 (50.0%)
Female	45 (50.0%)
Total	90 (100.0%)
Marital status Single	36 (40.0%)
Married	36 (40.0%)
Divorced/Widowed	18 (20.0%)
Total	90 (100.0%)
Education Elementary	9 (10.0%)
Secondary	27 (30.0%)
University	54 (60.0%)
Total	90 (100.0%)
Duration of treatment < 4	18 (20.0%)
> 4	72 (80.0%)
Total	90 (100.0%)
Duration of diagnosis < 4	9 (10.0%)
> 4	81 (90.0%)
Total	90 (100.0%)

SD, Standard Deviation; MS, Multiple Sclerosis.

With regards to these two clinical variables, it is observed in the below table that there are more patients who have less than 4 years of treatment, than patients who have less than 4 years of diagnosis. This difference is associated with the fact that 9 patients did not have to take medication when they were diagnosed with MS. Consequently, the time of diagnosis was different from the time that patients started to being treated. Descriptive sociodemographic and clinical data of the sample are presented in table 1.

Instruments

Measurements were conducted with the following instruments:

1   The World Health Organization Quality of Life instrument (WHOQOL-BREF) (WHOQOL Group, 2004) is a self - report generic QOL inventory of 26 items validated within Greek populations (Ginieri-Coccossis, Triantafillou, Antonopoulou, Tomaras and Christodoulou, 2003). These items fall into 4 domains: (a) physical health, (b) psychological well-being, (c) social relationships, and (d) environment.

Two of the items provide a facet measuring overall QOL/health. Higher scores indicate a better QOL.

2   The General Health Questionnaire (GHQ-28) is a widely used self - report measure of general health, developed by Goldberg in 1978 (Goldberg, 1978), and validated for Greek populations (Garyfallos, Karastergiou, Adamopoulou, Moutzoukis, Alagiozidoy and Mala, 1991). It may identify short - term changes in mental health and is often used as a screening instrument for psychiatric cases in medical setting and general practice. The 28-item version used in this study consists of four sub-scales: (a) somatic symptoms, (b) anxiety/insomnia, (c) social dysfunction, and (d) severe depression. Higher scores indicate a worse general health status.

3   The Multidimensional Health Locus of Control (MHLC) is a self-report tool measuring a patient's representations about control over health outcomes. The questionnaire has been translated into Greek and is under validation. However, we could say that in the present study, MHLC has adequate psychometric properties and presents satisfactory internal consistency (Cronbach's Alpha = 0.79). Health locus of control is one of the widely used measures of individuals' health representations and has been designed to determine whether patients are internalists or externalists. It includes three orthogonal dimensions (namely internal, chance, powerful others). A revised form of the MHLC further subdivides the powerful others scale into two separate scales: doctors and others (Wallston and Wallston, 1976). The brief description of the theory explores the fact that health locus of control is a degree to which individuals believe that their health is controlled by internal or external factors. Whether a person is external or internal is based on a series of statements. The statements are scored and summed to find the above. Externals refer to belief that one's outcome is under the control of powerful others (i.e., doctors) or is determined by fate, luck or chance. Internals refers to the belief the one's outcome is directly the result of one's behaviour (Wallston and Wallston, 1976; Wallston, Wallston and DeVellis, 1978). The 4 categories are not mutually exclusive and scores may weight in a particular direction. Higher scores indicate stronger presence of the specific dimension of representations.

Kolmogorov - Smirnov test was performed in order to check whether the values of the sample would fall within a normal distribution. Next, the analyses used aimed to investigate the relation between sexual functioning and mental health as well as health locus of control. Thus, correlation analysis was performed using Pearson's rho. Hierarchical regression analyses were also used to assess the above association in the total sample. A p - value of 0.05 or less was considered to indicate statistical significance.

All analyses were performed with the Statistical Package for the Social Sciences (SPSS 13.0 for Windows).

RESULTS

The values of the total cohort were found to pass the normality distribution test. Investigating the relation between sexual functioning and mental health, satisfaction about sexual life was associated negatively with two of the sub-scales of GHQ-28 questionnaire (*somatic symptoms, social dysfunction*) (table 2) as well as the total score. The results also indicated the positive relation of sexual functioning to *internal* locus of control and *important others* (table 2).

A hierarchical regression analysis was performed in order to investigate the afore mentioned association in the total sample. Specifically, satisfaction about sexual life was found to have a negative effect on all the sub-scales of GHQ-28 questionnaire (table 3). A positive association between sexual functioning and *internal* locus of control as well as *important others* was also observed (table 3).

Table 2. Correlations between sexual functioning and mental health as well as health locus of control in the total sample

| WHOQOL-BREF | GHQ-28 | | | | | MHLC | MHLC | MHLC | MHLC |
	Somatic Symptoms	*Anxiety /insomnia*	*Social dysfunction*	*Severe depression*	*Total score*	*Internal*	*Chance*	*Doctors*	*Important others*
Sexual functioning	-0.66**	-0.07	-0.54**	-0.16	-0.56**	0.34**	0.05	0.06	0.40**

**p<0.01; N=90.

WHOQOL World Health Organization Quality of Life, *GHQ* General Health Questionnaire, *MHLC* Multidimensional Health Locus of Control.

Table 3. Hierarchical Regression Analysis: Mental health and health locus of control affecting sexual functioning in the total sample

Dependent variable	Independent variables	Beta	p-value
Sexual functioning	GHQ-28 - Somatic symptoms	-0.92	0.00**
	GHQ-28 - Anxiety/insomnia	-0.38	0.00**
	GHQ-28 - Social dysfunction	-0.13	0.00**
	GHQ-28 - Severe depression	-0.59	0.00**
	MHLC - Internal	1.52	0.00**
	MHLC - Chance	-0.63	0.00**
	MHLC - Doctors	-0.67	0.00**
	MHLC - Important others	1.59	0.00**

**p<0.05; N=90.

GHQ General Health Questionnaire, *MHLC* Multidimensional Health Locus of Control.

DISCUSSION

The present study shows strong associations of sexual functioning with mental health and health locus of control in MS patients.

Concerning the relation between mental health evaluated by the GHQ-28 questionnaire and the variable of satisfaction about sexual life in the sample, it seems that a satisfactory sexual life is associated with less anxiety and depression as well as a more favourable evaluation from the patient's view concerning his/her status of general health. In the relevant literature, it has been suggested that increased sexual function in individuals with MS has the potential to positively affect outcomes through a number of mechanisms, including decreased levels of depressive affect and increased patient's perception of QOL (Theofilou, 2013).

Several limitations in this study warrant mention. First, sexual functioning was measured with a limited item from the WHOQOL-BREF questionnaire. Although future studies addressing similar questions should ideally use well established instruments that have proven reliable and valid, the reliability and validity of sexual functioning instruments that capture factors specific to MS and the lives of MS patients have not been established. Second, this research focused on the dimension of sexual functioning that relates to patients' satisfaction about their sexual life. Other dimensions of this variable (e.g., erectile function, sexual desire, orgasmic function etc.) merit additional study. Third, it was not possible to assess whether the levels of sexual dysfunction preceded or followed the initiation of MS, which should be viewed as a limitation especially for associations with adherence indicators and other outcomes assessed cross - sectionally at the initiation of the study. Sexual dysfunction may vary over time and may be important to consider at the initiation of MS.

There is also a need for future research to use prospective and longitudinal study designs to examine the interaction between sexual functioning and mental health in patients with MS.

Another methodological issue relates to the sample representativeness. Studies on the broader MS population and recruiting even larger samples to enable effective multi-group analysis should be pursued in future research.

Despite its limitations, the present study demonstrates the importance and the contribution of mental health and locus of control to the patients' evaluation of sexual functioning and specifically satisfaction about their sexual life.

ACKNOWLEDGMENTS

The authors would like to thank the patients for their participation in the study and acknowledge the support of the health professionals and administration personnel of the hospitals.

REFERENCES

Aronson, K. J. (1997). Quality of life among persons with multiple sclerosis and their caregivers. *Neurology*, 48, 74-80.

Braun, M., Wassmer, G., Klotz, T., et al. (2000). PDE-5 inhibition and sexual response: pharmaceutical mechanisms. *Int. J. Impot. Res.* 12: 305-311.

Brunet, D. G., Hopman, W. M., Singer, M. A., Edgar, C. M., and MacKenzie, T. A. (1996). Measurement of health-related quality of life in multiple sclerosis patients. *Can. J. Neurol. Sci.*, 23, 99-103.

Campagnolo, D. I., Foley, F. W., Sipski, M., et al. (2005). Sexual problems in persons with multiple sclerosis. *MS Quarterly Report.* Winter; 24 (4): 5-10.

Demirkiran, M., Sarica, Y., Uguz, D., et al. (2006). Sexual function in women with advanced multiple sclerosis. *Mult. Scler.* 12 (2): 209-214.

Foley, F. W., Werner, M. A. (2000). In: Kalb, R. ed. 2nd ed. *Sexuality: the questions you have-the answers you need.* New York: DeMoss Vermonde.

Fruewald, S., Loeffler-Stastka, H., Eher, R., Saletu, B., and Baumhacki, U. (2001). Depression and quality of life in multiple sclerosis. *Acta Neurol. Scand.*, 104, 257-261.

Garyfallos, G., Karastergiou, A., Adamopoulou, A., Moutzoukis, C., Alagiozidoy, E., and Mala, O. (1991). Greek version of the General Health Questionnaire: Accuracy of translation and validity. *Acta Psychiatrica Scandinavica*, 84, 371-378.

Ginieri-Coccossis, M., Triantafillou, E., Antonopoulou, V., Tomaras, V., and Christodoulou, G. N. (2003). *Quality of Life Handbook in reference to WHOQOL-100.* Athens: Medical Publications VITA.

Goldberg, D. P. (1978). *Manual of the General Health Questionnaire.* Windsor - England: NFER-Nelson.

Griswold, G. A., Foley, F. W., Helper, J., et al. (2003). Multiple sclerosis and sexuality: a survey of MS health professionals' comfort, training, and inquiry about sexual dysfunction. *Int. J. of MS Care.* Summer 5 (2): 37-51.

Hakim, E. A., Bakheit, A. M., Bryant, T. N., Roberts, M. W., McIntosh-Michaelis, S. A., Spackman, A. J. (2000). The social impact of multiple sclerosis--a study of 305 patients and their relatives. *Disabil. Rehabil.*, 22, 288-293.

Hauser, S. L. (1994). Multiple sclerosis and other demyelinating diseases. In: *Harrison's principles of internal medicine Edited by: Isselbacher, K. J.* McGraw Hill; 2281-2294.

Knight, R. G., Devereux, R. C. and Godfrey, H. P. (1997). Psychosocial consequences of caring for a spouse with multiple sclerosis. *J. Clin. Exp. Neuropsychol.*, 19, 7-19.

Kroencke, D. C., Denney, D. R. and Lynch, S. G. (2001). Depression during exacerbations in multiple sclerosis: the importance of uncertainty. *Mult. Scler.*, 7, 237-242.

Landtblom, M. A. (2006). *Expert review of neurotherapeutics; treatment of erectile dysfunction in multiple sclerosis.* June 6 (6): 931-935.

Moller, A., Weidemann, G. and Rohde, U. (1994). Correlates of cognitive impairment and depressive mood disorder in multiple sclerosis. *Actz. Psychiatr. Scand.*, 89, 117-121.

Murphy, N., Confavreux, C., Haas, J., Konig, N., Roullet, E., and Sailer, M. (1998). Quality of life in multiple sclerosis in France, Germany, and the United Kingdom. Cost of Multiple Sclerosis Study Group. *J. Neurol. Neurosurg. Psychiatry*, 65, 460-466.

Nortvedt, M. W., Riise, T., Myhr, K. M., and Nyland, H. I. (1999). Quality of life in multiple sclerosis: measuring the disease effects more broadly. *Neurology*, 53, 1098-1103.

Rothwell, P. M., McDowell, Z., Wong, C. K., and Dorman, P. J. (1997). Doctors and patients don't agree: cross sectional study of patients' and doctors' perceptions and assessments of disability in multiple sclerosis. *BMJ*, 314, 1580-1583.

Seidman, S. N., Roose, S. P., Menza, M. A., et al. (2001). Treatment of erectile dysfunction in men. *Am. J. Psychiatry* 158: 1623-1630.

Solari, A. and Radice, D. (2001). Health status of people with multiple sclerosis: a community mail survey. *Neurol. Sci.*, 22, 307-315.

The Canadian Burden of Illness Study Group. (1998). Burden of illness of multiple sclerosis: Part II: Quality of life. *Can. J. Neurol. Sci.*, 25, 31-38.

Theofilou, P. (2013). Sociodemographic and Clinical Determinants of Quality of Life and Health Representations in Greek Patients with Multiple Sclerosis. *Europe's Journal of Psychology*, 9, 33-50.

Wallston, B. S. and Wallston, K. A. (1976). The development and validation of the health related locus of control (HLC) scale. *Journal of Consulting and Clinical Psychology*, 44, 580-585.

Wallston, B. S., Wallston, K. A. and DeVellis, R. (1978). Development of the multidimensional health locus of control (MHLC) scale. *Health Education Monographs*, 6, 160-170.

Weinshenker, B. G. (1995). The natural history of Multiple Sclerosis. *Neurol. Clinic*, 13, 119-146.

WHOQOL Group. (2004). The World Health Organization's WHOQOL-BREF quality of life assessment: Psychometric properties and results of the international field trial. A report from the WHOQOL Group. *Quality of Life Research*, 13, 299-310.

EDITOR CONTACT INFORMATION

Dr. Frédérique Courtois
Université du Québec à Montréal
Department of Sexology
C.P.8888, Succ. Centre Ville
Montréal, Québec, H3C 3P8
Telephone: (514) 987-3000, Ext. 7713
Fax: (514) 987-6787
courtois.frederique@uqam.ca

INDEX

G

H

Q

R